T0327624

Dentistry in Rabbits and Rodents

Estella Böhmer Dr. med. vet.

Clinic of Small Animal Surgery and Reproduction
Center of Clinical Veterinary Medicine
Faculty of Veterinary Medicine
Ludwig-Maximilians-University
Munich, Germany

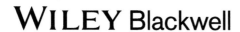

Library of Congress Cataloging-in-Publication Data
Böhmer, Estella, author.
   Dentistry in rabbits and rodents / Estella Böhmer.
      p. ; cm.
   Includes bibliographical references and index.
   ISBN 978-1-118-80254-0 (cloth)
   I. Title.
   [DNLM: 1. Dentistry–veterinary.   2. Lagomorpha.   3. Rodentia.   4. Tooth Diseases–veterinary.
5. Veterinary Medicine.   SF 867]
   SF867
   636.089′763–dc23
                                            2014017633
A catalogue record for this book is available from the British Library.

Wiley also publishes its books in a variety of electronic formats. Some content that appears in print may not be available in electronic books.

Cover images: Top right-hand rabbit image: ©iStock.com/jt1971. All other images courtesy of Estella Böhmer.

Set in 8.5/12pt Meridien by SPi Publisher Services, Pondicherry, India

Printed in the UK

Dedicated to my family

I would not have been able to accomplish this without the endless patience and active support of my husband and our four children.

Contents

Foreword, vi

Preface, viii

1 Dental Treatment of Small Mammals – Development and Aims, 1

2 Basics of Odontology, 5

3 Classification and Anatomical Characteristics of the Lagomorphs and Rodents, 21

4 Clinical Examination, 35

5 Radiographic Examination, 49

6 Computed Tomography, 88

7 Anesthesia and Analgesia, 90

8 Instruments for Examination and Treatment, 107

9 Diseases of the Incisors, 118

10 Changes of the Cheek Teeth, 153

11 Abscesses, 213

12 Periodontal Diseases and Caries, 242

13 Other Changes of the Jaw, 254

14 Follow-up and Prognosis, 260

15 Appendix, 267

References, 270

Further Reading, 276

Index, 280

Foreword

Small mammals, and among them rodents and lagomorphs, have been experiencing an increase in veterinary practice that is positively outstanding.

While livestock animals had still been the focus of veterinary work in the 1950s, the former large animal veterinary surgeries slowly turned into surgeries for small animals and became a women's domain. However, we are also witnessing revolutions within the small animal practices that the previous generation would not even have dreamt of. Small pets have reached the status of a beloved member of the family and significant expenditures are accepted in order to save, heal or prolong the life of a small pet.

The most astonishing thing, however, is the changing statistical structure of today's typical patient population in a small animal surgery: Where there used to be dogs as the center of attention, their frequency is currently decreasing as a direct consequence of politically motivated and objectively unjustified laws and regulations that mean an end to keeping a dog for many people that used to be enthusiastic owners. Hence smaller animals, which are also more low-maintenance, are fashionable, and it does not come as a surprise that the husbandry of cats and small mammals has been rising exponentially.

Only a few years ago, small mammals were considered low-budget animals and were not welcome in surgeries. They were mostly owned by children, were presented for treatment much too late and in an infaust condition, and were unpopular patients as they tended to compromise a surgery's reputation by spontaneously dying during examinations or treatments. That basic problem has not changed altogether, but the owners are now much better informed and have a good general awareness. The typical owner is not a child that is unable to cope with an animal's care but a single, "young urban professional." That kind of owner is well aware of the responsibility and feels the urge to take the best possible care of the animal and to keep it healthy and well for a long time. Fortunately, those kinds of animal keepers usually also have the financial means to consult a professional veterinarian in case of an illness of their animal.

The welcome increase in the number of small mammals, however, poses a new problem for surgeries in that they must first get accustomed to those species – some of which are entirely unfamiliar – and their specific illnesses. Competence in treatment of small mammals was not really promoted at all during the study of veterinary medicine – the more so as it might have been some years ago. Consequently, keen practitioners had to become acquainted with a multitude of very different disorders, which may also vary greatly between species. In addition, they were part of an international network and had to become accustomed to scientific exchange and coordination, in order to create standards for diagnostics and therapy. Numerous publications, congress papers and seminars serve to maintain a permanent exchange of views, and of course the study of diseases in small pets has also found its way into university research in the meantime.

A peculiarity in the veterinary medicine of small mammals is the frequency of tooth problems, which is above average. It remains to be clarified whether this is owing to a domestic feeding regime that is inappropriate for rabbits and rodents, which are used to meagre diets rich in raw fiber, or to the skeletal malformations of dwarf races bred for "cuteness." What is correct anyway is that dental disorders of rabbits and rodents represent an immense problem in their populations. Many tooth abscesses and tooth malformations are diagnosed too late and, consequently, they often require massive surgical interventions, some of which still lead to euthanasia in the end. Even less severe cases are often not curable but require – while the general condition is acceptable – lifelong corrections of the malpositioned teeth at regular time intervals.

The knowledge of the dental issues and their respective therapies has grown exponentially, and thanks for that are due to a significant extent to the author of this book, Dr Estella Böhmer, who has been focusing on those problems for almost two decades.

The present, comprehensive work represents the essence of her long-time efforts in tireless and dedicated research, as well as the acquisition of experience and the development of therapies and options for treatment, which, thankfully, she has been sharing with her colleagues in seminars and publications.

The book closes a big gap in the literature on pet animals and as far as I can see, it will be met with excitement from colleagues. Above all, however, it will help to alleviate the sufferings of the patients concerned.

Dr Peter Fahrenkrug

Preface

After having worked in the areas of orthopedics and soft tissue surgery of dogs and cats for almost 15 years, there was a sudden change. From now on I would be in charge of setting up and leading the small mammal (pet animal) ward of the Surgical Hospital. That was in 1996. While I had plenty of experience in orthopedics and soft tissue surgery in lagomorphs and rodents, and also knew how to treat dental disorders and jaw abscesses, I did not have a profound knowledge of the species-specific anatomy of the teeth and the gastrointestinal tract in different animals. Since there were hardly any books on the topic at that time, the challenge was to gain that knowledge by myself – step by step.

My biggest role model was Dr David Crossley in Manchester, UK, a man with an impressive professional knowledge starting from his PhD doctorate, who was able to impart that knowledge in such a clear and coherent way. Inspired and led by Dr Peter Fahrenkrug, the first seminar of the Bundesverband Praktizierender Tierärzte e.V. (National Association of Veterinary Surgeons) on dentistry in small mammals took place, and I had the chance to contribute as one of the main speakers. Pet odontology started to become my "hobby" and has remained so ever since. Dentistry in lagomorphs and rodents is a highly interesting field of work, with the diversity of different findings being particularly fascinating. As soon as one is familiar with the subject matter, it is simply out of the question to give up on a case until the cause of the problem has been found – even though an adequate therapy can often not be offered then because unfortunately the patient was presented for treatment too late. It is some consolation that even if patients eventually had to be delivered from pain, they would at least have been spared a lot of suffering beforehand.

With the present book, I would like to convey the knowledge accumulated over the years, and rather laboriously sometimes, to any interested reader. It is not only designed to help practitioners dealing with small animals in their everyday work but also students of veterinary medicine, if possible. It is supposed to be a manual for an in-depth look at rabbits and rodents with anorexia caused by dental problems, and easy to put into practice as well.

Writing a book is always a composite work of some complexity. The help of many people who support the project and provide valuable assistance is needed. First I would like to give many heartfelt thanks to my dear colleague at work, Carmen Blohm, who is a veterinary nurse. She was always there by my side during the treatment of patients and stayed on top of things even in stress situations. My sincere thanks are also due to all colleagues and staff in the X-ray department whose daily routine would have often been disturbed by my requests for "special views" ("Here comes that rabbit woman again!"). I would also like to thank the anesthetists who provided assistance whenever it was needed, as well as giving much valuable advice on how to optimize anesthesia in small mammals.

I would also like to give very special thanks to Prof. Dr Wolf Erhardt and associate professor Dr Christine Baumgartner for reviewing the anesthesia chapter.

Furthermore, my thanks are due to all staff across departments of the Hospital who have helped in providing loving care and attendance to pet patients in emergency cases as well as during weekend or holiday duties. Together with the nurses, interns and other apprentices, as well as students simply providing some help, they have made a significant contribution in the realization of this piece of work.

I would like to give my sincere thanks to Dr Marie Teltscher at Schattauer publishing house, who initiated the making of this book and always provided active support to me during the realization of this project. Her trust in my abilities as a writer was often much bigger than my own confidence in being able to realize the plan for the work.

Particular thanks are also due to my reader Dr Catharina Brandes, who provided significantly more structure and clarity to the contents of the book with her competent and patient revision of the manuscript.

Estella Böhmer
Munich, December 2010

CHAPTER 1
Dental Treatment of Small Mammals – Development and Aims

Eighty to a hundred years ago, the majority of a veterinary surgeon's dental patients were horses. They were primarily used as working animals and thus needed a healthy dentition. In the decades that followed, the number of dogs kept as pets rose significantly. Consequently, more dogs with dental conditions were presenting to general veterinary practices and to the increasing number of specialized small animal practices. From the 1970s on, the number of pet cats was also increasing, with a concomitant increase in the number of cats requiring dental treatment, particularly in urban areas. During the last 15 years, a focus of interest has been on small herbivorous mammals (rabbits, guinea pigs, chinchillas and degus) as pets.

Keeping small pets is becoming ever more popular, with lagomorphs and rodents in particular attracting attention as being "low-maintenance" animals – especially in urban areas. Nowadays, small pets comprise almost a quarter of patients in an urban veterinary practice, excluding those practices that focus only on small mammals. This is challenging for veterinarians, as they are presented with a great variety of animal species, and many of them must be treated in different ways due to their anatomical and physiological peculiarities. An ever-increasing knowledge in a variety of disciplines is required in order to make correct diagnoses and treat these patients appropriately. This is especially true in the area of odontology, as many small mammals have dental ailments.

One of the reasons for the high number of dental ailments presenting in small mammals is that some pet owners have an insufficient understanding of the dietary requirements of their herbivorous pets, which can lead to dental overgrowth with all of its possible consequences. This problem is compounded by the fact that for each species there is a vast multitude of foods available in specialist shops. In principle (and often contrary to the labeling), many of these are not suitable when given as a complete diet. The variety of feeds on offer is difficult to choose from for a pet owner who is not well informed. Consequently, the owner will often feed these pets – more or less randomly and uncritically – whatever seems suitable to them and whatever the animal prefers to eat. These kinds of high-energy grain mixtures often lead to gastrointestinal diseases, as well as resulting in insufficient abrasion of the incisors and cheek teeth, which keep growing during the whole lifetime of the animal. This will inevitably result in an acquired malocclusion.

Gastrointestinal disease tends to be readily recognized by the pet owner due to fairly obvious symptoms such as diarrhoea, abdominal pain or constipation. In contrast, dental problems may go unnoticed in their early stages by an animal's owner. Most animals that are starting to develop malocclusions continue to eat enough, although they may already be suffering from painful changes in their teeth and jaws. Their general condition may appear well, they may be lively, continue to groom and exhibit an interest in their surroundings, their owners or their conspecifics. Any weight loss may not be noticed early on unless the animal is regularly weighed. Early symptoms of malocclusion are also difficult to detect when the animals are kept in a group. For example, in the early stages of a dental disorder, many patients start to eat selectively, i.e. they prefer soft feeds and avoid harder feeds like hay. Such behavior may go unnoticed in animal groups. For these reasons, many patients do not present for treatment until they suffer

Dentistry in Rabbits and Rodents, First Edition. Estella Böhmer.
© 2015 John Wiley & Sons, Ltd. Published 2015 by John Wiley & Sons, Ltd.

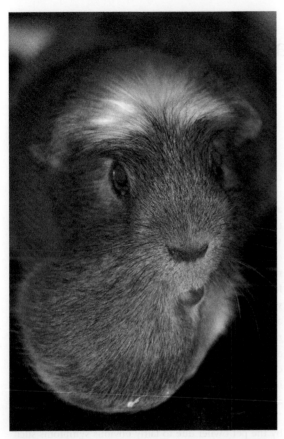

Figure 1.1 Abscess of the mandible as a result of chronic apical periodontitis of the first lower cheek tooth (P4) in a four-year-old guinea pig.

from quite advanced malocclusions or the formation of a tooth-associated jaw abscess which is clearly visible (Figure 1.1). Radiographs showing the extent of osseous changes that are already present are often met with amazement. How could the animals hide these painful conditions for such a long time?

In order to prevent situations like these arising, veterinarians should take every opportunity to describe early symptoms of dental disorders to an animal's owner and give advice about species-appropriate feeding and husbandry. Such opportunities include routine examinations, annual vaccinations, visits for neutering, clipping of claws and treatments for ecto- and endoparasitic diseases. Additionally, prophylactic dental examinations are generally recommended. The earlier malocclusions are detected, the better are the chances of curing them

with specific therapies, or at least having a positive impact on the course of the disease.

During the last three decades, not only has the way that corrections of the dental problems are performed changed but also the aims of these corrections. In the 1970s and 1980s, lagomorphs and herbivorous rodents with malocclusions would simply have had their elongated incisors clipped, and tips of teeth or spikes and spurs of the molars removed with a fine Luer bone rongeur forceps. Finally, the occlusal surface of the molars would have been "filed" a little. Little attention was given to the etiology of dental disorders, the anatomical and pathological peculiarities of the dentition of different species or to a possible prophylaxis of dental changes. In addition, there were no adequate instruments suitable to use for closer diagnostic examinations or therapies. Furthermore, radiographs of the head were generally taken in only one or two views, and almost always just for jaw abscesses, but not for so-called "uncomplicated" dental treatments. During recent years, dramatic changes have occurred concerning all of the aforementioned, and these changes require a re-definition of the aims of an optimal dental treatment.

Nowadays, the aim of correcting an occlusion involves more than re-establishing the best possible intraoral occlusion by simple trimming of the incisors and molars. Dental therapies are now looking to establish the primary causes of disorders of the jaw and teeth. If the cause of a disorder can be determined using adequate diagnostics (e.g. history taking, clinical and intraoral examinations, radiographic examination using a variety of positionings, etc.), it may then be possible to rectify it by means of a specific therapy. Often, a long-term cure may be feasible. Even if it is not possible to rectify the condition, then a treatment specific to the individual situation may at least delay progress of the pathological changes.

However, if diagnostics and therapy are limited to pathological changes that can be seen intraorally, as they were in the past, then hidden intraosseous processes will continue to progress unrestrictedly. One may sometimes wonder why a treatment has not been successful despite the correction of the dentition having been performed precisely according to the intraoral findings, not realizing that the pain is caused by intra-alveolar changes. A typical example of this is shown in Figure 1.2. This rabbit has an abscess of the lower jaw. Its cause is a longitudinally split lower mandibular cheek tooth (P3), with apical inflammation. A subtle

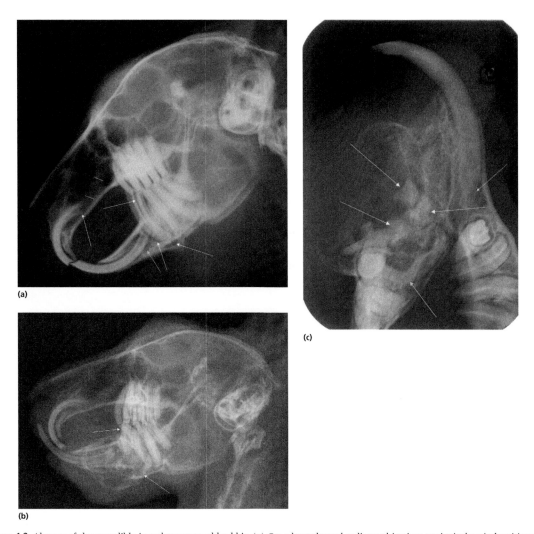

Figure 1.2 Abscess of the mandible in a three-year-old rabbit. (a) On a laterolateral radiographic view, periapical periodontitis and a longitudinal split of the first lower cheek tooth (P3; white arrows) can be seen. A slight distension of the ventral mandibular cortical bone with swelling of soft tissue is also clearly visible. Retrograde displacement of the apex of the lower incisor with periapical osteolysis (turquoise arrow), secondary malocclusion of the incisor with dental overgrowth and abnormal, blunt contact surface of the mandibular incisor as well as retrograde displacement of the maxillary incisor (yellow arrow) are also recognizable. The nasolacrimal duct is dilated (yellow lines). (b) Eight months after a simple abscess-related incision without tooth extraction, the laterolateral view shows a pronounced abscess of the mandible with a markedly distended, bony abscess capsule. A mandibular cheek tooth (P3) and a mandibular incisor are missing. The second lower cheek tooth (P4) is severely deformed intra-alveolar as well as extra-alveolar (white arrows). The clinical crown of the remaining mandibular incisor is markedly elongated (prognathic tooth position) and there are manifestations of apical inflammation. The maxillary incisors are elongated. (c) The intraoral radiographic image of the mandibles shows that the right incisor is missing and the adjacent first cheek tooth (P3) is only recognizable as an unstructured, multipart dentinoid (white arrows). There is a strong intra-alveolar deviation of the following second cheek tooth (P4; turquoise arrows) as well as extra-alveolar overgrowth and apical periodontitis of the left incisor (yellow arrow). The socket of the first left cheek tooth (P3) is slightly expanded.

overgrowth of the affected premolar dominates intra-orally. Secondarily, the infection has spread to the adjacent incisor. Unless the whole problem is identified correctly and both teeth causing it are extracted, the initially local infection will spread, leading to an area of lesion that is "inexplicably" not improving.

Misdiagnoses like these, as well as other complications, can be avoided by the use of well-founded radiographic diagnostics, and thus the majority of tooth and jaw diseases can now be treated more specifically and effectively. This should be our primary aim, in conjunction with an optimal correction of the dentition and providing the owners of small mammals with advice concerning diet and care of these animals. Diagnostics and therapy of tooth and jaw diseases in lagomorphs and rodents are highly complex and sometimes complicated areas of expertise. This, along with the variability and uniqueness of each individual case, makes this a fascinating area of work, one in which we face new challenges every day, with a variety of interesting problems to solve and decisions to make.

The relatively high frequency of malocclusions in these animal species is reflected in the scientific literature. A multitude of publications on this problem has appeared over the last few years. However, guinea pigs are largely omitted in the literature from English-speaking countries, despite being common pets in these countries. In addition to the literature, veterinarians who wish to expand their knowledge in theory as well as in practice may choose from a wide range of national and international advanced training courses. Concurrently, new instruments are being developed that are particularly suitable for dental treatment of pets. It is also possible to use teleconsulting via the internet, for example, when looking for help in interpreting X-ray images (e.g. www. curoxray.de). Given all these resources, one would hope that there will be no more insufficient diagnoses (e.g. diagnoses being made without radiographic examinations of the skull) or inappropriate therapies of malocclusions in small pets.

CHAPTER 2
Basics of Odontology

2.1 Evolution of teeth

In the animal kingdom, "true" teeth with dentin arose about 380 million years ago in the Devon age – their bearers having been the gnathostomous vertebrates (jawed vertebrates or gnathostomata). With this feature, whole new ways of feeding became accessible to the animals. The teeth of lower vertebrates (fish and reptiles) were arranged in rows, lacking dentin and cement and uniformly shaped (homodont). These animals had many teeth that were replaced continuously (polyodontia as well as polyphyodonty).

The further development of the dentition was dependent on the animals' method of feeding. The purpose of the teeth was simply to fix the food (carnivores) or to grind it down (herbivores and early carnivores). The transition from homodont to heterodont (diverse basic types of teeth) was not made until the earliest mammals appeared in the Mesozoic (Triassic, 245 to 208 million years ago), and the Cenozoic (Tertiary, 65 to 2 million years ago) saw the differentiation between carnivores, herbivores and omnivores (Gängler & Arnold, 2005). Some omnivorous mammals needed teeth with a better grinding capacity, so over time individual enamel cusps evolved into enamel ridges (lophodont teeth). Those primary enamel cusps cannot be directly detected any more in polylophodont teeth, whose occlusal surface is even more complexly structured owing to deep invaginations of the enamel into the body of dentin. This large variety of forms in the dentition of mammals was caused by the much higher energy demand of these warm-blooded animals, which forced them to exploit their food better by enhancing their chewing performance.

The basic biological pattern of odontogenesis is an invagination of the oral epithelium with a subsequent differentiation of that dental ridge into ameloblasts and a differentiation of the ectomesenchyme into odontoblasts and pulp cells. This primitive structure of teeth is always dome shaped. This basic pattern is then modified in the various species during the further development of the animal. The very different morphologies of the teeth depend not only on the species but also on the function of the tooth (cutting, gnawing, fixing, jabbing, grinding). Adult mammals have four different types of teeth: incisors, canines, premolars and molars. Rabbits and rodents lack canines; they possess only two functionally different types of teeth: incisors and cheek teeth. In these species, premolars and molars are morphologically and functionally identical in principle and can hardly be distinguished based solely on their shapes, so they are usually treated as the same (the so-called molarization of the premolars). There is a long gap devoid of teeth between the incisors and premolars, which is called the diastema. In lagomorphs and rodents, this zone contains a hairy mucosal fold, which often hampers intraoral examinations (Figure 2.1).

2.2 Anatomy and nomenclature of teeth

A good knowledge of the basics is necessary in order to understand the species-specific anatomy and the various pathological changes of the teeth and dentition of lagomorphs and rodents, and to choose a suitable therapy for the species concerned. That kind of knowledge is vital for a successful treatment because

Dentistry in Rabbits and Rodents, First Edition. Estella Böhmer.
© 2015 John Wiley & Sons, Ltd. Published 2015 by John Wiley & Sons, Ltd.

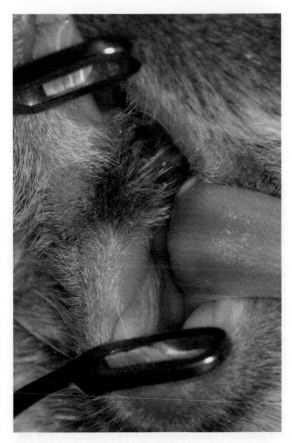

Figure 2.1 Hairy cheek of a rabbit (right).

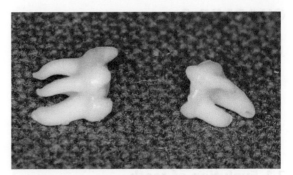

Figure 2.2 Multirooted, brachyodont cheek teeth of an approximately three-month-old rat with dental growth terminated (M1 left) and largely terminated (M3 right); differentiation of tooth crown including cusps are still clearly visible, with tooth neck and tooth roots.

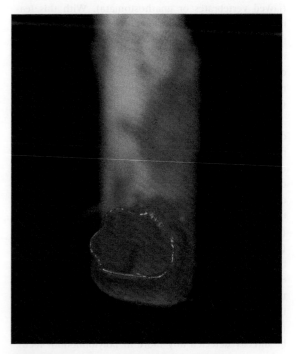

Figure 2.3 Apex of a hypselodont incisor of a rabbit.

dental and jaw disorders vary between species more than one would expect.

The basic anatomy of most teeth is divided into the crown (corona dentis), which protrudes into the oral cavity, and the root (radix dentis), consisting of the closed apical foramen and the tooth neck (collum dentis) (Figure 2.2). Elodont teeth, which keep growing during the whole lifetime of the animal, have a different anatomy. They consist of a single, elongated tooth structure which is homogeneous both extra-alveolarly as well as intra-alveolarly. Their apices remain wide open throughout life without forming any kind of "root" (aradicular teeth) (Figure 2.3). The germinal tissue (called pulp or apical dental sac), which is located at the apex continues to produce new tooth substance from ameloblasts, odontoblasts and cementoblasts. There is a differentiation between the clinical crown and the reserve crown. The clinical crown is the smaller, visible part outside the dental alveolus, whereas the reserve crown is the main part of the tooth, which is located subgingivally and thus intraosseously. Alternatively, these different parts can also be referred to as the extra- and intra-alveolar parts of the tooth. Both together form the long anatomical crown (corona anatomica) or the tooth body (corpus dentis).

In order to describe changes in teeth or jaw accurately, dentists make use of a special nomenclature (Table 2.1). This nomenclature also makes it possible to document the locations of teeth in relation to one another or in relation to other structures within the oral cavity. For example, occlusal is the term for the direction toward the occlusal surface of a cheek tooth (facies masticatoria). As for the incisors, the direction toward the cutting edge is called incisal. When looking at the tooth itself, coronal means directed toward the occlusal surface whereas apical means directed toward the apex. For rootless teeth, apical can also be referred to as basal. Lingual refers to the medial surface of a tooth (facies lingualis) for all lower cheek teeth, whereas palatal refers to the inner surface for all upper cheek teeth (facies palatinalis). Correspondingly, buccal refers to the outer surface of a tooth (facies buccalis), whereas the outer surface of the incisors is called labial (facies labialis). An alternative term for buccal as well as labial is vestibular (near the vestibulum oris=area between the teeth and lips or cheeks, which can also be called the vestibular fold). The terms interproximal and interdental are for spaces where adjacent teeth meet. Rostral is a general term for the cranial direction in the jaws, whereas distal marks the caudal direction. Alternative terms for these are mesial and distal. They are mainly used to describe those tooth surfaces within the dental arcade that face forward – meaning toward the middle of the dental arcade or toward the inner incisor – or backwards, i.e. toward the jaw joint (Baker & Easley, 2003).

Table 2.1 Terms for orientation in teeth and jaws.

Terminus	Description
Occlusal	Pertaining to the occlusal surface of the cheek teeth
Incisal	Pertaining to the cutting surface of the incisors
Coronal	Oriented toward the occlusal surface of a tooth
Apical	Oriented toward the apex of a tooth
Basal	The corresponding term for apical in rootless teeth
Lingual	Medial area of tooth in lower cheek teeth
Palatinal	Medial area of tooth in upper cheek teeth
Vestibular	Near the vestibulum oris=area between the teeth and the lips or Cheeks
Approximal, interdental	Areas where adjacent teeth meet one another
Rostral, mesial	Cranial direction of the jaw
Distal	Caudal direction of the jaw

2.3 Structure of teeth

In principle, the brachyodont and hypselodont teeth of lagomorphs and rodents consist of the same substances as the teeth of humans or other mammals. These substances are enamel, dentin, cementum and pulp (Keil, 1966; Thenius, 1989; Bishop, 1995; Hillson, 2005; Gorrel & Verhaert, 2006) (Figure 2.4).

2.3.1 Enamel
Enamel (substantia adamantina, enamelum dentis) has neither nervous tissue nor a blood supply. It is the hardest and mostly highly mineralized substance in the body of mammals. Dental enamel is made up of 96–99% inorganic material and is acellular; only approximately 1% of it is organic matter and water. The compressive strength

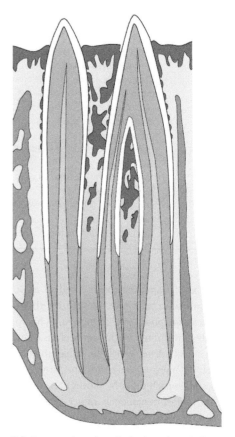

Figure 2.4 Cross-section of a trilophodont, hypselodont cheek tooth of a juvenile guinea pig (adapted from Cohrs, Jaffe & Meessen, 1958; originally published in Kotanyi, 1927); yellow=pulp, purple=dentin, white=enamel.

Table 2.2 Odontological terms.

Terminus	Description
Hypsodont	Long tooth body, long clinical crown
Mesodont	Medium–high tooth body
Brachyodont	Short, low crown
Elodont	Growing during the whole lifetime
Radicular elodont	Growing during the whole lifetime and forming a root
Aradicular elodont	Growing during the whole lifetime and not forming a root
Anelodont	Not growing during the whole lifetime, limited growth during tooth development
Hypselodont	Long tooth body and growing during the whole lifetime
Bunodont	Occlusal surface with low, rounded enamel cusps
Lophodont	Occlusal surface with transverse enamel ridges or folds ("lophs")
Loxodont	Occlusal surface resembling a washboard with multiple, parallel transverse ridges (elephant)
Bilophodont	Two transverse enamel ridges
Polylophodont	Several transverse enamel ridges
Selenodont	Crescent-shaped enamel ridges oriented mesiodistally (even-toed ungulates)
Lophoselenodont	Occlusal surface with longitudinal, crescent-shaped enamel ridges
Secodont	Cutting teeth
Monophyodont	Having only permanent teeth (deciduous teeth missing)
Diphyodont	Teething occurring (deciduous and permanent teeth)
Heterodont	Dentition including different teeth (shape, function)
Homodont	Dentition with uniform teeth

of human tooth enamel has been specified as 3000 N/ mm². The substance that is responsible for that special hardness is calcium phosphate in the form of hydroxyapatite crystals. It is formed by the ameloblasts. Individual apatite or enamel prisms, which are longer than those in bone or dentin (approximately 1600 nm), are closely and densely bound to each other by means of a cement substance. The prism orientation is rather different in the various species. The processes of the ameloblasts are called Tomes' fibers; they determine the exact direction of the orientation of the enamel prisms. In the area of the apex, the enamel is formed by the inner enamel epithelium, a single-cell layer of ameloblasts. These slender,

cylinder-shaped cells with a hexagonal cross-section lie close together and one of their narrow edges is in immediate contact with the newly formed enamel.

Amelogenesis occurs in two stages: the production and the maturation of the matrix. During production, an organic matrix is produced in which the thin crystallites are incorporated. This matrix has the same structural properties as complete mineralized enamel but consists of a third each of inorganic matter, protein and water. During maturation, water and protein are removed and the volume of the crystals is increased. The final product is mature enamel, with enamel prisms approximately 4–12 µm wide. Each ameloblast is responsible for a certain section of the enamel (see Section 2.11, enamel and dentin hypoplasia).

In rodents (except guinea pigs), the enamel is pigmented with iron oxides. These are stored within the enamel as tiny granules by the ameloblasts. Moreover, the enamel of rodents has a very peculiar structure, i.e. a species-specific and characteristically different orientation of the enamel prisms. This allows for a large number of rodent species to be exactly identified from an examination of the enamel of a single tooth (a so-called individual fingerprint). To enable this, the structure of the outer as well as the inner layer of enamel is evaluated. The different orientation of the individual enamel prisms and the type and amount of cement substance in between are of crucial significance for an identification of the species (Tomes, 1882).

2.3.2 Dentin

Dentin (substantia eburnea, dentinum dentis) is formed by the odontoblasts and represents the bulk and the frame of each tooth. It is less hard than enamel. Dentin is made up of approximately 70% inorganic material and about 18% organic material (mainly collagen) – the remaining 12% is water. The compressive strength or hardness of human dentin has been specified as 600 N/ mm². The inorganic part of the dentin consists mainly of calcium phosphate in the form of hydroxyapatite crystals, whose structure closely resembles the structure of cementum and bone but is packed more tightly. The hydroxyapatite crystals are smaller and more delicate than the corresponding structures in enamel and are 20–100 nm long. The crystals are embedded into a collagen matrix, which also resembles bone but does not contain osteocytes, osteoclasts or blood vessels.

Inside the enamel and dentin is the pulp, which is covered by a single-cell layer of odontoblasts which line the dentin. The latter are elongated, narrow cells resembling ameloblasts. The smaller, outer end of the cell is in constant contact with the predentin that is produced by these cells. The odontoblasts form fine processes (Tomes fibers), which lie in thin tubules (canaliculi dentales) and penetrate the dentin radially. In immediate proximity to the odontoblasts, the dentin contains fine sensory nerve fibers, which implicates a certain sensitivity to pain here and thus makes it a vital tissue. In rat incisors, the nerve ends are limited to the pulp and do not extend into the dentin tubules – as they do in the cheek teeth of rabbits and other species (Bishop, 1995).

Dentinogenesis occurs in two stages. During the first stage of development, organic material and the matrix is formed (predentin formation), with the matrix made up of collagen, glycoproteins and glycosaminoglycans. Subsequently the crystals are embedded (mineralization). Immediately adjacent to the odontoblasts is the predentin layer, while the proper layer of mineralization is located approximately 10–40 μm deeper. In teeth with a growth limitation (so-called radicular teeth), there is a differentiation between primary dentin, which is formed until root growth terminates, and secondary dentin, which is formed afterwards – during the physiological aging process of the tooth. The formation of tertiary dentin can be triggered by a stimulus, e.g. direct pulp capping. Hence, dentin can be formed throughout life if the pulp is vital.

In the jawbone, the dentin of brachyodont teeth forms one or several roots, which, when fully formed have a closed apical foramen (e.g. the molar of a rat) (see Figure 2.2). The volume of the secondary dentin of these types of teeth increases continuously until they are completely mature. As a consequence of this, the individual pulp cavities, which are initially relatively wide, become progressively narrower. In comparison, elodont teeth have only a very thin layer of dentin at their apical end and thus possess sharp apical edges (Figure 2.3). However, their coronal dentin becomes denser as a result of the continuous tooth growth. Odontoblasts continuously form new, regular secondary dentin in the area of the open apical foramen and the wall of the corresponding pulp cavity, respectively. That secondary dentin is deposited layer by layer from the inside (continuous apposition). Here the supragingival,

atubular dentin layers are no longer sensitive and susceptible to pain because the sensory nerve fibers degenerate and become a nonvital tissue.

2.3.3 Dental cementum

Dental cementum (cementum dentis, substantia ossea) is formed by the cementoblasts, resembles bone tissue and is avascular. Cementum is made up of about 61–70% mineral substances (calcium and phosphates), 21–27% collagen and 12% water. Here again precementum (cementoid) is formed first and later mineralized (mineralization). Although dental cementum resembles bone, it does not possess Haversian canals and thus is more compact than osseous tissue. Cementum is a crucial component of teeth as it supports both resorptive and reparative processes. However, resorption and build-up are significantly slower than in bone.

In herbivore teeth that grow throughout life, the cementum lies immediately on the outer surface of the tooth – a thin layer extending coronally from the apical end. In addition, the coronal cementum fills the outer enamel coat folds, extending into the dental tissue along the longitudinal axis of the tooth. The thickness of the cementum may vary between 20 μm and several millimeters. Coronal cementum is structurally different from the other cementum.

2.3.4 Desmodontium

Each tooth is positioned in a socket (alveolus) in which it is relatively firmly anchored in the alveolar bone by means of the periodontal ligament (thecodont dentition). The periodontium (periodontal fiber, periodontal ligament) comprises the gingiva, the dental cementum and fibers of connective tissue or fibrous collagen tangles (Sharpey's fibers) that fill the periodontal space. Those fibers run from the cementum to the alveolar bone and form a tight connection. They serve to attach the tooth firmly inside of the alveolus, yet they allow a small amount of physiological mobility of the tooth. In addition, the periodontal ligament contains very delicate blood vessels and nerves. The narrow gap between the mucosal surface of the gingiva and the corresponding lateral wall of the tooth is called the gingival sulcus. The gums (gingiva) normally fit closely to the tooth. A periodontal pocket forms when the gingival sulcus deepens due to inflammation.

In teeth that grow throughout life, the dentoalveolar syndesmosis is structured a little differently from the periodontium of normal teeth with a limited period of growth. The difference is in the more complex orientation of the periodontal fibers. The fibrous collagen tangles do not run straight from the bone to the cementum but run in various and constantly changing directions. They insert either on the alveolar bone or on the cementum and meet in the middle of the periodontal space, in an area called the intermediary plexus (plexus intermedius). It is then that they finally connect with each other in a complex fashion. Thus this plexus is made up of a large number of interweaving fibers, some of which are in parts almost parallel to the axis of the tooth (i.e. longitudinal instead of transverse). That plexiform arrangement of the fibers is the reason why a certain amount of longitudinal displacement of the tooth within the alveolus is possible. Individual Sharpey's fibers can come off the plexus intermedius relatively easily and then firmly reattach to it in another place. This special kind of fibrous lining in the alveolus allows unrestricted and permanent growth of the elodont teeth, with the intermediary plexus constantly being rearranged. The periodontal ligament also contains many blood vessels, which ensure an adequate supply of nutrients to the ameloblasts (Emmel, 1938; Keil, 1966; VanForeest, 1995).

2.3.5 Pulp

The pulp (pulpa dentis) is in the pulp cavity (cavum dentis), the hollow interior of a tooth. The pulp cavity contains mostly loose connective tissue with blood vessels, nerves, lymphatic vessels and undifferentiated mesenchymal cells. In multirooted brachyodont cheek teeth, there is a differentiation between the coronal pulp and the radical pulp of the respective roots. All individual pulp cavities are always connected with each other in the coronal area.

The pulp of teeth that grow throughout life has an elongated, conical shape. It is very wide in the area of the open apical foramen and becomes increasingly narrow coronally until it finally disappears entirely. The pulp chamber always ends slightly below the clinical crown, i.e. its outermost, coronal tip usually does not reach beyond the interdental gingival papilla – both in incisors and in cheek teeth (Figure 2.4). Teeth with enamel folds always have several pulp cavities that are connected with each other apically.

2.4 Classification and forms of teeth

When describing the teeth of lagomorphs and rodents, different technical terms may sometimes be used that can cause confusion if not applied properly. For example, "lophodont" is often equated with "having enamel folds," but brachyodont teeth can also be "lophodont" (in rats). Therefore, in the following section, the terminology (see also Table 2.2) is explained more closely (Thenius 1989, VanForeest 1995).

As for the anatomy and physiology of the teeth in mammals, there are two basic dental types: elodont (growing throughout life), which are mostly aradicular teeth, and anelodont, which are radicular teeth that are limited in time in their growth. Furthermore, there is a differentiation concerning dental morphology (relation between crown and root) between brachyodont teeth that have a short crown (Greek: *brachy* = short) and hypsodont teeth with long crowns (Greek: *hypsos* = high). The latter have an extremely long tooth body. This structure is typical of the incisors of rodents and lagomorphs as well as the cheek teeth of rabbits, guinea pigs, chinchillas and degus. Hypsodont molars are typical of animals that feed on very abrasive food. They are open wide apically and are typically also covered with enamel in the area of the alveolus. They can be either radicular (horses) or aradicular (rabbits, guinea pigs, chinchillas, degus). Only aradicular hypselodont teeth grow appositionally in length throughout life and thus exhibit a permanent tooth eruption that is in balance with the continuous tooth wear (Figure 2.3 and also Figure 2.5). Teeth with a medium crown length can also be called mesodont.

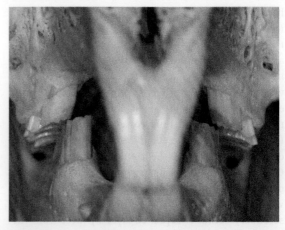

Figure 2.5 Normal occlusion and physiological anisognathism in a five-year-old rabbit (specimen).

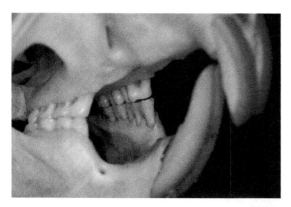

Figure 2.6 Slight malocclusion of the incisors in a one-year-old rat (specimen) with slight elongation of the incisors, isognathism and periodontitis-related loss of alveolar bone (lingually on the left).

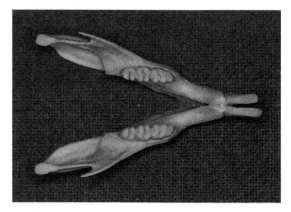

Figure 2.7 Normal occlusion in a one-and-a-half-year-old rat with molar occlusal surfaces worn down physiologically on both sides. The respective dentin bodies are partly exposed occlusally (mandible specimen).

Radicular teeth, which are often simply termed brachyodont, reach their ultimate shape and size relatively early in their development. During the subsequent maturation of the teeth, only the volume of the secondary dentin is changing. Those kinds of "normal" cheek teeth are found in humans and carnivores as well as some omnivorous rodents (e.g. rats, squirrels, hamsters, mice and gerbils). The radicular cheek teeth of small rodents are often defined as bunodont (Greek: *bunos* = hill), which is to say bluntly cusped, as their enamel cusps are relatively low and rounded. In young animals, the entire multicusped crown is covered by enamel. When food is ground, the jaws are moved predominantly in a vertical direction and only very slightly laterally. During this kind of movement, the cusps of a tooth slide exactly across the corresponding grooves of the antagonist, which makes the molars excellent tools for grinding (Figure 2.6).

In the course of evolution, a process during which simple dental cusps (cuspis dentis) were united and thus formed transverse or longitudinal ridges yielded what is termed the lophodont type of molar (Greek: *lophos* = ridge, crest), which has different forms: bilophodont teeth (two transverse ridges) and polylophodont teeth (several transverse ridges). An example of polylophodont teeth (pentalophodont in most cases) are the molars of myomorphic rodents, i.e. rats, mice, hamsters and gerbils (Thenius, 1989) (Figure 2.7).

Typical lophodont cheek teeth with long crowns – also termed lophelodont – and possessing multiple transverse occlusal enamel ridges or folds (so-called

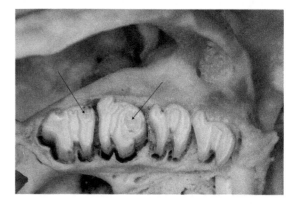

Figure 2.8 Early malocclusion of the right row of maxillary cheek teeth in a three-year-old guinea pig with structural changes of the occlusal surfaces of the last two cheek teeth (rostral dentin body of M2 and M3, respectively; black arrows) and significant expansion of the respective tooth sockets. The crown cement of the second cheek tooth (M1) is partly washed out whereas the first molar is physiological (specimen).

"lophs") are present in lagomorphs as well as chinchillas and guinea pigs. The complex structure of those polylophelodont teeth arises out of a deep invagination of enamel into the dentin. The enamel cusps, which in those teeth are also already present when they erupt, are quickly ground down postpartum by physical abrasion (Crossley & Aiken, 2004) (Figure 2.4). After that, the chewing surface is made up of layers of dentin, enamel and cementum of various thicknesses, which are arranged in a pattern that is specific for the respective species (Figure 2.8). Since enamel is worn down

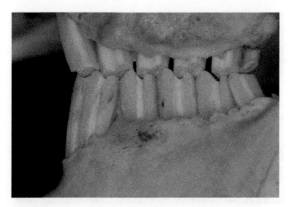

Figure 2.9 Buccal enamel ridges filled with crown cement in the lower jaw of a two-year-old rabbit (specimen; lateral view).

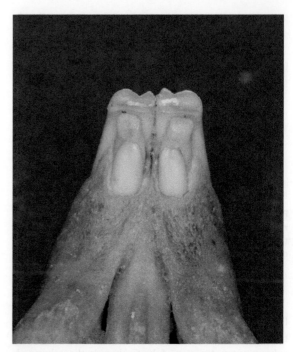

Figure 2.10 Teething in the maxilla of a five-month-old rabbit (specimen). Three incisors per jaw half can be seen (replacement of deciduous peg teeth).

less compared to dentin and cementum due to its extreme hardness, it forms a number of occlusal ridges, which give the occlusal surface a "corrugated" appearance. These enamel edges, which are always transverse in lagomorphs and herbivorous rodents, make chewing more efficient and thus reduce the functional abrasion of the cheek teeth.

A typical feature of enamel folded teeth are the folds (plicae) in the lateral walls of their crowns (Figure 2.9). Those folds extend across the entire height of the tooth and are reminiscent of the folds in a skirt. When the primary enamel cusps undergo occlusal attrition, the species-specific "pattern of folds" becomes visible when the dentin tissue is exposed. This structure is typical of the cheek teeth of rabbits, guinea pigs and chinchillas. In horses, the folding starts at the occlusal surface. These occlusal invaginations are termed infundibula (Latin: *infundibulum*=funnel). Infundibula may be found in isolation (solitary infundibulum on the incisor of a horse) or multiple instances (cheek teeth of elephants). They can also be partially connected to the corresponding lateral folds.

2.5 Teething

The occurrence of two generations of teeth is termed diphyodonty (two-time teething). During teething, the primary teeth (also called milk or lacteal or deciduous dentition; dentes decidui) are replaced by secondary teeth (so-called permanent dentition; dentes permanentes). European hares, for example, replace their deciduous dentition at the age of three of four weeks

(Keil, 1966). Rabbits who are altricial species do not finish that process before the age of four or five weeks (Tomes, 1882). On the 25th day of gestation, their foetuses have three deciduous cheek teeth and the deciduous peg tooth as well as the permanent incisor in each half of their maxilla. Their mandibles merely contain two deciduous molars as well as the permanent incisor (Horowitz, Weisbroth & Scher, 1973). The lacteal cheek teeth are – in contrast to the permanent molars – not elodont but anelodont and radicular (Tomes, 1882). They are partially worn in a process called bruxism (VanForeest, 1995). On the 31st day of gestation, the first permanent mandibular and maxillary molar, respectively, appear. Thus teething starts before birth, and postpartum both the tips of the permanent incisors and the first permanent molars are already present (Habermehl, 1975). In the period that follows there may temporarily be three incisors present in each half of the maxilla – they are the permanent incisors and the deciduous peg teeth to be replaced (Figure 2.10).

Although there should be no deciduous predecessors of the large incisors, two older studies show that in rabbits there is also an intrauterine replacement of the large incisors (Tomes, 1882). Those tiny deciduous teeth are built very simply as they do not develop further than a rudimentary stage. They have a simple conical shape, sit in the gingiva rather superficially and have a limited growth (Hirschfield, Weinrab & Michaeli, 1973). Although they are tiny they do feature the typical characteristics of a radicular tooth. The first typical hypselodont teeth are the following permanent incisors.

All rodents that possess only three permanent cheek teeth – rats, mice and hamsters – do not have a preceding deciduous dentition (true monophyodonty) (Tomes, 1882; Keil, 1966). However, there have been reports of deciduous incisors in guinea pigs and beavers (Keil, 1966). In rats, incisors erupt on the 10th day after birth, while the brachyodont molars do not appear before the 19th day. All permanent incisors and cheek teeth are clearly visible at 30 to 40 days postpartum, and their growth finishes at approx. 125 days after birth (VanForeest, 1995; O'Malley, 2008) (Figure 2.2).

In all rodents with more than three molars, the anterior cheek teeth are premolars that were preceded by a corresponding deciduous tooth (Tomes 1882). In guinea pigs and chinchillas, teething is completed before birth and the animals are born with a permanent, complete dentition (Berkovitz 1972). This phenomenon is called *intrauterine diphyodonty*. Their deciduous molars erupt intrauterinely between the 43rd and 48th day of gestation but have already been reabsorbed by the 55th day. They are very small when compared to the dentes permanentes (height about 1 mm) and possess a simpler clinical crown with cusps. The chewing surfaces of the lacteal cheek teeth undergo partial attrition intrauterinely (bruxism) and are replaced by permanent teeth before birth.

2.6 Dental formula

The original dental formula of higher order mammals is 3143 in the maxilla and 3143 in the mandible so there are three incisors, one canine, four premolars and three molars per jaw quadrant, a total of 44 teeth. However, there have been changes in the dentition as many animals have more specific dietary requirements. These changes relate not only to the structure of the teeth (more complicated patterns in the crown or a molarization of premolars) and the jaw (anisognathy) but also involved a degeneration or complete loss of individual teeth. Such dental reductions occurred mainly in a

mesiodistal direction. In addition, there may be individual variations from the species-specific dental formula (see Table 2.3). Typical findings are hypo- or polyodontia. For example, there is a report of a European hare possessing a double upper premolar on both sides (Hochstrasser, 2005). The same kind of polyodontia in a rabbit is shown in Figure 2.11. A differential diagnosis is a longitudinal splitting of a tooth, which can be clarified by means of a radiographic examination. However, such kinds of anomalies are rare in lagomorphs and rodents: only 4% of domestic rabbits are reported to exhibit these changes (Miles & Crigson, 2003).

Table 2.3 Species-specific dental formulas.

Species	Dental formula		Total teeth
	Upper jaw	Lower jaw	
Rabbit – deciduous teeth	2030	1020	16
Rabbit – permanent teeth	2033	1023	28
Guinea pig	1013	1013	20
Chinchilla	1013	1013	20
Degu	1013	1013	20
Rat	1003	1003	16
Mouse	1003	1003	16
Gerbil	1003	1003	16
Hamster	1003	1003	16
Chipmunk	1023	1013	22

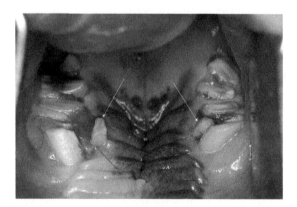

Figure 2.11 Polyodontia in the maxilla of a six-year-old rabbit. The first upper cheek tooth (P2) is present twice on each side (white arrows). On the left, a pronounced palatal displacement of the extra tooth body is apparent. The approximal areas are filled with food particles (chronic periodontitis).

2.7 Jaw relationship

The jaw relationship can be termed iso- or anisognathic (Thenius, 1989). Isognathy (Greek: *isos* = equal, *gnathos* = jaw) means that the upper and lower dental arch are equally wide (Figure 2.6). In this case the upper and lower jaws exactly oppose one another and the teeth will precisely meet one another along their entire occlusal surfaces when the jaws are closed (so-called central occlusion). An isognathic jaw relationship is typical for omnivores whose chewing action is predominantly a "squeezing" action (rats, mice, hamsters, gerbils). The majority of mammals, however, have anisognathic jaws, i.e. the width and length of their upper and lower jaws is different. For example, the mandibular arch of lagomorphs is narrower and shorter than their maxillary arch (Figure 2.5). By contrast, many smaller rodents with lophelodont teeth (guinea pigs, chinchillas, degus) have wider mandibles than maxillae , with the mandible also normally being shorter in these animals. In most cases the occlusal planes of the teeth are inclined differently as well (see Figures 3.20, 3.23 and 3.24b in Chapter 3).

2.8 Masticatory muscles

As well as the transition from isognathism to anisognathism, the temporomandibular joints and the masticatory muscles also changed continuously and species-specifically. In herbivores, the masseter muscle and the pterygoid muscle became especially strong chewing muscles. Both increase the chewing pressure, which helps to grind down fibrous foods more efficiently (Vollmerhaus, Knospe & Roos, 2001). This allows the animals to survive even in regions with very sparse vegetation. In lagomorphs and rodents, the masseter muscle and the medial pterygoid muscle are also the dominant muscles, whereas the temporal muscle is typically small (Thenius, 1989; Mickoleit, 2004). Three major forms of rodents can be distinguished based on their specific masseter muscles, i.e. the orientation of their superficial and deeper parts (Figure 2.12) (Mickoleit, 2004; Storch & Welsch, 2004):

Sciuromorphous type (representing squirrels). The ventral surface of the zygoma tilts and broadens into a zygomatic plate. The lateral masseter muscle extends forwards and origins on to this part of the rostrum as well as the superficial masseter muscle.

Hystricomorphous type (representing guinea pigs and chinchillas). The greater part of the medial masseter muscle origins on the lateral side of the rostrum and passes through an enlarged infraorbital foramen to finally insert on the mandible. The superficial masseter muscle originates on the front edge of the zygoma and the lateral masseter muscle extends over most of its length.

Myomorphous type (representing mice and rats). The medial as well as the lateral muscle belly of the masseter muscle are elongated and extend cranially. Just as in the hystricomorph type, the anterior bundles of the medial masseter muscle insert on the nasal bone and extend through the upper part of the infraorbital foramen (which is shaped like a keyhole). The anterior part of the lateral masseter muscle inserts on the infraorbital plate, which is positioned more vertically and expanded cranially.

2.9 Tooth attrition and abrasion

Attrition or parafunctional abrasion (bruxism) is the technical term for any immediate dental wear that is caused by the repeated rubbing and grinding on the opposite tooth while no food is being shredded (Thenius, 1989; Harcourt-Brown, 2002a). The teeth wear down each other, with the direction of scratches on the surface of the teeth depending on the direction of the jaw movement (Hillson, 2005).

A special form of attrition in rodents is the process which serves to actively sharpen the incisors (also named thegosis). The maxillary incisors are kept sharp by the sharp incisal edges of the mandibular incisors scraping past the former's caudal surfaces. Consequently, the mandibular incisors can be sharpened by bringing them in a prognathous position and having their caudal surfaces treated accordingly by the upper incisors (Miles & Crigson, 2003).

Animals that feed on large quantities of abrasive and low-energy food (such as grass, leafs, bark) are subject to a high continuous abrasion of the occlusal surfaces of their teeth. This functional abrasion is brought about mainly by the continuous contact of the teeth with the relatively hard and siliceous plant fibers (silica phytoliths, cellulose, lignine) and foreign matter contained in

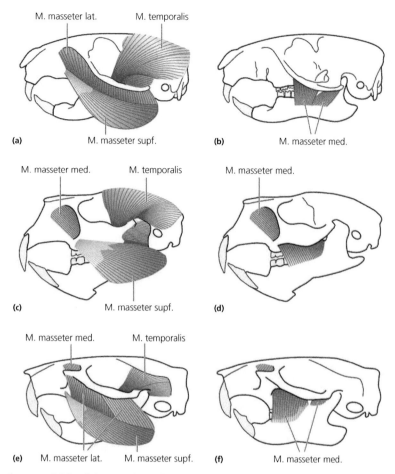

Figure 2.12 Jaw muscles, superficial and deep, in the (a, b) sciuromorph type, the (c, d) hystricomorph type and the (e, f) myomorph type of rodent (adapted from Starck & Wehrli, 1935; Vaughan, 1972, in Mickoleit, 2004. Reproduced with permission of Verlag Dr. Friedrich Pfeil and Elsevier).

these, such as sand or soil (Shadle, 1936; Ness, 1956; Hillson, 2005; Thenius, 1989). The continuous appositional growth of the teeth ensures that there is always just as much dental substance being formed as is being worn away occlusally. If this balance between eruption and abrasion is maintained, hypselodont teeth are theoretically indestructible and durable.

However, if animals with these kinds of specialized teeth experience a change in their diet, this may cause considerable dental problems. In horses that are fed in a species-appropriate way, cheek teeth grow 3 mm per year on average. However, if the animals are given food that is too rich in energy, the physiological abrasion will be reduced, resulting in malocclusions that require their teeth to be shortened regularly (Baker & Easley, 2003). This kind of situation is by far more problematic with

the elodont cheek teeth of rabbits, guinea pigs and chinchillas, which grow an average of 50 mm per year (Crossley & Aiken, 2004).

In order to avoid malocclusions, the balance between dental growth rate and abrasion, which is very prone to disturbances and varies greatly between species, must be maintained. The most important factors influencing it are the abrasiveness of the natural food and the length of time of feeding (Wolf & Kamphues, 1995). Both of these preconditions are not met whenever the animals are fed solely or mainly on dry pellets and high-energy compound feed. Contrary to this, wild rabbits, which spend most of the day feeding, hardly ever suffer from dental overgrowth. The consistent contact of the cheek teeth with the fibrous food ensures sufficient abrasion and prevents malocclusions (Figure 2.5).

2.10 Tooth growth

According to experimental studies, the incisors of rabbits, guinea pigs and rats grow at an average rate of 10–37 µm per hour or 300–1000 µm per day. However, the continuous tooth eruption of the maxillary incisors is slower than that of the mandibular incisors (Shadle, 1936; Matthews, 1972; Steedle, Profit & Fields, 1983, VanForeest, 1995; Wiggs & Lobprise, 1995a). Since dental abrasion is always proportional to dental growth, the consequence is a stronger physiological abrasion of the mandibular incisors (VanForeest, 1995). This could be either because they are used more and thus wear more quickly than the maxillary incisors or because they have a thinner enamel layer, which makes the teeth less resistant to abrasion in general. Of particular note is also that the incisors of hamsters grow especially quickly when compared with other animal species (see Table 2.4). The visible crown of the maxillary incisors is replaced entirely within a week; the mandibular incisors, which are longer, undergo that process in two and a half to three weeks (O'Malley, 2008).

In all animal species, the cheek teeth grow a little more slowly than the incisors. There are precise data for chinchillas, stating that their molars are physiologically worn down by an average of 1.0 mm per week, compared to approximately 3 mm for the incisors in the same amount of time (Crossley & Aiken, 2004).

Table 2.4 Average values for growth of incisors in lagomorphs and rodents.

	Average growth of incisors in mm in the upper jaw (and the lower jaw)		
	Daily	**Weekly**	**Annually**
Guinea pig	0.25–0,35	1.5	95–120
Rat	0.30–0.40	–	110–150
Golden hamster	0.2–0.8	–	73–280
Rabbit	0.35–0.40	2.0 (2.4–3.0)	120–150 (127–203)
Chinchilla	–	3.0	Approx. 60–80

Adapted from Shadle, 1936; Shadle, Ploss & Marks, 1944; Keil, 1966; Hamidur Rahman et al., 1983; VanForeest, 1995; Wiggs & Lobprise, 1995a; Harcourt-Brown, 2002a; Crossley & Aiken, 2004; O'Malley, 2008.

It is unclear just how exactly the continuous growth of (hyps-)elodont teeth is controlled. Many factors may play an important part in this process. For example, tooth abrasion is influenced by an animal's age as well as the individual occlusal pressure (Shadle, 1936; Ness, 1956). For an animal's body to be able to form the required quantities of enamel and dentin, its food must continuously contain sufficient calcium and other minerals, as well as vitamins. Any deficiency will inevitably lead to a qualitative degradation of the hard substance of teeth. Pregnancy also plays a certain role as the general increase in calcium demand causes the teeth to be less calcified temporarily and thus become softer.

Apart from this, the tooth growth is influenced by the blood flow in the periodontal tissue. Studies have shown that the production of tooth substance was temporarily halted or the tooth even sank deeper into the alveolus during such disturbances in blood flow (Matthews, 1972). On the other hand, tooth growth was enhanced by a local stimulation of the apex with low-intensity pulsed ultrasound (LIPUS).

However, what is really desired in the therapeutic treatment of recurring malocclusions of elodont teeth is a way of halting the constant tooth growth. At least in principle, this could be achieved by mechanically or chemically devitalizing or mummifying the pulp. For example, *para*-formaldehyde is said to kill off the germinal cells of the teeth concerned and thereby stop their growth (Wiggs & Lobprise, 1995a). Such an approach, however, has not yet been examined enough and proven to be feasible and scientifically proven for a larger number of animals. In addition, using formaldehyde is dangerous as it is not only cytotoxic but may also cause allergic reactions in rabbits and guinea pigs (Dold, 1924). Furthermore, formaldehyde has been demonstrated in animal experiments to have various systemic side effects and is absorbed into internal organs (Klimm, 2003).

The eruption velocity of the teeth is also influenced by the axial load of a tooth (Berkovitz, 1976). In an experimental study, rabbit incisors were put under varying kinds of pressure (Steedle, Profit & Fields, 1983). About two hours after a sustained load of 0.2 – 0.4 g was applied, eruption (approximately 34 µm/h) came to a halt. When a load of 2.5 g was applied, the teeth even intruded, i.e. a retrograde displacement of the apex occurred.

On the other hand, if there is no longer an axial load acting on an adult rabbit's incisor, its growth rate more than doubles temporarily (0.7 instead of 0.28 mm/day) (Augustin, 1937; Ness, 1956; Berkovitz, 1976). In rats, that rate even increases threefold (Schour & Massler, 1962). Hence, tooth eruption is markedly stimulated by a maximal shortening of the tooth. This is said to be true not only for the incisors of rabbits but also for their cheek teeth (Harcourt-Brown, 2002a).

If different loads are placed on the incisors of rabbits, this will not only affect their growth rate but also the thickness of their walls (Augustin, 1937). If after shortening of an incisor the remaining tooth acts as the sole antagonist for a pair of incisors, that tooth will automatically be abraded more. In response to this, the pulp chamber was found to end further away from the occlusal surface than the normal distance and the wall thickness of the tooth structure was found to have increased significantly (thickening of the dentin layer). By contrast, the dentin strength decreased very significantly in teeth that were shortened (making them temporarily functionless) – this may be because of the growth rate being doubled for a short time.

It seems that incisors exhibit eruption only when there is a certain amount of axial pressure relief. From this, it is possible to conclude that the incisors grow mainly during resting periods or at night. During the day, in contrast, they are used and abraded. The occlusal pressure during chewing inhibits a continuous tooth eruption (Mickoleit, 2004). However, if incisors or cheek teeth are in permanent contact (malocclusions with intraoral tooth elongation), no physiological tooth eruption is possible and the permanent axial load predisposes the tooth to a retrograde displacement of the apices.

It has not been proven experimentally if all the knowledge acquired from studies on incisors is also valid for the cheek teeth of rabbits and herbivorous rodents. Interestingly, however, in rabbits there is an initial uninhibited overgrowth of several (or all) molars in a jaw quadrant if their antagonists are extracted. However, according to the author's own experience, the longitudinal growth of those teeth usually ceases after a certain amount of time (three to five months on average) (Figure 2.13). This specifically applies to the maxillary cheek teeth of rabbits as more extractions are performed on mandibular teeth due to abscesses of the lower jaw. Without any loads acting on them, the maxillary cheek teeth of rabbits also tend to angle slightly buccally over time. Sometimes localized overgrowths of

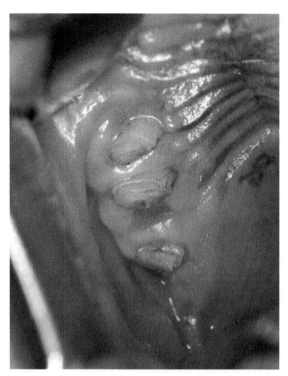

Figure 2.13 Four months after extraction of all lower cheek teeth, an intraoral hypodontia of the right maxillary arcade can be seen in a four-year-old rabbit. This is because some of the tooth bodies are located subgingivally and are not visible as a result of the secondary proliferation of the mucosa.

the gingival mucosa form and can indeed cover the molars in their entirety in individual cases.

Possibly, an inactivity-related low blood flow in the apical area may also cause a halt in tooth eruption. It seems that at least the cheek teeth of rabbits need a sustained formative stimulus in order to grow continuously. This is not the case for incisors, as can be seen in patients with brachygnathism whose incisors grow continuously despite a lack of tooth contact.

2.11 Enamel changes

Enamel defects are caused by local or systemic disturbances during enamel formation in the formative part of the periodontium. The surface enamel may either exhibit localized defects (grooves and nicks) or a generalized change of structure. In principle, there is a difference between enamel hypoplasia and simple hypocalcification of the "normal" enamel. Both kinds of changes can be found in isolation or in combination. A generalized enamel hypoplasia that affects all teeth can also be of genetic origin (amelogenesis imperfecta). However, those kinds of congenital defects do not seem to be an issue in rabbits and herbivorous rodents.

Generalized enamel defects are caused primarily by disturbances in mineral metabolism (particularly the calcium phosphate metabolism) (Miles & Crigson, 2003). This is reasonable as normal enamel is made up of more than 90% of mineral constituents, with calcium, phosphate, magnesium and iron playing the biggest part. The dental tissue is highly sensitive to any changes of the immediate availability of these minerals (Schour & Massler, 1962; Harcourt-Brown, 2002a; Mickoleit, 2004). This is particularly true for animals with elodont teeth because continuous tooth growth requires a steady provision of minerals (mainly calcium and phosphate) to ensure that dentin and enamel can be produced in sufficient quantities and of good quality.

It has been proven that alimentary calcium deficiency in young rats causes significantly decreased mineralization of enamel in their incisors (Lozupone & Favia, 1989). The normal quality of enamel was restored within 60 days by changing the animals' diet accordingly (Lozupone & Favia, 1994). Surgical removal of the parathyroid glands caused similar kinds of dental changes in rats (Erdheim, 1906). Due to a lack of calcification, newly formed incisors were very soft, exhibited structural changes and tended to fracture easily. At the same time, the laboratory animals suffered from severe periodontitis.

Multiple anomalies of the enamel structure may also be caused by various kinds of intoxication (fluoride or tetracycline in dogs or humans), endocrinopathies, febrile infections or systemic disorders. In pets, the most prevalent of these are chronic infectious diseases (Hillson, 2005; Harcourt-Brown, 2002a; Miles & Crigson, 2003). Apart from that, malnutrition may negatively affect the production of the enamel matrix because in such cases there will be an insufficient supply of vitamin A and proteins. Accordingly, structural – and mostly temporal – changes of the incisor enamel may sometimes be evidenced in dental patients that have undergone complicated surgery (e.g. an abscess revision). These enamel anomalies are a visible expression of the extreme strain of the procedure on the entire organism (Figure 2.14).

Enamel hypocalcification is described as a kind of enamel that has been formed in its normal thickness but has not been completely mineralized due to a disturbance

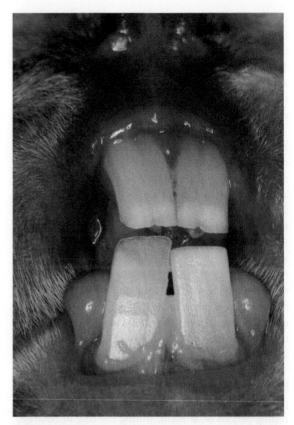

Figure 2.14 Changes of the incisors in a two-year-old rabbit with a hypomineralization of the tips of the maxillary incisors (whitish discoloration of the dental substance) and glass-like structure of the overlong incisal section of the right lower incisor.

in the maturation of the enamel. It is discolored in an atypical way and is significantly softer than normal enamel (Miles & Crigson, 2003). Clearly visible clinical evidence of a decreased mineralization of the enamel are chalky white and murky stains within the transparent enamel of the affected teeth.

By contrast, hypoplastic enamel defects are a result of a disturbance in the matrix production of the enamel that is the actual process of enamel formation. The thickness of the enamel (substantia adamatina) is changed, although this layer, which is often very thin, is usually normal hard because the enamel is well mineralized. Often only one tooth is affected by hypoplasia, which indicates a localized irritation of the germinal tissue (ameloblasts). Such an irritation may be a local infection or a trauma (Miles & Crigson, 2003). For example, experimentally damaging the germinal dental

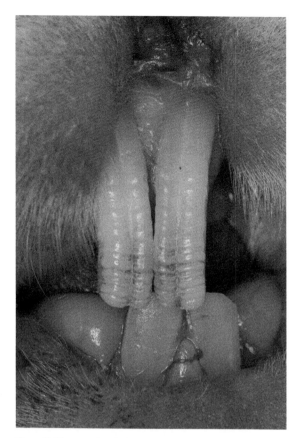

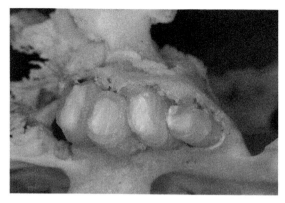

Figure 2.16 Severe enamel and dentin hypoplasia of the left maxillary cheek teeth in a seven-year-old rabbit with a distinct segmentation of the respective dental bodies: a central dentin lamella (white) and a peripheral enamel coat (yellow). Folding of teeth is lacking.

Figure 2.15 Enamel and dentin hypoplasia of the maxillary incisors in a three-year-old rabbit with typical transverse grooves in both incisors and an extra-alveolar dental overgrowth. The lower incisors are nonphysiologically short.

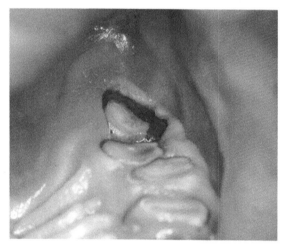

Figure 2.17 Recurring malocclusion in a seven-year-old rabbit with severe enamel and dentin hypoplasia of the second-to-last right upper cheek tooth (M2) and a typical segmentation of the tooth body: a central dentin lamella (yellow) and a peripheral enamel coat (red brown). The last cheek tooth (M3) is lacking.

tissue of newborn guinea pigs (needlestick) could cause an enamel hypoplasia – apart from other pathological changes of the dental tissue (Santone, 1937).

Clinically, enamel and dentin hypoplasia is marked by multiple fine transverse grooves that give the enamel surface a washboard-like appearance (Figure 2.15). However, there can also be a solitary, wider notch. These changes are clearly visible in rabbits' incisors whose enamel is normally smooth and shiny. Transverse grooves are often the first signs of an acquired malocclusion developing. If mineral deficiency is causing the defective enamel formation, a new production of healthy, smooth enamel can be induced by supplementing calcium accordingly (Harcourt-Brown, 2002a).

In the early stage of an enamel hypoplasia, tooth shape and eruption remain largely unchanged.

Eventually, structural changes of the teeth occur, accompanied by progressive damage of the germinal cells. Fully functioning hard enamel is no longer produced, being replaced by a dental substance that is rather soft and brittle (Figure 2.16). The maxillary incisors lose their rabbit-specific physiological groove in the longitudinal direction and the affected cheek teeth also lose their typical enamel folds. At the same time, the enamel, which usually is uniformly white, turns dirty yellow and becomes totally transparent in the same way as glass. The entire dental substance becomes very fragile and there are multiple crazes on the surface or even enamel fractures. As long as there is still atypical enamel being formed, it surrounds a dentin body that is completely altered pathologically in terms of structure and shape (Figure 2.17). The latter is also very soft, discolored a dirty yellow and is often thickened. Teeth with such kinds of changes are hardly functional and tend to fracture intra-alveolarly. It can also often be rather difficult to therapeutically trim such molars because the soft dental material will easily enter the surface pores of the bur, rendering the process less effective. In an advanced stage like this, the pathological processes in the area of the formative cells are irreversible and thus cannot be affected any longer. Finally tooth growth will cease entirely (Harcourt-Brown, 2002a).

CHAPTER 3

Classification and Anatomical Characteristics of the Lagomorphs and Rodents

The classification of lagomorphs and rodents is given in Figure 3.1.

3.1 Lagomorphs

3.1.1 General

The lagomorphs comprise two families: the *Leporidae* (rabbits and hares) and the *Ochotonidae* (pikas). Their classification can be seen in Figure 3.2. A typical feature of both families is a third pair of upper incisors, which remains small and is positioned behind the maxillary incisors: the so-called peg teeth. It is due to these additional teeth that the order of the lagomorphs is also called Duplicidentata. The two mandibles are firmly connected to each other via a bony symphysis.

The oral cavity is very narrow and elongated, and the tongue is massive and has a distinct torus linguae. Lagomorphs have a split upper lip, a long, toothless diastema and a heterodont dentition with hypselodont, lophodont molars. Both the incisors and the cheek teeth are white as their enamel does not contain pigments. The cheek teeth occlusion is anisognathous, i.e. the row of teeth in the mandible is narrower than the maxilla (see Figure 2.5 in Chapter 2). As a consequence of this, only the teeth of one jaw will occlude immediately with each other at a given point in time during the grinding of food. Yet whilst chewing, the teeth in occlusion will switch approximately 120 times a minute (O'Malley, 2008).

The sled-shaped temporomandibular joint is oriented rostrodistally and is slightly wider but distinctly shorter than in rodents (Figure 3.3). This causes the mandibular condyle, which is positioned very high, to be guided less tightly in the area of the processus zygomaticus ossis temporalis. At rest, the condyle, which is shaped like a rice grain, rests on a small step in the rostral section of the mandibular fossa (rostroventral prominence); in a way it is displaced rostroventrally (Crossley, 1995a). Only during this phase should the incisors be in contact, whereas the cheek teeth should be approximately 1 mm apart (healthy dentition) (Figure 3.4). The mandible is displaced slightly rostrally at this point; hence the mandibular row of cheek teeth is also shifted slightly forward (approximately half a tooth's width) with respect to its maxillary counterpart.

During gnawing, the condyle shifts even further in front of that small joint step such that the incisors assume the typical rodent position. For chewing, however, the mandible is displaced slightly caudally from its resting position. During the lateral grinding movement, the condyle is now located caudally from the concave temporomandibular joint groove. In this way, the incisors are in a distant position with no contact to each other, whereas the cheek teeth are in occlusion.

In most domestic rabbits, however, the mandibular incisors are in occlusion with the upper peg teeth in a pathological fashion during chewing. This causes the occlusal edges of the incisors to be also worn down during the lateral/sideward grinding movement (Harcourt-Brown, 2002a). Partly as a result of this, they receive their typical chisel-shaped biting edge. However, this does not conform to a normal occlusion (see above).

Excursions of the jaw during chewing are predominantly laterolateral (ectental jaw movement), with the multiple molar enamel ridges reaching exactly into the interdental gaps of the antagonists positioned opposite them. During that chewing movement and while immediate pressure is

Dentistry in Rabbits and Rodents, First Edition. Estella Böhmer.
© 2015 John Wiley & Sons, Ltd. Published 2015 by John Wiley & Sons, Ltd.

Class: Mammalia (mammals)
Subclass: Theria (live-bearers)
Infraclass: Eutheria (Placentalia – higher mammals with a potent
        placenta)
Superorder: Glires
Order: Lagomorpha (lagomorphs – hares, rabbits, pikas)
        Duplicidentata: 2 families, 13 genera and 60 species
Order: Rodentia (rodents)
        Simplicidentata: largest order of mammals; 7 suborders,
        31 families, 344 genera, more than 300 species),
        among them:
Suborder: Sciuroidea (squirrels, groundhog, beaver)
Suborder: Myomorpha (rats, mice, hamsters, gerbil)
Suborder: Hystricomorpha/Hystricognathi (guinea pig, chinchilla,
        degu and other South American rodents)

Figure 3.1 Taxonomic classification of the lagomorphs and rodents.

Order: Lagomorpha
Family: Leporidae (leporids – rabbits and hares)
Subfamily: Leporinae
Genus: *Oryctolagus* (rabbits)
Species: *Lepus europaeus* (European hare)
Family: Ochotonidae (pikas)
Subfamily: Ochotoninae
Genus: *Ochotona*
Species: *Ochotona princeps* (pika)

Figure 3.2 Classification of the lagomorphs.

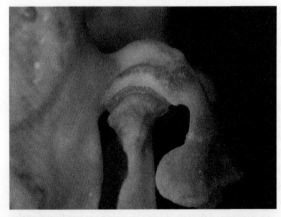

Figure 3.3 Temporomadibular joint specimen of a two-year-old rabbit, with a meniscus between the mandibular fossa and the mandibular condyle (caudal view).

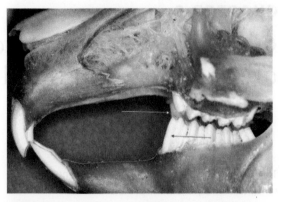

Figure 3.4 Resting position of the jaws of a wild hare (specimen). The incisors are in contact whereas the cheek teeth are slightly apart (white arrow). The mandible is displaced slightly rostrally (red arrow).

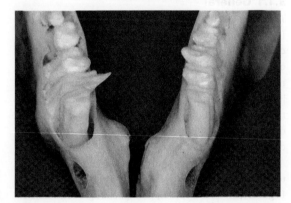

Figure 3.5 Malocclusion in a two-year-old rabbit (mandible specimen). There is a pronounced lingual deviation and a secondary formation of dental spurs in the second right cheek tooth (P4) and a lingual tipping of the third cheek tooth (M1). Moderate enamel and dentin hypoplasia of all premolars and molars (on the right) and a generalized periodontal disease with a severe expansion of the tooth socket and marked loss of the lamina dura (more pronounced on the right than on the left) are apparent. Furthermore, there is a slight lingual spur of the third left cheek tooth (M1).

applied to the food, a slight angulation of the occlusal planes causes the mandible to always be guided back into its median starting position (see Figure 2.5 in Chapter 2). The typical chewing movement seems to be largely independent of the kind of food, but the chewing pressure rises proportionally to the hardness of the food. Those kinds of forces acting on a mandibular molar that is sloped or curved inwards with respect to its longitudinal axis will increasingly displace this tooth lingually or deform it even more (Figure 3.5). Consequently, the maxillary cheek teeth will be curved buccally. A simultaneous rostrodistal shift of the mandible is prevented by the exact laterolateral movement of the jaws (Harcourt-Brown, 2002a; Crossley & Aiken, 2004).

In rabbits, the roughness of the molar occlusal surface is maintained by the regular attrition (Harcourt-Brown, 2002a). Rabbits often exhibit that kind of thegosis during periods of rest. If the occlusal surface is observed more closely, the effects of attrition and abrasion can be easily distinguished:

> Dental wear due to bruxism results in surfaces on the hard substance of the tooth that seem to be polished (these are always present in rabbits with a healthy dentition), whereas dental wear due to abrasion causes the surface of the teeth to be scratched accordingly (Harcourt-Brown, 2002a; Hillson, 2005).

This is an important aspect in evaluating the dentition during a thorough intraoral examination.

If physiological, abrasive food is consumed, the occlusive force acts mainly horizontally and barely vertically on contact of the cheek teeth during grinding. With their specially designed occlusal surface, the molars are perfectly equipped for that lateral cutting function and thus excellently suited for grinding fibrous plant parts. However, if the food is thicker and harder than hay or lush grass (e.g. grains or pellets), vertical forces are predominant during grinding. Those forces increase the curvature of the cheek teeth that is already present physiologically. The consequence is a typical formation of dental spurs (Figure 3.5).

Due to the horizontal grinding movements, the mandibular cheek teeth of healthy domestic and wild rabbits or hares always exhibit slight lingual spurs – particularly in the middle section of the mandibular row of teeth (P4–M2) (Figure 3.6). These "dental spurs" are physiological and must not be filed – which one is fooled into doing easily when experience is lacking.

3.1.2 Incisors

In principle, the large incisors of rabbits serve to bite off and chop up food. The precise function of the rudimentary peg teeth, however, is unclear. They are located palatally from the large incisors, are much smaller and stand out only a few millimeters beyond the gingival margin. Their cross-section is circular, they are almost straight or are slightly curved intraalveolarly and they lack a typical cutting surface; they mostly have a blunt end. Some animals do not have any peg teeth – possible reasons for this are a hereditary hypodontia, a failed

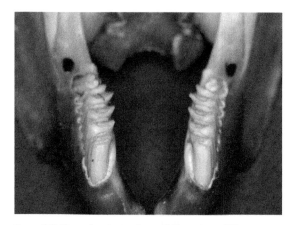

Figure 3.6 Normal occlusion in a wild hare (mandible specimen) with physiological lingual spurs of the middle cheek teeth.

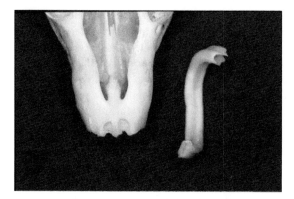

Figure 3.7 Rostral maxilla with a spirally twisted upper incisor in a five-year-old rabbit (specimen).

eruption of the tooth that is present (tooth retention) or a traumatic loss of very small peg teeth. Due to recessive inheritance, peg teeth can also be doubly present (VanForeest, 1995). That polyodontia vera must be distinguished from a polyodontia falsa, which occurs during the physiological loss of deciduous peg teeth (see Figure 2.10 in Chapter 2).

The lagomorphs' large incisors are aradicular hypsodont and elodont. They have different radii of curvature intraalveolarly: the maxillary incisors are always more strongly curved than the mandibular incisors. In addition, there is a slightly spiral lateral deviation in the maxillary area in many rabbits (Figure 3.7). The maxillary incisors feature a relatively deep, vertical enamel groove (sulcus) running across the entire length of their labial surface, which, apart from this, is smooth. That enamel and dentin invagination approximately divides the tooth into two areas of different sizes: the medial part, which is always a little smaller, and the larger outer part of the tooth (see Figure 2.14 in Chapter 2). The cross-section of the maxillary incisors is rectangular with rounded corners. The mandibular incisors have a smooth frontal surface and appear to be a little more rhombic in their cross-section. The apical area of the maxillary incisors is situated approximately at the level of the middle of the diastema, a few millimeters above the palatine bone. The intraalveolar part of the mandibular incisor is in the ventral half of the mandible and ends with the apex positioned just mesial to the first molar (see Chapter 5, Radiographic examination).

Both the large incisors and the peg teeth are uniformly white as they are covered with nonpigment enamel on all surfaces. The enamel layer is much stronger on the labial surface than it is on the lingual or palatal surfaces, especially in the maxillary incisors. Contrary to rodents, the enamel is made up of only one layer. That particular enamel distribution causes the palatal surface of the maxillary incisor, which is made up predominantly of softer dentin, to be worn more on contact with the mandibular incisor's harder edge, which allows for the formation of the typical chisel-shaped incisal edge (Keil, 1966; VanForeest, 1995; Hillson, 2005).

> Contrary to rodents, rabbit incisors are sufficiently abraded if the animals are fed species-appropriately (involving dental abrasion due to the gnawing or lateral cutting of fibrous plant material). Hence any special material for gnawing is not necessary primarily (VanForeest, 1995).

In rabbits with normal occlusion, the maxillary and mandibular incisors are in direct contact only at rest (incisal occlusion), whereas the cheek teeth are apart from each other. In that situation, the tips of the mandibular incisors are usually between the maxillary incisors and the peg teeth, or slightly caudal from that contact site (immediately on the peg teeth) (Figure 3.4). The occlusal plane of the teeth is horizontal when seen from the front, with upper and lower incisors being of equal length (the length ratio of the visible crowns is 1:1).

Rabbits do not "gnaw" like rodents, except when they suffer from problems concerning their cheek teeth that affect the normal chewing procedure (Crossley, 1995a).

The mandibular incisors are mainly used for biting off things. During that process, the sharp edges of the mandibular incisors glide sideways between the maxillary incisors and the peg teeth, cutting off a little piece of food in the way a pair of scissors does (Thenius, 1989; Crossley, 1995a). Since rabbits do not use their incisors primarily for grasping food, the incisors can be removed without causing too many problems – provided the indication is correct. After that, the animals are able to take in food by means of their lips, but they are no longer able to chop it into smaller pieces. Hence fresh food must be offered in appropriate smaller pieces (O'Malley, 2008).

However, the incisors of the lagomorphs can also be used for gnawing. For this, the sharp biting edges of the mandibular incisors repeatedly glide along the caudal occlusal surface of the maxillary incisors. These rostro-distal jaw excursions result in "scraping" movements (Harcourt-Brown, 2002a). As – contrary to the Rodentia – both the maxillary and the mandibular incisors are used during gnawing, there is typically a fourfold gnawing imprint in the wood below the bark that was consumed (Hillson, 2005).

Rabbits have a partially haired buccal mucosa (inflexum pellitum) in the area of labial angle or on the inside of the lip commissure (see Figure 2.1 in Chapter 2). During gnawing, the animals are able to retract these furry cheek folds into the diastema in such a way that they touch each other behind the incisors and above the tip of the tongue. In this way, the oral cavity is divided into two isolated sections: an anterior gnawing section (containing the incisors) and a posterior chewing section. This separation enables the animals to gnaw on hard material without a risk of sharp-edged splinters getting into their oropharynx and being swallowed inadvertently (O'Malley, 2008).

3.1.3 Cheek teeth

The enamel-folded, aradicular hypselodont cheek teeth of lagomorphs form, in their entirety, a relatively long, contiguous, rough occlusal plane. Due to the species-specific "interlocking" of the cheek teeth, it is optimally suited for chopping up fibrous food components into the finest pieces (Keil, 1966; Michaeli, Hirschfield & Weinreb, 1980; Hillson, 2005). Indeed, with the multiple, sharp, transverse enamel ridges as well as the extensive laterolateral jaw movement, the food is basically more cut up than ground up (contrary to the herbivorous rodents, whose chewing surfaces grind up the food) (Miles & Crigson, 2003; Harcourt-Brown 2002a). Although there are six maxillary and five mandibular cheek teeth occluding in rabbits, the length of the occlusal plane is almost the same (Figure 3.4). If only the dentin bodies of the cheek teeth are considered, there are 10 molariform dentin lamellae occluding – 10 of the maxillary cheek teeth contacting 10 of the mandibular cheek teeth (Harcourt-Brown, 2002a). Since the middle four teeth in the maxilla are much wider in shape (transverse oval) than the corresponding first and last molars, the middle part of the maxillary occlusal plane shows a slightly convex curvature to the buccal side, whereas the cheek teeth lie in a row medially (palatal) (Figure 3.8). The teeth of picas are smaller and the maxilla lacks one cheek tooth each on both sides (Hillson, 2005).

Both the mandibular and the maxillary cheek teeth of rabbits are arranged in a straight row that is oriented rostrodistally. If seen from the front, however, the cheek teeth are slightly curved – concave to the outside in the maxilla and concave to the inside in the mandible (Figure 3.9). Due to the anisognathism, there is only partial contact between the mandibular and maxillary cheek teeth when the jaws are closed; i.e. the buccal edge of the mandibular cheek teeth is barely in contact with the palatal edge of the maxillary cheek teeth (rostrocaudal view). The occlusal plane is approximately 10–15° oblique (see Figure 2.5 in Chapter 2). While in most domestic rabbits the intraoral part of a cheek tooth,

which extends beyond the alveolus (clinical crown), is white, it is rather brown in wild rabbits or rabbits that feed mostly on grass and other plants, due to herbal pigments (Figure 3.10).

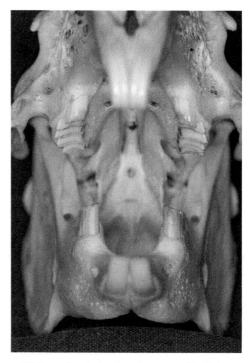

Figure 3.9 Normal occlusion in a three-year-old rabbit (specimen) with a physiological length of cheek teeth and occlusal surface (approximately 10° tilt).

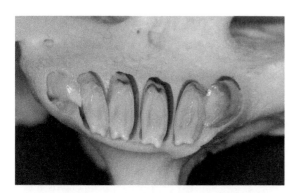

Figure 3.8 Normal occlusion of the left maxillary row of cheek teeth (specimen) in a one-year-old rabbit, with a physiological occlusal surface, bilophodonty of the middle cheek teeth (P3-M2) and a more simple structure of the first (P2) and last cheek tooth (M3) (a one-fold dentin lamella with an enamel coat).

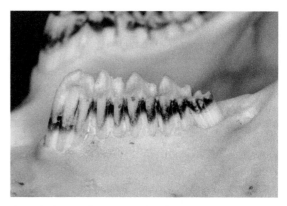

Figure 3.10 Normal occlusion of the left mandibular row of cheek teeth in a wild rabbit (specimen). The clinical crowns of all cheek teeth are partly colored by plant pigments. The occlusal surface is zigzag-shaped physiologically.

The structure and the dental pattern of lophodont cheek teeth is fairly complex. In the area of the dental body, they have deep enamel folds and there are sharp-edged enamel ridges on the occlusal surface. Premolars and molars are built almost identically (molarization of the premolars) (Hillson, 2005). The shape of the maxillary molars is predominantly transverse oval, whereas the mandibular cheek teeth have a mostly square cross-section (Figure 3.10). All cheek teeth have approximately the same length and structure of the tooth body. Together they represent a functional unit, the chewing surface. Both in the maxilla and in the mandible the most anterior and posterior cheek teeth prop up against the middle molars such that there is a slight slope of the teeth toward the middle of the occlusion (Figure 3.4). These marginal teeth are not only different from the others in terms of orientation and size, but are also composed in a less complicated way. Among them are the miniaturized last molar both in the maxilla and the mandible (M3) as well as the first maxillary cheek tooth (P2), which is also smaller. Those teeth are structured more "primitively," with the third molar in the maxilla being the smallest. The first mandibular cheek tooth (P3) is also anomalous in that it is much stronger and thicker compared to the rest of the cheek teeth (see Figure 2.9 in Chapter 2).

The basic structure of the lagomorph cheek teeth is made up of two lamellae, the anterior and posterior lobus, whose dentin bodies or dentin columns are circularly surrounded by enamel. This kind of structure is termed bilophodonty (Thenius, 1989). The two lamellae are firmly connected with each other via a thin layer of crown cementum; additionally there is a buccal enamel bridge in the maxilla and a lingual one in the mandible (Figure 3.8). While that connection is relatively thick in the maxilla (enamel and dentin bridge), there is only a significantly narrower enamel layer between the two dental bodies in the mandible. This predisposes the mandibular cheek teeth to split longitudinally in case of malocclusions with an apical irritation or an infection of the germinal cells. The mandibular premolars (P3/P4) are a prime example of this.

In summary, each cheek tooth consists of a more or less oval enamel cylinder including a dentin core, and the tooth is separated into two parts by a deep intradental fold that's visible from the outside in the mandible and a deep fold visible from the inside in the maxilla (see Figure 2.9 in Chapter 2).

The intradental enamel fold of the middle four upper cheek teeth is built a little more complexly than the folds in the rest of the molars (Figure 3.8). Its mesial wall is more folded, forming a relatively acute, denticulated ridge. That kind of enamel structure resembling a saw blade fits exactly in between the distal or mesial transverse outer lamellae of the two antagonists. Thus the transverse ridges and invaginations of the occlusal surface continuously alternate in the rostrodistal direction. They form a zigzag line on radiographs in a laterolateral view that is typical for the cheek teeth of rabbits (Harcourt-Brown, 2002a) (Figure 3.11).

The molars, being composed of two pieces, also have two pulp cavities, one each per dentin body (lamella dentis). The two converge in the area of the apex and form a common cavity there. Both pulp cavities become narrower as they get closer to the occlusal surface until they are finally closed completely by secondary dentin. The dentin also changes its structure toward the occlusal surface. What has initially been tubular dentin increasingly becomes thicker, atubular dentin, which is also denser radiographically. The outer surfaces of the cheek teeth are made of enamel that is covered intraalveolarly by a layer of acellular cementum

Due to the enamel folding, there are also longitudinal grooves and protrusions of various depths in the outer walls of the mandibular and maxillary cheek teeth. They are especially prominent buccally in the maxilla and rather lingually in the mandible. They fit exactly into corresponding bulges of the dental alveolus

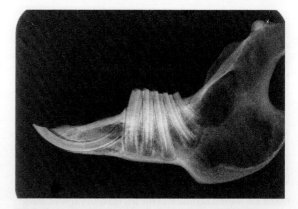

Figure 3.11 Normal occlusion in a one-year-old rabbit in a laterolateral projection. Mandible with clearly visible periodontal lamina dura and intradental enamel fold of the cheek teeth. The incisor has a physiological length (the mandibular plate merges directly with the cutting plane).

(Harcourt-Brown, 2002a). Another peculiarity of lagomorphs are the different heights of the alveolar walls. While the mandibular cheek teeth are positioned equally far out of the alveolus buccally and lingually, the maxillary molar alveolar walls extend as far up as the occlusal surface buccally whereas they terminate well below the chewing surface palatally (see Figure 2.5 in Chapter 2 and Figure 3.9).

As in all enamel folded cheek teeth, the softer dental substances (crown cement and dentin) are worn more quickly than the harder enamel in the area of the occlusal surface. This causes the latter to form a centrally arranged, sharp, transversal double ridge running across almost the entire width of the occlusal surface of each individual molar (Figure 3.10). Since each cheek tooth is covered with an enamel coat peripherally, slightly elevated edges consisting entirely of enamel also form there. In summary, the occlusal surface of rabbits is made up of a number of sharp-edged enamel ridges that are oriented linguobuccally and palatobuccally.

The individual intradental folds can be identified as radiopaque lines on radiographs of the mandible in a laterolateral view. Those lines divide the cheek tooth into a rostral and a distal section (Figure 3.11). That kind of structure is missing in the first and last maxillary cheek teeth, which are structured more simply. Both of those teeth are made up of a simple dentin core that is covered by an enamel layer on all sides. Their cross-section is circular to oval (Figure 3.8).

3.2 Rodents

3.2.1 General

Rodents represent the largest order of mammals. They comprise more than 2000 species and approximately 30 families. There are species of very different sizes (capybaras, beavers, porcupines, coypu, squirrels, chipmunks, chinchillas, guinea pigs, rats, mice, gerbils, hamsters and harvest mice).

The *Sciuromorpha* (squirrels and relatives; Figure 3.12) are found in a variety of habitats, from forests through to steppes and deserts. They are distributed worldwide, except for Australia, and there are approximately 250 species with sizes ranging from mice to groundhogs. There are climbers and gliders, while others live in subterranean burrows. Their cheek teeth are bunodont.

Order: Rodentia
Suborder: Sciuromorpha (squirrels and relatives)
Subfamily: Sciurinae (flying squirrels and some tree squirrels)
Genus: *Sciurini* (tree squirrels)
Species: *Sciurus vulgaris* (red squirrel)
Genus: *Tamias* (chipmunks)
Species: *Tamias striatus* (Eastern chipmunk)
Species: *Eutamias sibiricus* (Burunduk, Siberian chipmunk)

Figure 3.12 Classification of the Sciuromorpha (squirrels and relatives).

Order: Rodentia
Suborder: Myomorpha (mice and relatives)
Family: Muridae (true mice)
Subfamily: Murinae (Old World rats and mice)
Genus: *Mus* (mice)
Species: *Mus musculus* (house mouse)
Genus: *Rattus* (rats)
Species: *Rattus rattus* (house rat)
Species: *Rattus norvegicus* (common rat)
Subfamily: Cricetinae (hamsters)
Genus: *Mesocricetus*
Species: *Mesocricetus auratus* (Syrian hamster)
Subfamily: Gerbillinae (gerbils)
Genus: *Meriones*
Species: *Meriones unguiculatus* (Mongolian gerbil)

Figure 3.13 Classification of the Myomorpha (mice and relatives).

Comprising more than 1200 taxa, the *Myomorpha* (mice and relatives; Figure 3.13) are the most speciose group of rodents. They have bunodont to lophodont cheek teeth and lack premolars, and their infraorbital foramen is located in a deep indentation of the rostrum.

The *Hystricomorpha* or *Hystricognathi* (porcupines and relatives; Figure 3.14) have aradicular hypsodont, lophodont cheek teeth. They used to be called Caviomorpha.

The Rodentia live in the most diverse of habitats. Depending on the different ways of feeding and the food supply of their environment, many anatomical variations of cheek teeth have arisen over time. A uniform feature of rodents are their typical gnawing teeth and a largely flexible symphysis made up of connective tissue (e.g. in rats, mice, hamsters, gerbils and chipmunks). In some rodents, however, the, mandibles are permanently fused (bony symphysis in guinea pigs, chinchillas and degus).

Order: Rodentia
Suborder: Hystricomorpha/Hystricognathi (porcupines and relatives)
Family: Chinchillidae (chinchillas and relatives)
Subfamily: Chinchillinae
Genus: *Chinchilla*
Species: *Chinchilla laniger* (Chinchilla)
Family: Caviidae (guinea pigs and relatives)
Subfamily: Caviinae
Genus: *Cavia* (true guinea pigs)
Species: *Cavia porcellus* (guinea pig)
Family: Octodontidae (octodontids)
Subfamily: Octodontinae
Genus: *Octodon* (degus)
Species: *Octodon degus* (common degu)

Figure 3.14 Classification of the Hystricomorpha or Hystricognathi (porcupines and relatives).

Rodents have a heterodont dentition (VanForeest, 1995). There is a long, toothless diastema between the incisors and the cheek teeth; canines are missing. At first, rodents seem rather confounding and difficult as a group because of the high degree of variability that exists in their cheek teeth. Omnivorous rodents, which feed mainly on high-energy food and thus do not need a highly specialized dentition (rats, mice, hamsters, gerbils and chipmunks), have cheek teeth that are primarily brachyodont or bunodont. However, there is a tendency toward lophodonty in those anelodont, radicular molars (Keil, 1966; Hillson, 2005) (see Figure 2.2 in Chapter 2).

Rodents that feed on fibrous food (herbivorous species like guinea pigs, chinchillas and degus) have molars that are aradicularly hypselodont as well as lophodont. The formation of enamel folds increases the proportion of resistant enamel of the occlusal surface. Since the transverse enamel ridges wear down much less than the adjacent dentin and the crown cement deposited in the folds, they protrude beyond the occlusal surface as a system of multiple, transverse and very sharp-edged ridges in adult animals. These are optimally suited for grinding down the food very finely within the context of propalinal-ectental jaw movement; in total, they act in a similar way to a file (Hillson, 2005). Other than in rabbits, the folding structures of the maxillary and mandibular cheek teeth of herbivorous rodents (guinea pigs and chinchillas) do not match. Hence in these animals there are no enamel ridges that lock into the corresponding grooves (as in the lagomorphs).

In rodents, gnawing or chewing of the food is always done with different jaw positions (Mickoleit, 2004). For

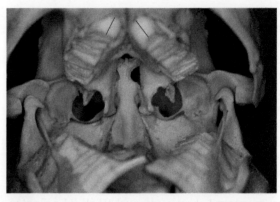

Figure 3.15 Tooth bridge formation in a four-year-old guinea pig (specimen, rostrocaudal view) in the area of the mandibular premolars and asymmetrical wear of the maxillary cheek teeth (clinical crown on the left is longer than on the right; black lines). The sled-shaped temporomandibular joints are without pathological findings.

gnawing, the mandible is shifted forwards, whereas for chewing and grinding of food, it is shifted backwards. The food of myomorph rodents is chopped up by means of propalinal jaw movement as well as simultaneous orthal motion components (vertical force application), with the food being chewed either on one side or two sides. The possibility of lateral excursion is usually restricted. During gnawing, rostrodistal jaw excursions are also made.

The sled-shaped temporomandibular joint consists of a bony longitudinal groove that is parallel to the longitudinal axis of the skull. It is open rostrally and caudally and has a medial and lateral ridge. The mandibular condyle, which is cylindrical and also oriented rostrocaudally, slides in that groove. Thus the joint guidance is very tight and does not allow much lateral jaw movement (Figure 3.15).

Whenever the mandible is shifted forwards for gnawing, the condyles rest in the middle of the mandibular fossa. This allows for expansive propalinal jaw movement, whereas lateral excursion is restricted (Miles & Crigson, 2003). Whenever the lower jaw is shifted backwards, into the so-called gnawing position with the cheek teeth immediately occluding, the head of the condyle comes to rest predominantly in a fibrous area that is located behind the bony fossa. This also allows lateral jaw movement. However, it does not apply to guinea pigs and chinchillas, where the condyle is in the area of the caudal fossa.

In rodents whose occlusal surfaces converge toward the rostral end (e.g. guinea pigs), the chewing action is rather diagonal (propalinal–lateral jaw movement) and only one-sided. An imaginary point in the area of the lower jaw could be seen tracking a circular arc in the frontal plane, an arc that is open at the distal end (by contrast, in rabbits, with their expansive sideways grinding movement, that point would track a straight, transverse line). At rest, the condyle, which is shaped like a rice grain and oriented rostrodistally, lies in the caudal area of the fossa mandibularis. During mastication, the head of the condyle moves rostrally in a longitudinal direction. During grinding of the food, one condyle slips forwards while simultaneously the contralateral one moves backwards (and vice versa). The jaws are not opened during that grinding movement, only the teeth move against each other. While the teeth on one side are grinding, those on the other side are moving apart. Thus new food can be placed between the chewing surfaces in order to be ground correspondingly. Mastication is accompanied by some typical grinding noises that are caused by the reciprocal rubbing of the cheek teeth. During grinding, the mandibular incisors carve transverse grooves out of their antagonists in the maxilla (this would not be possible with a purely propalinal grinding movement). The fact that the cheek teeth shift longitudinally against each other during mastication keeps the occlusal surface even. As a consequence of that very specific mastication, a pathological "step formation" of the occlusal plane is almost impossible in guinea pigs.

During gnawing, a two-sided rostral shift of the mandible occurs. That movement always involves an associated opening of the jaws, which is necessary for biting off and gnawing. When the mouth is closed, the jaws slide backwards again (Ganzer, 1908).

Another thing typical of rodents is the fact that the mandible can be passively shifted easily into a prognathous position due to the particular orientation of the temporomandibular joints. This most often happens with smaller rodents whose fur is grasped in the neck when trying to fix them (neck grip), causing the mandible to displace rostrally.

Small rodents with a bunodont dentition like rats, mice and hamsters have an isognathous jaw relation – they "crush" their food – whereas larger rodents with lophodont molars exhibit anisognathism, i.e. the mandible is wider than the maxilla (see Figure 2.6 in Chapter 2 and Figure 3.15). Independent of this, the cheek teeth of rodents occlude immediately with each other at rest, while at the same time the incisors are

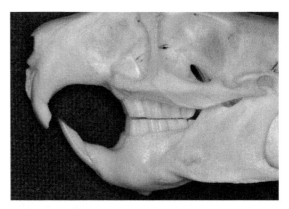

Figure 3.16 Normal occlusion of the cheek teeth in a three-year-old degu (specimen) and slight elongation of the incisors.

apart which is typical for rodents. The incisor's tips, however, are always level with each other in normal occlusion. Hence it seems that the lower jaw of rodents is in a physiological retrognathous position (Figure 3.16).

3.2.2 Incisors

A common feature of all rodents are the incisors, which are characteristic for this order. They are rather large and strong in some species and are used as a highly specialized tool for gnawing, so they are also called gnawing teeth (see Figure 2.6 in Chapter 2 and Figure 3.16). Since rodents have only one incisor in each jaw half, this order is also called Simplicidentata. The gnawing teeth lack roots (aradicular hypselodont), are curved in a semicircle, smooth on the surfaces and have a chisel-shaped cutting edge. The maxillary incisors are always more markedly curved than the mandibular ones. Depending on the species, there can be an additional spiral curvature of the teeth. Both incisors are deeply anchored within the bone for approximately two-thirds of the length of their entire tooth structure. Depending on the species, the apex of the maxillary incisors is located at different positions (in the region of the diastema). In the mandible, the apical area of the incisors is located either lingually or distally from the row of cheek teeth (see Section 5.6 in Chapter 5, Radiographic examination, normal occlusion).

The ratio between the visible parts of maxillary and mandibular incisors is approximately 1:2 to 1:3 at the maximum (rats). Only the labial (frontal) sides of the incisors are covered by a thick layer of enamel, which occupies a large part of the cross-section, making the teeth much more stable. The enamel cover becomes continuously thinner on the lateral surfaces until it cannot even be verified on the lingual/palatal side. The enamel consists of two layers on top of one another, the outermost of which is thicker. In rats, that enamel cover, which is more compact, represents approximately a third of the entire substance of the incisors. This results in a particular high strength of the teeth.

In healthy rodents, the labial surface of the gnawing teeth is colored in a species-specific way (yellow, orange, brown, red) – the exception being guinea pigs whose teeth are completely white. This coloration is brought about by an incorporation of iron pigments in the superficial enamel layer (Keil, 1966). Apically from the so-called hardening zone of the enamel, the pigment layer can be simply wiped off because it is only laid out on the soft enamel, which is still immature. The intensity of the enamel coloration increases with advancing age. The pigmentation of rodent teeth is very sensitive to metabolic disturbances and can therefore be regarded as an indicator of metabolic processes (Keil, 1966). Depigmentation may occur in cases of vitamins A, B, D and E, iron, calcium or magnesium deficiency, as well as in (experimental) overdoses of fluoride, cadmium or strontium. Depigmentation also results from experimental removal of the parathyroid glands (Keil, 1966). Hence any atypical pigmentation of incisors may indicate a primary vitamin or mineral deficiency. However, color changes of the incisors may also be caused by local infections, trauma of the teeth, various systemic disorders, increased dental growth or any combination of these factors. Most affected teeth exhibit typical white patches or remain totally unpigmented (Figure 3.17).

The lingual and palatal aspect of the incisors consists predominantly of dentin. During gnawing, that softer material is abraded more quickly than the hard labial enamel edge (or gnawing edge) that scrapes it. This is what forms the species-specific sharp, chisel-shaped gnawing edge. In addition, the rostral part of the dentin – the part that lies immediately below the labial enamel layer – is harder than the caudal dentin layer in rodents. This contributes to the formation of the typical gnawing tooth's shape (Tomes, 1882). The physiological length of the incisors is maintained by their steady use as well as thegosis (Hillson, 2005). That is the reason why rodents always need appropriate material for gnawing (suitable things are wood, twigs, bark, nutshells, etc.). In addition,

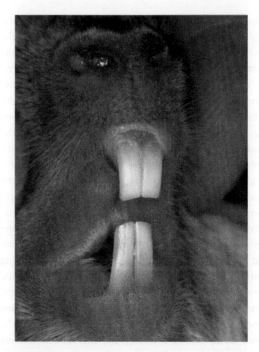

Figure 3.17 Mineral deficiency with insufficiently pigmented enamel of the incisors in a six-month-old chinchilla with an increased propensity for cramps. A subtle longitudinal groove can be seen on the labial surface of the right mandibular incisor.

> In summary, species-appropriate husbandry plays a major part in the maintenance of normal occlusion in rats, hamsters and mice.

it is also very important for their well-being. To offer suitable food is not enough to ensure a physiological dental abrasion – contrary to the lagomorphs.

During gnawing, the maxillary incisors are pressed into the object to be gnawed. They serve as a kind of support for the lower incisors that scrape against the upper incisors (Keil, 1966). During this, the lower jaw repeatedly executes rostrocaudal movements. The lateral cheeks are moved to fit into the diastema from the side, dividing the oral cavity in two sections. That division results in the posterior part of the oral cavity being protected during gnawing (O'Malley, 2008).

Rats, squirrels and groundhogs are able to twist the two halves of the lower jaw which are firmly connected against each other (Keil 1966). In this way the incisors can be used for gripping and splitting, too. In addition,

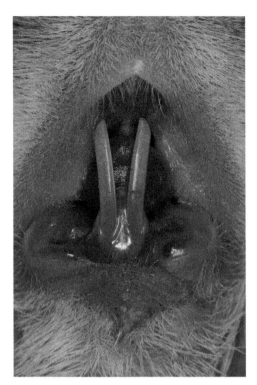

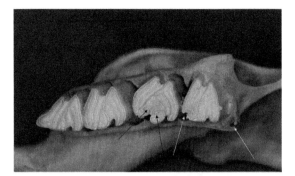

Figure 3.19 Early malocclusion of the right mandibular row of teeth in a two-year-old guinea pig (specimen), with a pathological occlusal surface of the third cheek tooth (M2; black arrow), a secondarily dilated desmodont, a subtle carious defect in the area of the mesiolingual edge of the last cheek tooth (M3; yellow arrow) and an expansion of the distal tooth socket with a small area of osteolysis of the caudal alveolar wall (white arrow).

Figure 3.18 Mandibular incisors spread apart in a one-year-old mouse: physiological finding due to an active contraction of the musculus transversus mandibulae (flexible symphysis).

the mandibular incisors of some rodents (groundhogs, squirrels, rats, mice and hamsters) can be spread like a pair of tweezers in the area of the tips of the teeth (Keil, 1966; Thenius, 1989). Squirrels use that mechanism to burst nuts (Figure 3.18). This is achieved by an active contraction of the transverse mandibular muscle, which circumnavigates both mandibles caudally from the symphysis. The incisors of rodents can also be simply pressed against each other vertically, just like in offensive biting.

3.2.3 Cheek teeth

Guinea pigs have four cheek teeth in each of the jaw quadrants. Those teeth are aradicular hypselodont and consist basically of two long, intraalveolarly curved lamellae or enamel prisms – a feature termed bilophodonty (Figure 3.19). The mesial, oval-elongated dentin body of each cheek tooth is significantly smaller than the distal one, which is triangular. The two lamellae are connected with each other via a relatively narrow dentin bridge, which is lingual in the mandible and buc-

cal in the maxilla. There is no enamel cover of the cheek teeth in that area (Hunt, 1959; Moriyama et al., 2006). Each of the distal dentin bodies has a relatively small buccal notch in the upper jaw or a corresponding lingual one in the lower jaw. A tendency toward polylophodonty in the form of a caudal spur is present only in the last maxillary and mandibular molar (M3). There are deep enamel folds filled with crown cement between both dentin prisms. The enamel fold runs from the buccal almost to the lingual end in the lower jaw and correspondingly palatal to buccal in the upper jaw. These enamel folds give rise to multiple zigzag-shaped, sharp-edged ridges on the occlusal surface.

The mandible is wider than the maxilla (anisognathism) and the two rows of teeth diverge markedly toward the caudal end. The cheek teeth face each other directly, with the two occlusal planes having approximately the same length. The occlusal surface, which is always smooth in normal occlusion, is tilted by approximately 40° (rostrocaudal view), angled toward the buccal side in the upper jaw and the lingual side in the lower jaw (Figure 3.20). The long tooth structures are strongly curved intraalveolarly, i.e. concave to the outside in the upper jaw and concave to the inside in the lower jaw.

Chinchillas also have four cheek teeth in each of the jaw quadrants. Those teeth are aradicular hypselodont, with each of them consisting of three transverse, stretched or slightly curved dentin lamellae that are

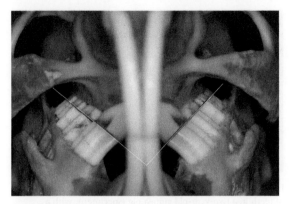

Figure 3.20 Normal occlusion in a four-year-old guinea pig (specimen, rostrocaudal view), with a physiological length of the cheek teeth, a 40° tilt of the chewing surface and anisognathy.

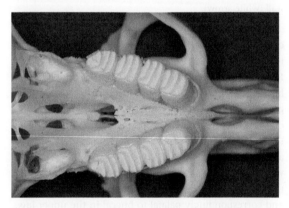

Figure 3.21 Mild malocclusion of the maxilla in a five-year-old chinchilla (specimen), with a mild elongation of the clinical crowns of all cheek teeth, a dilatation of the periodontal ligament space in the area of the anterior two cheek teeth (P4/M1; more pronounced on the right than on the left) and clearly visible folding of the tooth bodies (trilophodonty).

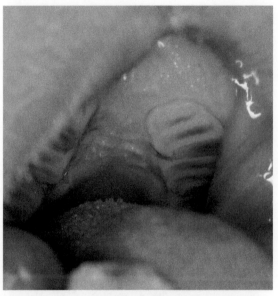

Figure 3.22 Early malocclusion of the left maxillary row of cheek teeth in a two-year-old chinchilla, with physiological length of the first cheek tooth (P4) and slight intraoral elongation of the remaining molars.

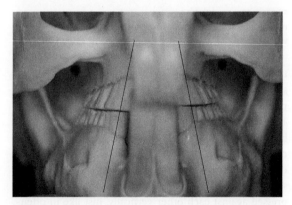

Figure 3.23 Malocclusion in a two-year-old chinchilla (specimen), with distinct elongation of the clinical crowns of all cheek teeth (more pronounced in the upper jaw than in the lower jaw) and a mild intraoral overgrowth of the mandibular incisors.

closely adjacent to each other and connected by crown cement. This is termed trilophodonty (Hillson, 2005) (Figure 3.21). The first mandibular cheek tooth has a triangular shape whereas the rest of the molars are rectangular. Clinical intraoral findings show the maxillary molars to be significantly shorter than those in the mandible. In normal occlusion, they are flush with the mucosal border whereas the teeth in the mandible protrude approximately 2–3 mm (Figure 3.22). When looking at prepared specimens of skulls or radiographs of healthy animals, however, the whole structure (dentin lamellae) of the mandibular and maxillary

cheek teeth have an identical length. The mandible is a little wider than the upper jaw (anisognathism) and the rows of teeth diverge toward the distal end, with the chewing surface being horizontal and physiologically smooth. The cheek teeth are slightly tilted with respect to the jaw – 10° buccally in the maxilla and the same angle lingually in the mandible (Figure 3.23).

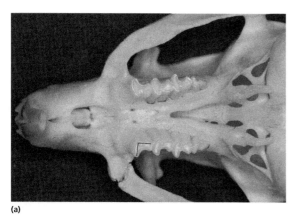
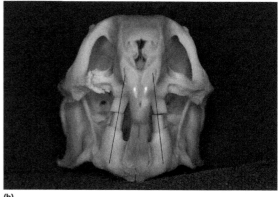

(a) **(b)**

Figure 3.24 Normal occlusion in a two-year-old degu (maxilla specimen). (a) View from below: physiological shape of the clinical crowns and occlusal surfaces of all cheek teeth, and an older fracture of the right zygomatic process. (b) Rostrocaudal view: physiological length and position of the cheek teeth. The fracture of the zygomatic process can also be seen here.

Degus also have four cheek teeth that are aradicular hypselodont in each of the jaw quadrants (Figure 3.16). The occlusal plane of the mandibular molars is shaped like a basin, having a slightly elevated outer enamel edge that resembles a figure of eight. The maxillary cheek teeth of adults are rather L-shaped as each tooth has a lateral spur rostrally (Figure 3.24a). Like chinchillas (but more subtle), the cheek teeth are slightly tilted with respect to the jaw – buccally in the upper jaw and lingually in the lower jaw. The occlusal plane is planar (Figure 3.24b).

Mice and rats have three molars in each of the jaw quadrants (see Figure 2.6 in Chapter 2). The radicular cheek teeth are brachyodont and exhibit enamel cusps, but also occlusal enamel folds in adult animals (Hillson, 2005). The main cusps are oriented in buccolingual or buccopalatal rows and connected by lower ridges. In the maxillary molars, each row has three cusps, with the middle being the largest. In the mandible, each row has two cusps of equal size. Some cheek teeth exhibit additional enamel cusps. Individual enamel cusps can only be distinguished as long as the tooth is not abraded, which is the case in juvenile animals.

With advancing age, physiological abrasion brings about the formation of enamel ridges that continuously get larger – so-called lophs, which connect the individual cusps on a larger scale. The dentin on the chewing surface of the teeth (which are polylophodont by then) is exposed unprotected between the multiple enamel ridges (O'Malley, 2008) (see Figure 2.7 in Chapter 2). This predisposes the teeth to caries.

The maxilla and mandible are equally wide in principle (isognathism), but the rows of teeth in the maxilla are slightly closer to each other. During chewing, there is usually only contact on one side. The size of the teeth decreases from rostral to caudal. The largest are the first mandibular and maxillary molars, which are multirooted (mostly five apices). The rest of the cheek teeth are three-rooted.

Hamsters have three molars in each of the jaw quadrants. The radicular, brachyodont cheek teeth of the Cricetidae are those with the shortest crowns of all small pet rodents. They are termed bunodont molars (Hillson, 2005). The first molar in the upper and lower jaw has six main cusps, which are oriented in two typical mesiodistal rows, whereas the second and third molars have four cusps each, which are positioned in a rectangle. In adult animals, the occlusal surface increasingly wears off and various rhomboid, zigzag-shaped ridges that connect the individual cusps are forming. The dentin of the teeth (which are polylophodont by then) is exposed occlusally, rendering the teeth more susceptible to carious defects. In hamsters the size of the teeth also decreases from rostral to caudal, just like the number of apices (Figure 3.25). The jaws of hamsters can be opened wide, by approximately 180°. Hence the oral cavity can be inspected relatively well, making hamsters interesting subjects, particularly for caries research, and making intraoral examination much easier for the veterinarians concerned.

Gerbils also have three molars in each of the jaw quadrants. The cheek teeth of the Gerbillinae or Meriones are also radicular and brachyodont, but relatively high-crowned compared to the hamsters and relatives

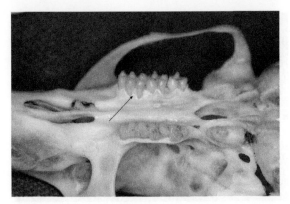

Figure 3.25 Normal occlusion in a six-month-old hamster (maxilla specimen): partially worn down occlusal surface with some enamel cusps still clearly visible and a mild loss of the palatal alveolar wall in the area of the first cheek tooth (M1; black arrow).

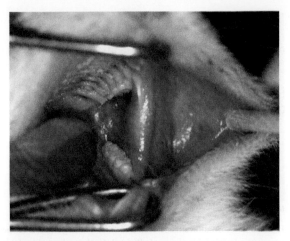

Figure 3.26 Normal occlusion in a one-year-old chipmunk: left mandibular and maxillary occlusal surfaces with partially worn-down enamel cusps.

(Hillson, 2005). In adult animals, there is a species-specific formation of three transverse enamel ridges on the first molar, the so-called lophs (trilophodonty). On the second cheek tooth, only two of those can be identified (bilophodonty) and only a corresponding structure remains present in the third molar. Hence there is unprotected dentin exposed in the area of the occlusal surface in older animals (due to ridge abrasion). In gerbils, also, the size of the cheek teeth as well as the number of roots decreases from rostral to caudal.

Squirrels have five molars in the upper jaw and four in the lower jaw. The cheek teeth are radicular and short-crowned (buno-brachyodont). The upper cheek teeth have four transverse buccopalatal ridges that run transversely across the occlusal surface (Hillson, 2005). The primary tooth cusps are lower on the palatal side and higher on the buccal side. The mandibular molars are shaped like a basin, with high mesial and buccal edges (Figure 3.26).

CHAPTER 4
Clinical Examination

4.1 History

All examinations of dental patients start with the "signalment" (breed, age, sex). For example, rabbits with an acquired malocclusion of cheek teeth are mostly presented for treatment for the first time when they are one to three years old. In guinea pigs and chinchillas, that average age of three to four years is significantly higher. Subsequently, a detailed history is taken in which more precise questions are asked concerning the housing and nutritional conditions as well as earlier illnesses and individual habits of the owner's animal. This will give the most exact impression of the environment and living conditions of the patient. Questions should not only concern the teeth, but consider all organ systems. An important question about nutrition would be whether the food that is offered comprises customary mixed or compound feeds and pellets as a principal food apart from hay. Are grass and hay the essential components of daily feeding? Is the animal offered vegetables and fruits, and, if so, in what quantities? Are there any treats offered (e.g. yogurt drops)?

Of particular importance is the question about pre-existing dental disease or pathology associated with the jaws. Have there already been any dental treatments or treatment of abscesses (with or without tooth extractions; number of teeth extracted)? How often and at what intervals? Were the treatments successful? Is the patient currently undergoing treatment with medication? How has the weight of the patient changed recently (weekly weighing) and how much food does the patient still consume by itself? Reduced feeding or even anorexia can be pain-related or a functional defect of the dentition. Has the owner noticed anything regarding feeding? Are there any

History

- Signalment (breed, age, sex)
- Housing, feeding, placement
- Previous dental treatment (type, frequency, therapy success)
- Medication
- Weight (normal, reduced, cachexia)
- Eating (normal, reduced or anorexia)
- Change in (selective) feeding behavior
- Change in food intake and atypical chewing movements
- Character changes
- Bruxism (rabbits)
- Atypical (empty) chewing movements
- One-sided "wiping off" of the mouth with the paws (guinea pigs, chinchillas)
- Recurrent wide opening of the mouth during eating (guinea pigs)
- Incomplete closing of the mandibles ("mouth is open")
- Hypersalivation (secondary dermatitis)
- Amount and consistency of faeces
- Digestion problems (e.g. colic, diarrhoea, obstipation, ileus)
- Caecotrophy
- Water uptake
- Urination
- Changed grooming behavior (unkempt fur, tangles in hair)
- Asymmetry or swellings of the head or jaw
- Halitosis
- Nasal discharge (runny nose, sniffing)
- Eye changes (epiphora, chronic infections, bulb protrusion or exophthalmos)

Dentistry in Rabbits and Rodents, First Edition. Estella Böhmer.
© 2015 John Wiley & Sons, Ltd. Published 2015 by John Wiley & Sons, Ltd.

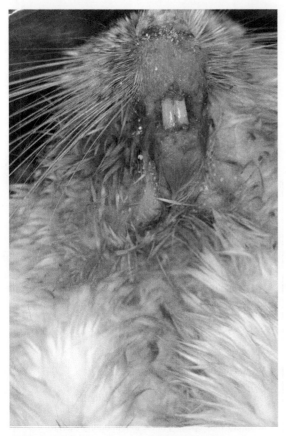

Figure 4.1 Malocclusion in a five-year-old chinchilla with hypersalivation ("slobbers").

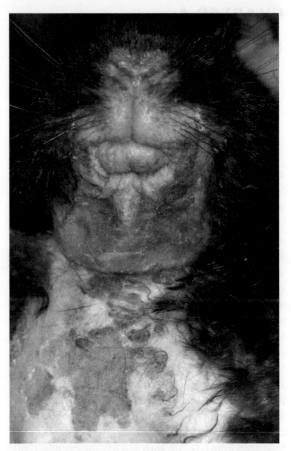

Figure 4.2 Malocclusion in a seven-year-old rabbit with chronic dermatitis and alopecia around the chin and throat, due to persistent hypersalivation.

changes in feeding behavior, e.g. a preference for soft food or a staunch refusal of hard food? Is the food consumed and chewed in a normal way or are there any changes in gnawing or mastication, e.g. does food that has already been chopped up fall out of the mouth again?

Have there been any noticeable changes in character or behavior? Are there any hints of pain-related aggression or is there more of a reduction in general well-being, or even apathy? Do rabbits grind their teeth (bruxism) or do they sometimes make atypical or "empty" chewing movements? Do the animals (particularly guinea pigs and chinchillas) frequently wipe their lips with a paw whilst opening their mouths extremely wide as if something had been stuck between their teeth?

Sometimes the patients are not able to close their mouths correctly due to generalized tooth elongation, which may be the time when owners finally realize that the incisors might be too long. Often the animals also

salivate more (Figure 4.1). Hypersalivation ("slobbering") may also be an indication of painful lesions of the oral mucosa (from the lingual or buccal tips of teeth) or problems swallowing (e.g. mandibular tooth bridge with tongue entrapment in guinea pigs). The animals concerned have a chin and chest fur that is sticky from the saliva. Over time a local moist dermatitis develops, which can also involve the front limbs when the mouth is repeatedly wiped with the inside of the paws (Figure 4.2). In the case of persistent hypersalivation, electrolyte imbalances must also be considered (e.g. an acidosis may result).

Questions should be asked regarding the fecal production – how much, what shape and what is the consistency? Digestive problems are quite common in dental patients due to insufficient grinding of the food or a rough fiber deficiency – the latter being a result of hay no longer being eaten. The animals may suffer from tympany, dysbacteriosis and diarrhoea or obstipation accompanied by the formation of small, dehydrated fecal pellets. Recurrent colics are also particularly frequent. In certain cases, there is a danger of an acute intestinal obstruction due to swallowing larger food particles; insufficiently chopped up pieces of carrot pose a particular risk. In the case of anorexia, defecation may temporarily be suspended completely. Associated with the digestive problems is the fact that most diseased animals do not drink enough, resulting in symptoms of dehydration. Furthermore, particularly dental patients with lingual or buccal spurs often refuse to drink water from bottles, because the repeated tongue movements that are necessary for this cause pain when the tongue rubs against the spurs.

Along with the history and physical examination, the anogenital region should be inspected. If the caecotrophes are not ingested as a consequence of a painful malocclusion, the 'night faeces' will often stick onto the fur in the anogenital area. This can lead to perineal dermatitis. The owners may suspect that their animal has diarrhoea or the feces seem to be softer. A consequence of this local dermatitis may be problems with urination with pain-related colic-like symptoms. Furthermore, the animal's grooming behavior may change due to malocclusion, resulting in the fur becoming scruffy and even matted as the affected animals may not be able to groom their fur sufficiently and remove the dead undercoat. This is predominantly an indication of primary or secondary malocclusions of incisors.

Many owners do not consider a possible dental problem until the animals have developed extensive jaw swellings (abscesses) and start to smell of pus or until the animals start to suffer from chronic disorders of the eyes or the nasolacrimal duct, which are resistant to treatment (Figure 4.3).

During discussion with the owners, their commitment and understanding of the responsibility to the animal are also evaluated. Treatment for malocclusions is often tedious and therefore can be frustrating. It can only be successful if the owner is prepared to bear the costs of repeated diagnostic and therapeutic measures, which are often substantial. Furthermore, the owner should be capable of looking after the patient appropriately at home following clinical treatment (assisted feeding with syringes, nutritional adjustments, daily weighing, regular checks, etc.). Having been thoroughly

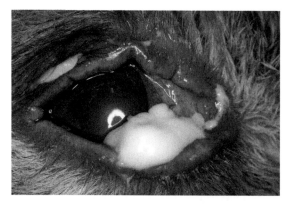

Figure 4.3 Purulent dacryocystitis in a four-year-old rabbit, due to a compression of the nasolacrimal duct caused by retrograde elongated maxillary incisors and a severe blepharitis.

informed, the owners should be allowed to decide how much to expect from their animals and whether they would like to discontinue treatment for reasons of animal welfare. Thus, they will be involved in the decision, take some responsibility and be prepared to carry out instructions from the veterinarian in charge as consistently as possible.

4.2 General clinical examination

After taking a full history, a thorough general clinical examination should be performed. This will determine the way to proceed. Surprisingly, the body temperature of herbivorous rodents is rarely elevated, even in cases of severe tooth or jaw infections. The clinical examination will determine whether thorough dental examination under anesthesia can be planned in the short term, immediately followed by treatment, or if the patient must first be stabilized (infusions, assisted feeding, etc.). In order to preclude or verify concomitant diseases of various organ systems or other primary causes of the anorexia, abdominal and thoracic radiographs should be taken if necessary. Additionally, a blood analysis may be considered Hematogenous, intrathoracic or intra-abdominal abscesses are not uncommon, particularly in cases of chronic, tooth-associated osteomyelitis (Figure 4.4a and b).

Blood analyses are rarely helpful for an immediate diagnosis of jaw abscesses because acute infections involving pyogenic bacteria do not lead to leucocytosis

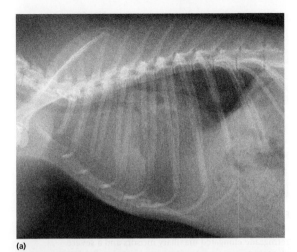

(a)

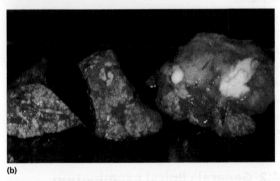

(b)

Figure 4.4 Intrathoracic abscess in a five-year-old rabbit. (a) Visible on laterolateral view as a solid radiodensity the size of a child's fist, located caudally from the heart in the fifth through eighth intercostal spaces. (b) Open pulmonary abscess the size of a child's fist and purulent pneumonia after the hematogenous spread of a chronic purulent osteomyelitis of the mandible.

or neutrophilia in rabbits and guinea pigs (Toth & Krueger, 1989; Harcourt-Brown, 2002b; Hein & Hartmann, 2003a, 2003b; Jenkins, 2008). Both species have a blood differential with a high lymphocyte count with hardly any banded neutrophil granulocytes present, so there is no "left shift" which would be typical for infections. In the case of infections, there is usually more of a shift toward the granulocytes (increase in pseudoeosinophil granulocytes). Hence a relative pseudoeosinophilia and a lymphopenia are indications of a chronic infection or an abscess (Hinton, Jones & Festing, 1982; Harcourt-Brown & Baker, 2001), or sometimes a mild monocytosis or an anemia (Harcourt-Brown, 2002b; Ward, 2006).

4.3 Specific clinical examination

4.3.1 Visual Inspection

Specific examinations of the dentition start with an examination of the head. Particular attention should be paid to the maxilla and mandibles as well as the area surrounding the eyes. Any asymmetries or local swellings are palpated. Swellings of the facial structure, maxilla or mandible may be indications of abscessation or a severe retrograde displacement of individual tooth apices. Neoplasia is also possible, but relatively rare in these pets. Hypersalivation in rabbits is thought to be caused by lingual or buccal tooth spurs, whereas in guinea pigs it may rather be the consequence of the formation of a tooth bridge with tongue entrapment that prevents the normal swallowing of saliva. A consequence of an apically displaced or infected maxillary incisor in a rabbit may result in a patient that presents with a chronic unilateral purulent discharge of the nostril due to a compression of the nasolacrimal duct running nearby, and a subsequent chronic infection and secondary dilatation of the canal. If the purulent infection spreads to nearby regions or even perforates into the nasal cavity, then the patient exhibits symptoms of a unilateral rhinitis (Figure 4.5).

Frequent consequences of a chronic infection of the nasolacrimal duct are ocular symptoms like unilateral epiphora, (kerato-)conjunctivitis or dacryocystitis. However, if a subtle bulb protrusion with a secondary prolapse of the nictitating membrane or even an

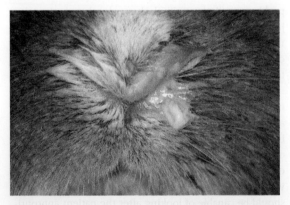

Figure 4.5 Left-lateral nasal discharge in a four-year-old rabbit with a chronic purulent infection of the nasolacrimal duct, due to an acquired incisor malocclusion with a retrograde displacement and elongation of the left maxillary incisor.

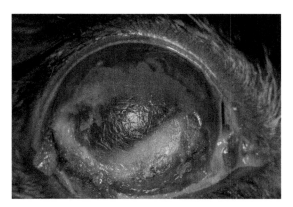

Figure 4.6 Right-sided protrusio bulbi in a four-year-old rabbit with an incomplete closing of the eyelids and a secondary corneal desiccation as well as a severe exposure keratitis with a fluorescein-positive corneadefect ulcer, all due to a tooth-associated retrobulbar abscess.

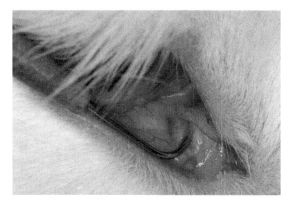

Figure 4.8 Area of the canthus of the right eye in a one-year-old rabbit. The rigid nasolacrimal cannula is in the punctum lacrimale, with the opening located approximately 4–5 mm away from the eyelid margin.

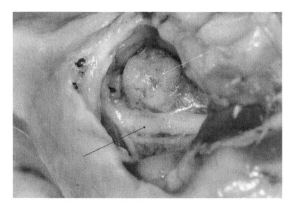

Figure 4.7 Left orbit of a three-year-old guinea pig after removal of the eye. Malocclusion with a severe retrograde growth of the second last maxillary cheek tooth (M2; white arrow) and lateral displacement of the nervus maxillaris (black arrow). In the area of the canthus, both lacrimal puncta are visible.

exophthalmos with an associated exposure keratitis is present, it is a sign of a severe retrobulbar infection (Figure 4.6). In rabbits, this kind of infection results from pathological changes of the last four maxillary cheek teeth (P4 – M3), whereas in guinea pigs and chinchillas the last two maxillary molars are primarily affected (M2/M3). Differential diagnosis includes retrobulbar neoplasia or suppuration of the tear glands caudal to the globe (hematogenous spread of infection in chronic infectious diseases). If there are nasal as well as ocular symptoms, an extreme retrograde elongation of the maxillary cheek teeth may also play an important

part, particularly in chinchillas and guinea pigs (Figure 4.7).

In rabbits with a secondary, chronic dacryocystitis, pus can often be expressed from the tear sacs when pressure is applied to the lower eyelid area near the canthus (Figure 4.3). If in such cases there is a suspected obstruction or infection of the nasolacrimal duct, then irrigation of the canal should be performed during further diagnostics. Using local anesthetic eye drops, this is possible without sedating the animal. In rabbits, there is only one small lacrimal punctum, which is located approximately 4–5 mm away from the edge of the eyelid positioned near the canthus on the inner aspect of the lower eye lid (Figure 4.8). Very delicate metal nasolacrimal cannulas can be used for flushing the duct, or alternatively the plastic part of a pediatric intravenous catheter could be used. Guinea pigs and chinchillas have two lacrimal puncta per eye, which are located near the canthus on the edges of both eyelids, which is similar to dogs. They are, however, so small that irrigation is usually not possible (Figure 4.7).

4.3.2 Palpation

Palpation focuses on swellings, asymmetries or deformations of the jaw bones and the periorbital region. Particularly the species-specific predilection sites for an ectopic displacement of the tooth apices are palpated (ventromedial and ventrolateral margins of the mandible, the base of the zygomatic process, preorbital maxilla). If palpable changes are present, a certain localized pain can be provoked by applying small

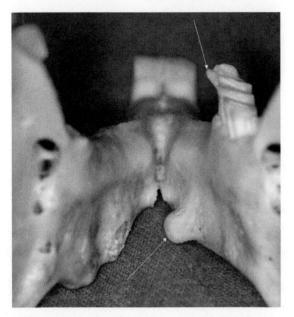

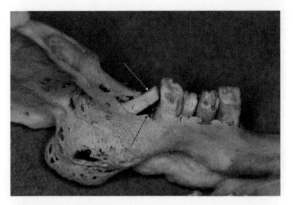

Figure 4.10 Left mandibular row of cheek teeth (specimen, medial view) of a six-year-old rabbit with malocclusion: mesial tilt of the last cheek tooth (M3; white arrow) with an enlarged approximal area (black arrow); periapical, mediodistal distension of the jaw (abscess); severe enamel and dentin hypoplasia of the remaining cheek teeth along with a loss of the lamina dura.

Figure 4.9 Malocclusion in a six-year-old rabbit (mandibular specimen, caudorostral view) with a retrograde apex displacement and lingual tooth spur formation of the second cheek tooth (right P4; white arrow). All clinical crowns of the left cheek teeth are missing; significant retrograde destructive processes of the ventromedial cortical bone of the mandible can be identified here. The pathology seen on the left side would be considered "end-stage" malocclusion.

amounts of pressure but they can also be entirely indifferent to palpatory stimuli. If painful, this usually indicates that the sensitive periosteum has been perforated.

Jaw neoplasia may palpably vary between hard and soft depending on the kind of tumor, whereas "classic" jaw abscesses generate rather softer, mostly fluctuating lumps. If pressed lightly pus may sometimes discharge straight into the oral cavity via the alveolus, which prompts the animals to perform certain chewing and swallowing and exudes a typical smell (halitosis). However, if the abscess capsule is calcified or consists of severely deformed, distended jawbone, then the abscesses feel hard and solid when palpated. Likewise, purulent infections feel rather sturdy and therefore "tumor-like" when they are located below the masticatory muscles (masseter muscle especially). This is often the case when apical abscesses of the last two mandibular molars are present in rabbits and guinea pigs.

Rostral mandibular distensions are usually a consequence of purulent apical or peridental infections

---

Systematic examination

History

General clinical examination (including fur and anogenital area)

Specific clinical examination

- check for: asymmetries, swelling, hypersalivation, nasal discharge, epiphora, conjunctivitis, keratitis, dacryocystitis, prolapse of the nictitating membrane, exophthalmos
- Palpation: asymmetries, swelling, local pain, pussy discharge
- Smell: halitosis, typical "smell of pus"
- Examination of the incisors (retracting the lips)
- Initial examination of the oral cavity and the cheek teeth (otoscope, endoscope)
- Flushing of the nasolacrimal duct

---

of the incisors. Often pus can be expressed from the infected tooth's alveolus when light pressure is applied to the swollen area of the jaw. In rabbits and guinea pigs, the inner aspect of the mandible is also always palpated thoroughly as the retrogradely displaced tooth apices of the anterior and posterior mandibular cheek teeth preferentially erupt medially (Figure 4.9). Consequently, abscess formations often originate on the inner aspect of the caudal mandibular area, which is easily overlooked during clinical examination (Figure 4.10).

4.3.3 Intraoral examination

Restraining the patient

For the examination of the oral cavity and the teeth, it is a good idea to have the animal held by its owner as experience has shown that the patient does not resist as much or not at all. This is particularly true for rabbits, guinea pigs and chinchillas. More defensive animals or smaller rodents (rats, mice, hamsters), however, should be restrained by an experienced assistant. The result of specific examinations of unsedated animals varies greatly. It depends mainly on the species and the individual willingness of the patient to cooperate and also on the experience of the examiner. In general, all small pets are typical prey species and therefore are always ready to flee; sudden defensive reactions and biting must always be reckoned with.

Rabbits in particular must be restrained firmly and securely for examination as they tend to kick their hind legs explosively. In so doing, they are in danger of injuring their spine (fracture or luxation) simply by contracting their powerful back muscles. The following method of restraint has proven itself in practice, as it can be quickly demonstrated to owners and then be performed by them without a problem:

> With the animal sitting on a table, its front legs are immobilized by means of the left hand; this is achieved by gripping both paws just above the carpus between the index and middle finger or by clasping both with the thumb and index finger. The person restraining the patient then bends down slightly over the animal and lifts its anterior body including the fixed paws in such a way that the rabbit's thoracic spine is pressed against the assistant's sternum. At the same time, the flexed stifles are covered by the palm of the right hand and pressed firmly against the belly and against the assistant (Figure 4.11). This ensures that the animal's backbone is optimally secured because the rabbit will not be able to kick its legs in that position.

This method of restraint can also be used for guinea pigs and chinchillas. Contrary to rabbits, these two species are very skillful at shoving the otoscope or endoscope aside with their little paws during intraoral examination – hence one must be mindful of a particularly good immobilization of the front legs. Alternatively, the animal can be completely wrapped in a towel.

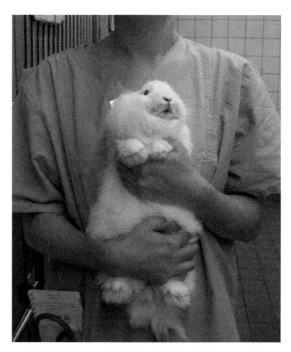

Figure 4.11 Immobilization of a rabbit for examination of the oral cavity.

If the animal starts to panic, the result can be an increased release of catecholamine with a dramatic rise in blood pressure and a tachycardia. Via a secondary arrhythmia, the latter can lead to sudden death due to stress within a very short time. In rabbits, an indication of that kind of stress reaction may be a sudden bilateral exophthalmos associated with a secondary protrusion of the nictitating membrane (Figure 4.12). The eye is pushed out of the bony orbital cavity simply by mechanical force, due to an increased blood flow in the retroorbital venous plexus. This causes the part of the sclera near the cornea to become visible as a white ring – any manipulations on the animal should be finished immediately and the patient should be given an opportunity to recover quickly (rest, dimming of light). The examination is then performed under sedation at a later time.

In order to restrain small rodents like rats, mice and hamsters, which are less susceptible to stress but more able to resist, the neck grip is best suited. The animal is first placed on a nonslip surface (e.g. flokati rugs) before one hand is used to fix it on the base of its tail such that the hind legs are lifted slightly off the ground. As the rodent is trying to run away, its entire body is pressed

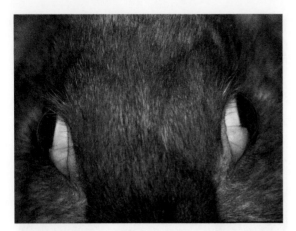

Figure 4.12 Stressed rabbit with a protrusion of the eyes on both sides and a prolapse of the nictitating membrane due to increased blood flow in the retrobulbar venous plexus.

When immobilizing pets, excessive or unnecessary coercive measures should generally be avoided as the animals (particularly rabbits, guinea pigs, chinchillas and degus) are extremely susceptible to stress.

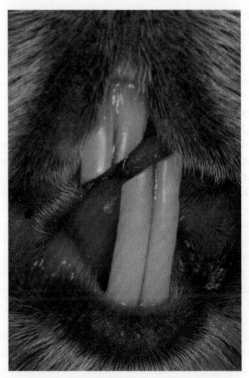

Figure 4.13 Secondary, acquired incisor malocclusion and hypersalivation in a three-year-old guinea pig with an abnormal oblique occlusal plane and a lateral displacement of the mandible due to primary cheek teeth problems.

down flat with the second hand (immobilization) and then grasped by the neck by means of the thumb and index finger. In this way, the patient can be picked up and at least a visual examination can be performed while it is lying safely in the palm of one's hand. Intraoral examination for an overview is possible with calmer animals. More aggressive rodents can be totally covered with a small towel or handkerchief, which is then pressed down flat. They are then picked up in the way described, with the neck being grasped along with the towel.

Incisors

For an examination of the incisors of lagomorphs and herbivorous rodents, the lower lip is pulled down by means of the thumb and index finger of the left hand; correspondingly, the upper lip is pulled up (and, in rabbits, aside at the same time) by means of the thumb and index finger of the right hand, coming from dorsally. Thus the entire extra-alveolar section of the tooth, the so-called clinical crown, can be seen. An evaluation is made of the species-specific occlusion of the incisors in the resting position as well as their shape, length and thickness, the quality, surface structure and color of

their dental substance and the state of the occlusal edge. If the latter is no longer chisel-shaped and not oriented horizontally when examined from the front, but instead is blunt and oblique, and if the incisors occlude in a pathological way in a resting position (lateral displacement, prognathy, etc.), then it is a clear case of primary or secondary incisor malocclusion (Figure 4.13).

More severe tooth deformations as well as primary structural changes of the tooth substance are likely to be indications of primary incisor problems. It is advisable to always check the outer enamel layer carefully by running a fingernail across it, because subtle pathological findings (as tiny horizontal grooves) are often difficult to detect solely by visual inspection – particularly when dealing with the uniformly white teeth of rabbits and guinea pigs (Figure 4.14). Alternatively, the teeth can be viewed more closely from the side with a darker background. While primary disorders affecting the incisors of rabbits, guinea pigs, chinchillas and degus are rather rare, secondary and acquired malocclusions of

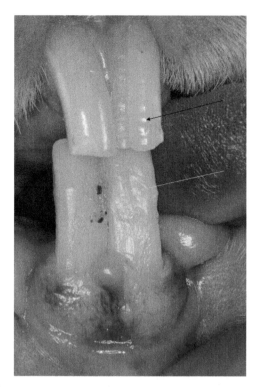

Figure 4.14 Incisor malocclusion in a one-year-old rabbit with subtle enamel grooves on the labial surface of the left upper incisor (black arrow), structural irregularities on the labial enamel surface of the left mandibular incisor (turqoise arrow) and mild overgrowth of both lower incisors.

Evaluation of the incisors

Occlusion (position of the incisors with respect to one another)

Occlusal surface (chisel-shaped, blunt, pointed, oblique)

Form

Length

Thickness

Structure/surface (enamel defects, horizontal grooves, fissures, chip fractures, splits)

Color

Deviation

Pathological changes of the peg teeth

Mouth gags and cheek dilators on nonanesthetized patients must never be used as there is always a great danger of injury to the soft tissue of the mandibles due to the defensive movements of the animals (the leverage effect caused by lateral jaw excursions). This relates particularly to the gingiva around the incisors, where local pressure necrosis together with periodontitis as well as iatrogenic loosening of teeth are possible (Figure 4.15).

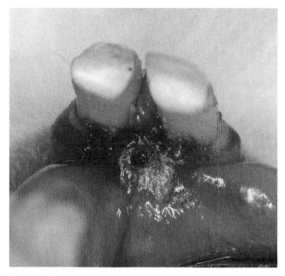

Figure 4.15 Mandibular incisors of a two-year-old rabbit (dorsal view) with gingival lesions of the mucosa after using a mouth gag without sedation of the patient.

Oral cavity and cheek teeth

It is not possible to view and evaluate the cheek teeth of herbivorous pets without any instruments because the jaws of the animals cannot be opened wide enough manually and the cheeks bulging far into the oral cavity also obstruct the view. Thus an initial examination of the oral cavity and the cheek teeth for orientation purposes is performed by means of an otoscope equipped with a rigid cap (ear speculum) as wide as possible and suitably sized or, even better, a suitable endoscope. Alternatively, a small spreadable speculum may be used.

The practicality of a conscious intra-oral examination depends on the size of the animal species as well as the individual character of the patient. When dealing with very uncooperative small rodents or ones that are susceptible to stress, the intraoral examinations are always

the incisors are fairly common (Figure 4.14). The latter are always an indication of a primary cheek teeth problem. On the other hand, it must not be assumed that the cheek teeth will be normal if there is correct occlusion of the incisors.

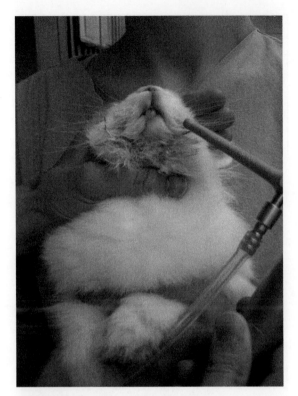

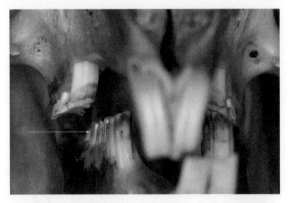

Figure 4.17 Mild elongation of the clinical crowns of all cheek teeth in a wild rabbit (specimen, rostrodistal view), with the left mandible having been shifted for a better view of the right maxillary molars (white arrow).

Figure 4.16 Immobilization of a rabbit's head for intraoral examination using an endoscope. The thumb is placed ventrally across both mandibles, while the remaining fingers clasp the roof of the skull.

done under anesthesia. When using an otoscope, the view into the oral cavity depends on the diameter of the chosen ear speculum (plastic or metal) as well as on the experience of the examiner. Particular changes of teeth or soft tissues that are deep inside the oral cavity are likely to be overlooked during this examination, which is performed more for orientation purposes. The final intraoral examinations, which are crucial for the choice of therapy to be initiated, are usually performed under general anesthesia along with the specific radiographic examination.

In order to restrain the head of a rabbit, the thumb of the left hand is placed below each mandible while the remaining fingers grip the top of the skull. The right hand holds the otoscope or the endoscope. The scope is carefully introduced into the oral cavity in the area of the toothless diastema, from the lateral aspect at a rather acute angle (Figure 4.16). It is during that kind of manipulation in particular or when the sensitive whiskers

are touched that the animal may make defensive movements. Many patients are highly sensitive around the entire head area and therefore try to elude any touch. That kind of behavior is usually a result of chronic pain or from the experience of previous tooth trimmings that were performed incorrectly or without sedation, leading to a generally over anxious patient.

During the intraoral examination, the jaws can be pressed gently but firmly against each other if necessary, such that the mouth remains closed in the resting position. This allows an evaluation of individual teeth without the constantly moving tongue obstructing the view via the otoscope. In rabbits, the jaws can be shifted slightly to the left or right with an additional lateral shear movement, with the direction depending on which of the maxillary or mandibular rows of cheek teeth are to be examined more closely (Figure 4.17).

A major advantage of the endoscope is the fact that the animal's owner is able to see the pathological intraoral findings on the monitor. This makes it easier to explain the findings and to discuss possible therapeutic approaches. In addition, working with up to a twenty-fold optical magnification – particularly in the context of the subsequent examination under anesthesia – allows detection of even the smallest changes of the mucosa and the teeth without any difficulty (Hernandez-Divers, 2008).

In order to get a good overview of the oral cavity, and also to prevent the patient biting into the delicate, rigid cap of the endoscope, the left index finger is introduced into the oral cavity via the right diastema during the intraoral examination. With that finger placed between the tongue and hard palate, the animal will not be able to close its mouth entirely. Yet the possibility is still there to press the jaws against each other with the thumb on the lower jaw and the remaining fingers on the top of the skull when immobilization is desired.

Neither an endoscope nor an otoscope will allow each individual tooth to be evaluated accurately from all sides. Particularly the lateral surfaces of the distal cheek teeth are not seen optimally, and small buccal tooth spurs may easily go unnoticed without a subsequent examination under anesthesia. In addition, the oral cavity is often filled with food remains or the patients exhibit an excessive production of saliva (this specifically applies to guinea pigs and chinchillas with secondary lesions of the mucosa), which may hamper intraoral examination or even make it impossible. In such cases the oral cavity must first be cleaned grossly. This can be done most easily by means of a delicate cotton swab that is introduced into the cheeks when the jaws are closed and then moved blindly between the teeth a few times with the jaws slightly opened. This is repeated a few times. In order to prevent intraoral accumulation of food, the patient should not be fed for approximately one to three hours before the planned examination.

During the examination, the length, form, position and structure of each cheek tooth should be noted. Furthermore, the occlusal surface is evaluated with respect to the species-specific shape and structure of its surface as well as its angulation. If there are buccal or lingual tooth spurs or tippings of single or various individual teeth, the adjacent soft tissue is inspected more closely (Figure 4.18). Intraorally visible bloody saliva or pus are indications of advanced malocclusions of cheek teeth with secondary soft tissue lesions or periodontal pathology resulting in mobile teeth. Particularly in guinea pigs that do not show any signs of malocclusions at first glance, each individual tooth's occlusal surface must be evaluated carefully. Subtle structural irregularities of the occlusal surface or the entire visible tooth structure may already indicate severe change of the subgingival tooth structure, and this can mostly be confirmed by means of good radiographic examination (see Figure 3.19 in Chapter 3). If the occlusal surface of single or various teeth is darkly discolored, it is primarily an indication of decreased dental wear and the (usually painful) cause of this must

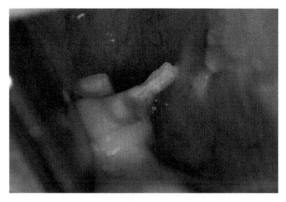

Figure 4.18 Right mandibular row of cheek teeth of a four-year-old rabbit with malocclusion: lingual tipping and overgrowth of the abnormally worn down second cheek tooth (P4). A secondary ulceration of the tongue can be identified rostrally (blurred).

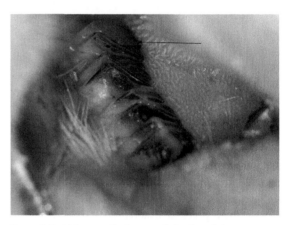

Figure 4.19 Right mandibular row of cheek teeth in a three-year-old rabbit with malocclusion: structurally changed occlusal surface of the last molar (M3; black arrow) and dark discoloration of the chewing surface of all cheek teeth, indicating insufficient dental wear (which is mostly pain-related).

be identified by means of radiographic examinations (Figure 4.19).

There is often a marked discrepancy between the findings of an intraoral examination on the one hand and the clinical symptoms on the other. For example, it is not unusual to discover intraoral signs of a malocclusion in rabbits, e.g. subtle curvatures of teeth with early stages of tooth spurs, a slight step formation or enamel hypoplasia and dentin hypoplasia, while the animals lack clinical symptoms. Conversely, the intraoral

If any doubt, radiographic examination should always be performed subsequent to any clinical examination that showed no intraoral pathology.

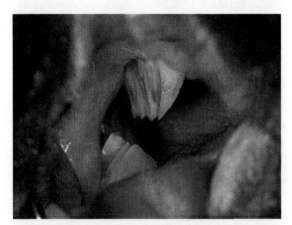

Figure 4.20 Right maxillary row of cheek teeth in a four-year-old guinea pig with malocclusion; vertical chewing surface of the right maxillary cheek teeth (P4/M1) indicating intraalveolar tooth problems in the right maxilla or mandible.

examination can be widely normal while the patient suffers from tooth-related anorexia. In most of these cases, there are relatively pronounced intraosseous changes that cannot be seen directly but are well defined radiographically.

This is crucial, especially when examining chinchillas, because early stages of malocclusions may go undetected in merely intraoral examinations (depending on the experience of the examiner). Malocclusion would then be diagnosed only when clearer clinical symptoms like anorexia or epiphora are found as the result of an advanced retrograde displacement of the apices of the maxillary cheek teeth – and the great pains associated with these processes – or when the teeth start to show an overgrowth that can be detected intraorally.

Although intraoral examinations without anesthesia usually allow only the front part of the oral cavity to be seen sufficiently well, a good impression of the entire dentition is still obtained. For example, in guinea pigs atypical angulation or asymmetries of the occlusal plane are indications of massive intraosseous findings that should be further clarified radiographically (Figure 4.20). However, even if the changes are less dramatic there are usually at least some indications as to which half of the

Intraoral examination for an evaluation of the cheek teeth and soft tissue

Occlusion: position of the cheek teeth with respect to one another, total height

Occlusal surface: species-specific or atypical shape and tilt, steps

Overall symmetry of the dentition

Number of cheek teeth: hypo- or polyodontia

Occlusal surface of individual teeth, particularly in guinea pigs

Shape of individual teeth: pathological curvature, deformation

Length of individual teeth

Thickness of individual teeth

Surface: enamel defects, transverse grooves, fissures, chip fracture, split, fracture

Structure: enamel and dentin hypoplasia, tooth demineralization, soft dental substance

Resorptive tooth changes: caries-like lesions in chinchillas and smaller rodents

Color of the tooth and the occlusal surface

Formation of plaque or calculus, more often in smaller rodents

Tipping/deviation: malformation of single or multiple teeth

Tooth surface: spurs, lingual or buccal tooth spikes, sharp edges

Oral mucosa: soft tissue lesions, ulcers of tongue, cheeks, palate or floor of the oral cavity

Intraoral pus: diffuse or localized

Gingiva: color, inflammation, swelling, hyperplasia (chinchilla), bleeding tendency, lesion

Signs of periodontitis : enlarged, inflamed periodontal pocket; local or diffuse

Impaction of hairs or foreign bodies (plant fibers) in the periodontium or interdentally

Possible mobile teeth

Exposed bone in fractures

Intraoral swelling due to an abscess, neoplasia or local inflammation

jaw or what jaw quadrant is the concern. Sometimes there may be only one suspicious tooth but, due to the pains it causes, it is the actual reason for the advanced malocclusion.

If a suspected malocclusion of cheek teeth is confirmed by additional radiographs of the head without anesthesia (in four views, if possible), then the findings and the further approach can be discussed and planned with the owner. Regardless a thorough examination of

Rabbit dental assessment chart

Owner's name						
	Reference Code or Address					
Animal's name	Breed	Age	Sex	Weight	Date	

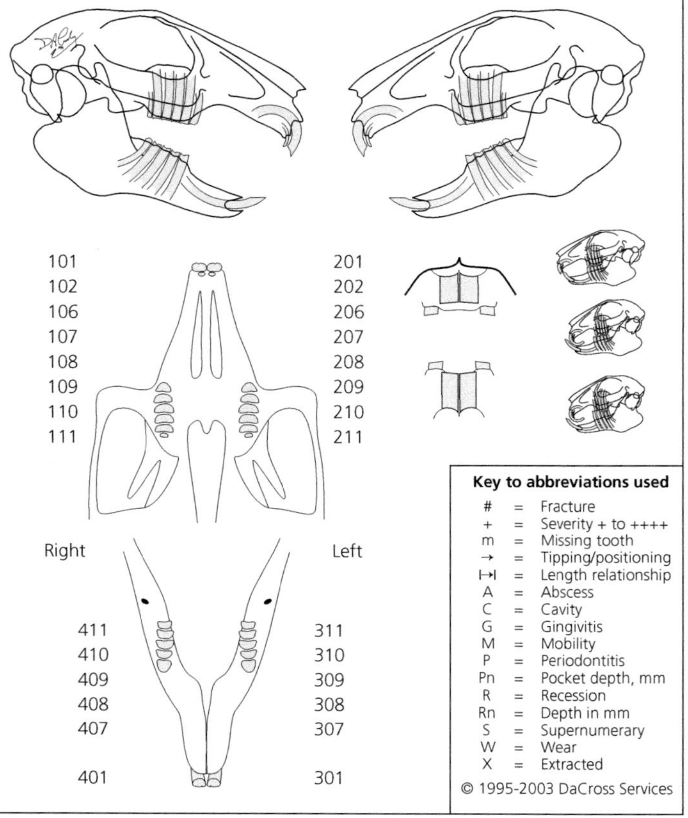

101
102
106
107
108
109
110
111

201
202
206
207
208
209
210
211

Right

411
410
409
408
407

401

Left

311
310
309
308
307

301

Key to abbreviations used

\# = Fracture
\+ = Severity + to ++++
m = Missing tooth
↑ = Tipping/positioning
|—| = Length relationship
A = Abscess
C = Cavity
G = Gingivitis
M = Mobility
P = Periodontitis
Pn = Pocket depth, mm
R = Recession
Rn = Depth in mm
S = Supernumerary
W = Wear
X = Extracted

© 1995–2003 DaCross Services

Dental procedures

Performed		Required
{ }	Pre-anesthetic checks	{ }
{ }	General anesthesia	{ }
{ }	Radiography	{ }
{ }	Occlusal assessment	{ }
{ }	Supra-gingival scaling	{ }
{ }	Subgingival scaling	{ }
{ }	Root planing	{ }
{ }	Polishing	{ }
{ }	Gingival lavage	{ }
{ }	Gingival surgery	{ }
{ }	Extraction	{ }
{ }	Periodontal splinting	{ }
{ }	Crown height reduction	{ }
{ }	Endodontic therapy	{ }
{ }	Restoration	{ }
{ }	Orthodontic treatment	{ }
{ }	Oro-facial surgery	{ }
	Homecare program	{ ✓ }

Assessment by quadrant

(graded +, ++, +++, ++++)

	1 (RU)	2 (LU)	3 (LL)	4 (RL)
Plaque	...	...	...	...
Calculus	...	...	...	...
Gingivitis	...	...	...	...
Periodontitis	...	...	...	...
Occlusion	...	...	...	...
Tooth wear	...	...	...	...

Other comments

Routine Home Dental Care

Herbivores naturally wear their teeth by prolonged chewing. To compensate for this the teeth continue erupting. If they do not have enough natural food the teeth get longer and develop sharp spikes which injure the cheeks and tongue. Chewing exercise is also beneficial as it stimulates natural tooth cleaning and protection mechanisms. In general hard and artificial chewing objects are not a good idea as many animals damage their teeth and gums on them, and swallowed pieces can cause serious problems.

Provide the bulk of the diet as growing grass or hay. Avoid feeding soft sticky foods and never give items containing sugar or oil/fat.

Specific Instructions

Figure 4.21 Documentation sheet for recording pathological changes of teeth and jaws in rabbits (reproduced by kind permission of David Crossley).

the oral cavity under anesthesia should be carried out, as well as other specific radiographic examinations (special projections) if necessary. Only then is the definitive therapeutic approach determined.

4.4 Documentation of pathological changes of the teeth and jaws

In order to evaluate the course of a malocclusion as accurately as possible, and to be able to recognize changes to the teeth and jaws of patients quickly and precisely when the animals are re-examined, the findings are recorded in suitable documentation sheets. Those sheets were prepared by David Crossley for the most relevant animal species. A sample of the dental chart sheet for rabbits is pictured in Figure 4.21. The corresponding documentation tools for other species can be obtained as a download via the following internet link: http://www.vetdent.eu/cpd/cpd.html#chartsandthesis.

Findings can be accessed quickly and easily if those completed sheets assigned to the respective patients are directly included in the practice medical records along with the radiographs with the reference lines drawn in. Digital photographs of the intraoral or intraoperative findings and endoscopic video recordings can also be added.

CHAPTER 5
Radiographic Examination

In general, radiographic examinations should be carried out for all dental patients, as they are an essential – if not the most important – part of the diagnostics of tooth and jaw disorders in lagomorphs and rodents. It is the only way to identify the whole extent of hidden, intraosseous changes of teeth and bones, something that is essential for an exact evaluation of malocclusions. Those hidden changes may remain unidentified in even the most careful clinical examinations (Gracis, 2008). Notably, disorders of that kind amount to an average of 80% of all pathological processes (Crossley & Aiken, 2004). The intraalveolar part of a tooth, as well as the entire periodontium and the adjacent jawbone and the nasolacrimal canal, are all located extraorally. Hence any intraosseous changes in these structures can only be identified with specific radiographic examinations (see Figure 1.2a in Chapter 1).

Apart from what is mentioned above, radiographic examination is a vital tool for choosing the ideal therapy in each individual case and provides crucial information needed to correctly make a long-term prognosis. In addition, a veterinarian may be able to use radiographic examinations in explaining diagnoses to the patient's owner. Clear illustrations of hidden findings can help to improve understanding of an overall situation that is often problematic. The therapeutic approach can then be explained step by step and a possible prophylaxis of dental and jaw disorders can be discussed with the owner.

> More than 90% of all abscesses in the head area are a consequence of infected incisor teeth and/or cheek teeth. These abscesses may go undetected for a long time unless there is an appropriate radiographic examination.

A further 5–8% of all cases are due to a nasolacrimal duct that is primarily dilated and secondarily infected, causing intranasal abscessations that are also usually not detected early in general clinical examinations. If such an intranasal infection is allowed to spread unnoticed, the maxilla is often perforated outwardly in the area of the cribriform plate. In such an instance, the abscess will become clinically visible due to an increasing facial swelling (Figure 5.1). Any infected teeth and early stages of jaw abscesses can usually be detected by means of good radiographic diagnostics, and an ideal treatment considering all findings in the individual case can then be implemented rather quickly.

5.1 Indications

Apart from persistent anorexia, any kind of asymmetry, lump or abscess of the head and jaw, as well as any malocclusion in general, are indications for a radiographic examination of the skull, particularly if one is unfamiliar with the patient. Radiographs are also indicated if metabolic bone disorders such as osteodystrophy or secondary hyperparathyroidism are suspected (Figure 5.2).

Another indication is a periodontal infection of individual teeth, which are often identified during intraoral examination due to their increased pain or mobility. Such kinds of suspicious incisors or cheek teeth should be projected preferably in isolation (intraoral images). If the suspicion of an intraalveolar infection is confirmed, the affected tooth should be extracted – there is no alternative (see Figures 1.2a in Chapter 1 and 3.19 in Chapter 3).

Dentistry in Rabbits and Rodents, First Edition. Estella Böhmer.
© 2015 John Wiley & Sons, Ltd. Published 2015 by John Wiley & Sons, Ltd.

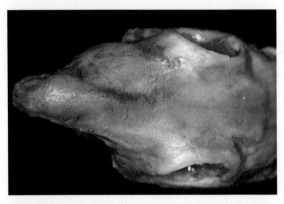

Figure 5.1 Intranasal abscess in a three-year-old rabbit (postmortem preparation, dorsal view) with a clear protrusion of the maxilla in the area of the cribriform plate, due to a tooth-associated infection of the nasolacrimal duct caused by obstruction (retrograde elongation of the right maxillary incisor).

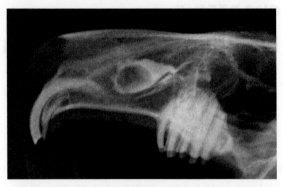

Figure 5.3 Intranasal abscessation in a three-year-old rabbit (radiograph of the maxilla, laterolateral view, postmortem specimen): contrast medium shows the abscess that originated from a chronically purulent nasolacrimal duct. The nasolacrimal duct was filled with 0.5 ml Solutrast® via the punctum. A retrograde displacement of the maxillary incisor apices with a slight protrusion of the palatal bone plate is visible.

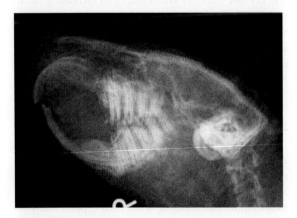

Figure 5.2 Generalized osteodystrophy with pain-related anorexia in a three-year-old guinea pig (laterolateral view). The consequences are a moth eaten bone structure and marked demineralization of the entire skull. The structure and shape of all cheek teeth is pathologically changed. Intraoral dental overgrowth and a thickening of the wall of the tympanic bulla are visible.

Tooth extractions are also much easier to plan and perform with the aid of radiographs because projections with at least two planes will provide an exact view of the intraalveolar area as well as the shape of the tooth concerned.

Other indications for a radiographic examination are structurally altered teeth (e.g. enamel and dentin hypoplasia, longitudinal splitting, thickening, etc.) and more marked deformations or displacements of teeth. Radiographic imaging is also indicated in chronic

infections of the nasolacrimal duct or a unilateral exophthalmos.

Furthermore, in the case of missing teeth the dental alveolus in question should be examined more closely with the aid of radiographs. This will clarify whether the entire tooth is missing or merely a part of the tooth structure has been lost as a consequence of an infection-related intraalveolar fracture. This differentiation can be essential for long-term prognoses.

Larger cavities caused by abscesses can be made visible with a contrast agent to evaluate their extent well in advance of any surgery. However, before using a contrast agent, pus must be drained away – at least partly. This technique has proven successful, particularly in intra-nasal abscesses, where the contrast agent (e.g. Solutrast®) can usually be introduced into the abscess area simply via the nasolacrimal duct (Figure 5.3). Prior aspiration of the infection site is usually not necessary.

Radiographic imaging also may help in critically evaluating and possibly adjusting current therapy for an abscess, tooth extraction or tooth trimming. In addition, radiographic documentation of the healing process over time is useful for teaching purposes; in this way objective evaluations of the condition and objective recommendations for treatment can be made. Radiographic examination is not to be omitted; it may be challenging, but is one of the keys to success – along with the selection of the appropriate treatment.

5.2 Radiographic techniques

The sharpest and best possible radiographic projections that allow detection of the finest bone and tooth structures are a necessary prerequisite for good examination of the jaw of lagomorphs and rodents. Non-screen dental X-ray films, which have a very good fine-detail reproduction, are particularly suitable for this. However, their routine use – especially for overview images of the head without anesthesia – is not only impractical but also obsolete because of problematic X-ray protection when using them as high exposures are required. Instead, metal cassettes are still used for radiographic examinations of malocclusions, but with only one intensifying screen (so-called mammography cassettes with mammography films). Much lower radiation energies are needed when using these single-screen films instead of non-screen films. The depicted image, however, is slightly less sharp because of the grain of the intensifying screen/film. Standard radiographic projections that are taken with customary X-ray cassettes are not recommended because of their poor image quality. They contain two intensifying screens, which will not show fine bone details with sufficient precision.

Unfortunately, using digital radiographic techniques for pets (by means of direct data transfer or storage media) does not yet offer the desired image quality – at least when using the kind of radiographic equipment that is common in veterinary practice. Particularly in views of the head with its delicate bone structures, the desired fine-detail reproduction is lacking and very important information may thus be lost. Certainly this problem will be solved within the next few years as the technology of the equipment improves.

5.3 Positioning

The most important prerequisite for a correct interpretation of radiographic images is a careful, symmetrical positioning of the patient. This may well be achieved without sedation or anesthesia (at least in rabbits, guinea pigs and chinchillas, and for overview images) provided that the animals do not resist too much. Radiographic examinations under anesthesia are preferable, of course, but many patients are too weak or unstable to allow this in the first instance. It is therefore important to obtain a general view of the overall dental situation in order to proceed with the approximate diagnosis and to estimate prospective costs for the pet's owner.

While positioning the patient, one must adhere to all mandatory measures for personal radiation protection, including the compulsory use of lead gloves. Those measures have been omitted in figures showing each of the special projections in order to depict the patient's corresponding immobilization in a better way. Positioning can be made accordingly in anesthetized patients without the need for manual support; immobilization tools such as foam rubber cushions or adhesive tape may be used.

5.4 Various projections

First the patient's head is projected in at least two planes – in a laterolateral and a dorsoventral view. However, pathological changes often cannot be attributed with certainty to a definite side or a quadrant of the jaw because structures of the two halves of the jaw superimpose each other, and more subtle findings may even go unnoticed. Hence a primary diagnosis in four planes is recommended. For this, additional views of the skull are obtained – right and left side oblique with a 40° tilting of the head. With such a relatively strong tilt of the head, not only the apical area but also the majority of the intraalveolar sections of the mandibular cheek teeth may be depicted (Figure 5.4). With these kinds of projection, however, radiographic examination of the maxillary cheek teeth will only be possible to a limited extent.

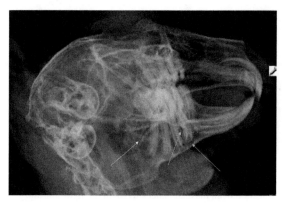

Figure 5.4 Malocclusion in a three-year-old rabbit (oblique projection of the left mandible) with a longitudinal split of the last molar (M3; white arrow) and periapical pathology of the first cheek tooth (P3; turquoise arrows).

Of these four standard projections, the most important basic information – always depending on the individual case situation – is gained from a perfectly positioned lateral projection, because here reference lines that are essential for prognoses can be drawn according to Böhmer and Crossley (see Section 5.6). Projections of the head in a dorsoventral view are sometimes omitted as they tend to offer little additional information (Gorrel & Verhaert, 2006). This may be true for individual cases, but especially the intra- and periorbital areas (the last four upper cheek teeth apices in rabbits), as well as the lacrimal bone, the surroundings of the temporomandibular joint and the caudal branch of the mandible, are often evaluated correctly only with this additional projection (Figure 5.5).

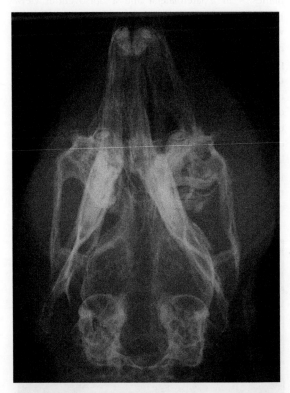

Figure 5.5 Right-sided exophthalmos in a five-year-old rabbit (dorsoventral view) with severe retrograde displacement and elongation of all maxillary cheek teeth on the right side and marked malformation of the tooth structures as well as extensive osteolysis of the tuber faciale maxillae. A bullous bony growth can be seen in the rostral orbital area.

Other special radiographic projections that often require species-specific positioning allow certain features to be depicted separately without any superimpositions. Those features include a variety of bone areas, various incisors or cheek teeth, the mandibular joints or intranasal structures. Additional projections are not made on a routine basis but rather are targeted precisely whenever specific issues arise. They usually require the patient to be anesthetized.

An additional examination of the head in a rostrocaudal view is also indicated if there is reason to suspect a pathological change in the temporomandibular joints. Furthermore, in rabbits individual incisors or cheek teeth can be examined in closer detail by means of intraoral radiographic examination, without unwanted superimposition of other teeth. Each tooth may even be depicted in full length if the head is tilted slightly for the projection (see Section 5.7). Thus intraoral radiographic images are particularly critical for precise diagnoses whenever an exact evaluation of pathological changes of the dental alveolus, the intraalveolar tooth body or the adjacent bone is needed. However, those images must never be interpreted in isolation, but only in the context of corresponding standard and oblique views. Otherwise the overall dental situation and malocclusion could be misinterpreted. Exceptions to this rule are short-term rechecks, e.g. the area of an abscess, a tooth extraction, a wound healing complication or dentinoid formation.

In guinea pigs and chinchillas, there are two more projections (according to Böhmer, 2001a) that allow for an isolated view of both mandibles and the maxilla. By positioning the patient correctly not only the mandibular incisor teeth but also every individual mandibular cheek tooth can be projected in its full length. The same applies for the upper jaw. The entire intraalveolar tooth structure can be depicted almost without any superimposition if the head is slightly rotated at the same time (as in the intraoral image). This depiction includes the entire alveolar bone, the periodontium and the apex. Those two special kinds of positioning have become prevalent as an alternative as well as a complementary measure to intraoral radiographic examination, although these can also be used in guinea pigs and chinchillas. However, intraoral images are still the best choice for quick and easy checks in the area of the incisors of these animals.

5.4.1 Standard projections
Laterolateral skull view

Of the four standard projections, the view of the head in a laterolateral view is the most important. This is particularly true in chinchillas because in this species the cheek teeth do not appear to be elongate during an intraoral examination, despite clearly visible radiographic findings indicating the opposite. In such cases a marked hypertrophy of the maxillary gingiva gives the impression of a physiological length of the maxillary cheek teeth. However, by drawing the appropriate basic reference lines on the standard lateral projection of the skull prior to therapy the extent of intraosseous findings may be evaluated presurgically much better. This is just as essential in other species, although in these the suspected intraoral findings will often coincide more closely with the radiographic changes.

In order to immobilize and properly position the patient, a single person maximally extends the front limbs toward the caudal end of the animal and then fixes them firmly with both hands to the ventrolateral part of the thorax (see Figure 5.9 later). The head can be adjusted to the desired position by rotating or tilting the entire body of the animal on the X-ray table (rabbit, guinea pig, chinchilla, degu). The caudal extension of the front limbs also helps to stretch the hind legs a bit, which – in combination with the thumbs pressing down on the thoracic and lumbar spine – will usually be

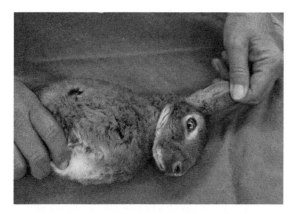

Figure 5.6 Positioning of a rabbit by a single person for a radiograph or X-ray. The author acknowledges that hand-held positioning of conscious animals for radiography is against radiation safety regulations in the UK and thus advises that alternative positioning is used.

sufficient to prevent the animal from lunging (kicking) out. In small patients, one hand will be enough to fix the limbs to the thorax if the thumb is directed across the animal's back in the proper way. The other hand can help in positioning the head by carefully pulling the tips of the ears (Figure 5.6).

If two assistants are on hand, one of them immobilizes the animal in the rump area by pressing the pelvis firmly toward the X-ray table with one hand. It is not necessary to hold on to the hind legs near the paws with the other hand. Such an immobilization would only increase the risk of iatrogenic injuries to the hip joints as a result of sudden defensive movements of the patient, e.g. kicking the legs. The second assistant grasps each of the patient's ears or front limbs with one hand and then pulls them in opposite directions (180°). Desired positioning is then achieved by inclining the head accordingly.

Whenever animals are positioned for lateral projections, it is essential to ensure that the head is oriented absolutely horizontally. This can cause considerable problems in guinea pigs whose skulls are relatively wide in their caudal part or if lumps in the area of the jaw (abscesses) are present (see Figure 1.1 in Chapter 1). In such cases the side with the swelling should always be on top. During inspection, the vertical alignment of the two eyes provides a pair of useful points of orientation as the globes should be aligned in views from above or from the front. Alternatively, the ventral margins of the two mandibles can be palpated as the two should be exactly opposite each other. The most common mistake with this kind of positioning is a ventral slope of the nose. As a result of such incorrect positioning, a guinea pig's zygomatic process may appear to be a significant dental overgrowth with a formation of "spurs" (Figure 5.7). Adhesive tape can be useful for correct positioning, as can small wedges or rolls of foam rubber placed under the tip of the nose. Alternatively, the head is inclined or rotated toward the correct position by carefully pulling one of the auricles.

For the lateral view, the mouth can be kept open for a few millimeters by placing a small piece of cork or cotton wool between the incisors. With the cheek teeth moving slightly apart as a result, the occlusal surface can be evaluated better – particularly in rabbits, but also in other species (Harcourt-Brown, 2002a). The reference lines may still be drawn as described in Section 5.6.

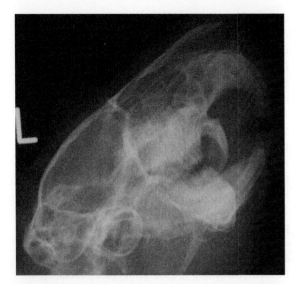

Figure 5.7 Incorrect positioning of a two-year-old guinea pig in a laterolateral beam path. The nose is tilted toward the table, causing the zygomatic process – being a bony process rostral from the cheek teeth – to interfere with interpretation and possibly be confused with a maxillary spur formation. All cheek teeth are superimposed and can thus hardly be evaluated.

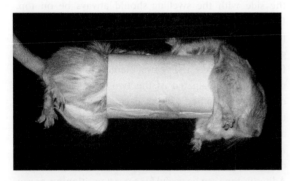

Figure 5.8 Positioning of small rodents for radiographic examinations. A suitably sized cardboard roll is opened lengthwise, placed around the patient's thorax and abdomen and closed again by means of sticky tape; knees and elbows of the patient remain outside the roll.

For standard projections of their heads in a laterolateral view, it will be almost impossible to restrain degus, hamsters, mice or rats securely by their neck coat. In order to immobilize these animals, a suitably sized cardboard roll that is cut lengthwise and fixed together again by adhesive tape may be used (Figure 5.8). This method is also useful for standard dorsoventral views.

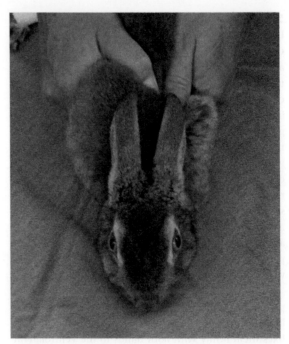

Figure 5.9 Positioning of a rabbit by a single person for a dorsoventral skull radiograph. The author acknowledges that hand-held positioning of conscious animals for radiography is against radiation safety regulations in the UK and thus advises that alternative positioning is used.

Dorsoventral and ventrodorsal skull view

For radiographic projections in a dorsoventral view, the positioning of the head does not usually pose a problem. The animal's neck must be stretched maximally and then both mandibles – laid out flat in full length on the X-ray table – must be aligned symmetrically underneath the central beam (Figure 5.9). If positioned by a single assistant, the patient's front limbs are extended toward the caudal end and fixed to the thorax. In so doing, the animal's body will usually hover slightly above the table top, which helps to extend the neck. If two assistants are present, one of them places the animal on the table in ventral recumbency while the other assistant grasps the tips of the ears on both sides and positions the head by pulling the ears downwards and sideways.

Positioning is again checked exactly by means of the positions of both eyes, which should lie in one horizontal plane. In order to obtain images that are diagnostically conclusive and can be compared to others, the patient's neck must be as close as possible to the table top. If it is not pressed down properly, the head will be depicted

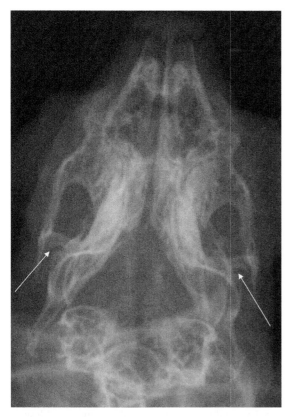

Figure 5.10 Incorrect positioning of a four-year-old rabbit for a dorsoventral radiograph. .The neck is insufficiently overextended. There is a good view into the temporomandibular joint on both sides (white arrows).

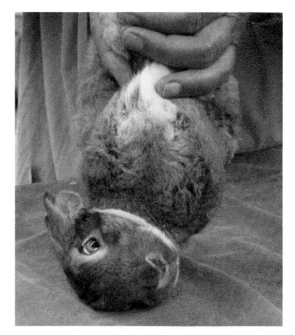

Figure 5.11 Positioning of a rabbit by a single person for a right-sided oblique projection of the head. The author acknowledges that hand-held positioning of conscious animals for radiography is against radiation safety regulations in the UK and thus advises that alternative positioning is used.

with a ventral tilting of the head with an angle of about 30–45° in what is more of a caudorostral view, resulting in an image that will be difficult to analyse because of superimposition (Figure 5.10). If the focus is on intranasal structures, correspondingly lower values for exposure level and time are chosen.

Positioning of the head can be difficult whenever there are abscesses in one or both mandibles, as the skull tends to tip sideways when the patient is in ventral recumbency. In such cases the radiographic projection is made in a ventrodorsal view (with the patient in dorsal recumbency). In order to properly analyse this kind of projection – just like dorsoventral views – and to compare it with the latter, the nose must be supported slightly with a foam wedge so that the area of the ventral lower jaw (mandibular branch and mandibular body) is in one horizontal plane.

Oblique views (head tilted approximately 40°)

Standard views in two planes are often not sufficient to define certain changes radiographically or to locate them precisely. Slightly oblique lateral projections of each mandible (right and left oblique views of the skull) help to differentiate findings in such cases. For this, the head is primarily positioned laterally and then rotated by approximately 40°, with the area to be examined closest to the table (Figure 5.11 and also Figure 5.4). With this relatively marked rotation of the head, each individual cheek tooth in the mandible can be depicted in isolation in its full intraalveolar length. In this way the findings on both sides can be ideally compared. With a smaller rotation of the skull (approximately 20°), by contrast, the ventral sections of the mandibular cheek teeth will be projected.

In this kind of positioning, the tympanic bullae should lie exactly in one line above each other – independent of species. In rabbits, they will then form a figure of eight in the X-ray image. The first cheek tooth in the lower jaw (P3) may sometimes appear to be slightly curved intraalveolarly (Figure 5.4). If that same premolar is to be projected in

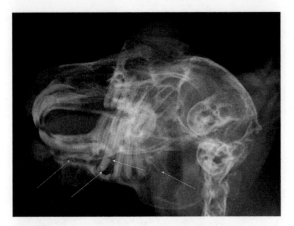

Figure 5.12 Abscess of the mandible in a five-year-old rabbit (right-sided oblique projection) and periapical pathology associated with the first lower cheek tooth (P3). There is an apical dentinoid as well as a transverse fracture of the tooth located further occlusally (white arrows). Also visible are a structurally altered right mandibular incisor with expansion of its alveolar socket (turquoise arrow) and a retrograde elongation of the last mandibular cheek tooth (M3) with periapical osteolysis (yellow arrow), an apical radiolucency around the second last lower molar (M2) and a retrograde elongation of the second mandibular cheek tooth with a partial perforation of the ventral mandibular cortical bone.

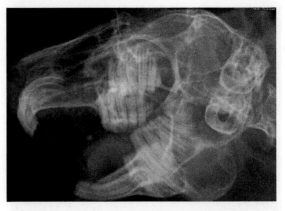

Figure 5.13 Normal occlusion in a three-year-old rabbit (right-sided oblique projection, with the jaws held open using a syringe placed between the incisors, and the tip of the nose slightly lifted). There were no pathological findings of the right maxillary molars that were to be imaged.

detail in its full length, then the tip of the nose is lowered a bit toward the table top, causing the tympanic bullae to shift slightly against one another (the upper bulla will then be just in front of the lower one) (Figure 5.12). If the diagnostic focus is on the caudal mandibular molars, the nose can be supported by means of a small foam wedge.

The maxillary cheek teeth on each side of the jaw can be evaluated relatively well and without any superimposition by means of oblique views with an angle of about 40° (evaluations should preferably be done by comparing the two sides). In this kind of projection, however, the teeth will appear to be markedly shortened and partially deformed. If the right mandibular area is depicted by means of a right oblique projection, the tooth structures of the left maxillary molars can be identified on the X-ray image as well (they are located far dorsally). Accordingly, the right maxillary cheek teeth are depicted in left oblique views. With intubated rabbits, positioning should be made such as to ensure that the tube will not interfere with important pathological findings in any of the radiographic projections.

In rabbits, the maxillary molars may be projected better if the jaws are kept open for taking oblique views

(Figure 5.13). The side whose cheek teeth are to be depicted in isolation should be closest to the table. In order to avoid superimpositions of the mandibular cheek teeth on the opposite side, the tip of the patient's nose is raised a little more from the table. Positioning is achieved by means of two gauze bandages that are placed around the rostral areas of the upper and lower jaw. It is best to hook the gauze up among the incisors to prevent it from slipping off. In this way, the mouth may be kept open wide enough (just like in a dog). Alternatively, a suitably sized piece of cork may be placed as a wedge between the incisors. A syringe body that is cut out and shortened appropriately may also be used if all sharp edges are smoothed carefully or padded with gauze (Figure 5.14). In contrast to normal oblique views, however, these kinds of projections can only be taken with the patient under sedation or anesthetic.

Guinea pigs' cheek teeth can be depicted in isolation by means of lateral oblique projections of the head if the animals' skulls are rotated as explained above or even more (approximately 40–45°). This method will also allow for a depiction of the long, sled-shaped temporomandibular joint and the physiologically even chewing surface that is located on the same level species-specifically (Figure 5.15). Having correctly positioned the head, the tip of the nose will be slightly above the table surface and the two tympanic bullae, which are exactly one above the other (in a line), will form a figure of eight on the X-ray image – similar to the same situation

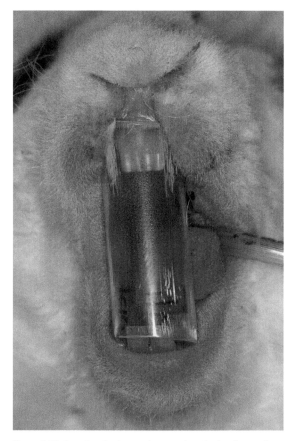

Figure 5.14 Opening the jaws using a syringe body. Sharp edges must be carefully polished or angled in order to avoid injuries to the mucosa. Alternatively, a suitable piece of cork can be used.

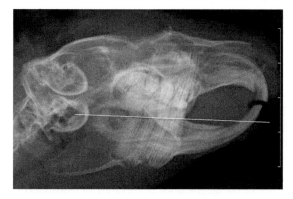

Figure 5.15 Slight malocclusion in a two-year-old guinea pig (left-sided oblique projection), with a mild retrograde displacement of the apices of the mandibular cheek teeth as well as an elongation of the clinical crowns of both mandibular incisors; otherwise there is normal occlusion. Temporomandibular joint and mandibular chewing surface are level.

in the rabbit. However, an evaluation of the upper molars will be almost impossible with this kind of positioning, as the cheek teeth will interfere with the opposite side as well as the zygomatic process.

It may be possible to obtain oblique views of both sides (left and right oblique views) without anesthesia if patients are relatively calm. In order to immobilize the animal, the front limbs are stretched toward the caudal end of the patient and pinned to the thorax with both hands, as described for the rabbit. The patient's body is then raised and rotated in a 45° angle toward the table such that the head is properly positioned without any further immobilization (similar to Figure 5.11). After a short period of complaining with some species-specific squeaking that may accompany repeated lifting of the head (simply wait for it to end), most guinea pigs will surrender and remain in the desired position for a moment. If necessary, positioning may be optimized by rotating the animal's entire body. This technique will also be of used for laterolateral and dorsoventral views. Should it be impossible because of vigorous defensive movements of the animal or should an exact positioning of the head be very difficult because of jaw abscesses, further diagnostics should be made under anesthesia – immediately prior to surgical and dental treatment.

5.4.2 Specific projections

All standard projections of the head in four planes (laterolateral, dorsoventral or ventrodorsal views as well as oblique views of both sides) that have so far been described can usually be taken without sedation or anesthesia in the majority of herbivorous pets. When using X-ray cassettes, a film can be subdivided into four sectors by means of blinding out certain quadrants, and then each of the four parts of the film can be exposed separately with one kind of positioning. Specific problems can be solved by means of further positioning (some of which are species-specific), as well as other radiographic techniques (intraoral images). All of these projection techniques are taken under anesthesia immediately prior to treatment – not on a routine basis, but as needed.

Rostrocaudal view

Specific changes in the caudal area of the head are usually examined in practice by means of a rostrocaudal view. This projection technique yields particularly good images of the temporomandibular joint (its longitudinal axis) and the tympanic bulla, which is close by. Those

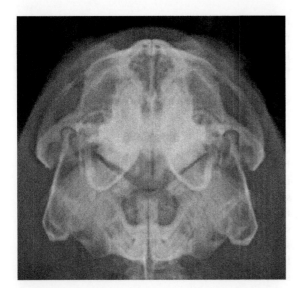

Figure 5.16 Caudal, left-sided abscess of the mandible in a four-year-old guinea pig (rostrocaudal view). The temporo-mandibular joint and occlusal surface are without pathological findings. A slightly blurred structure of the bone is visible in the area of the last mandibular cheek tooth (M3 on the left). There is a suspected osteomyelitis and this would be an indication for an isolated image of the mandible.

structures are depicted in isolation and with a good comparison of both sides. In addition, the species-specific angulation of the molars' occlusal planes may be verified and the ventrolateral margin of the mandible evaluated accordingly (Böhmer, 2001a) (Figure 5.16). In order to take this kind of radiographic projection, the patient is placed in dorsal recumbency with the nose pointing vertically upwards. This kind of examination can also be attempted without sedation in very tolerant animals – in dorsal recumbency, with the front limbs extended caudally and fixated to the body (thorax). In so doing, however, a perfectly symmetrical positioning of the head will only very rarely be achieved, and this will greatly reduce the validity of the images. Hence it is more advisable to take this specific projection under general anesthesia.

For positioning, the patient is placed in dorsal recumbency. Adhesive tape is placed across the nose and fixed on both sides of the thorax (laterally) on the table such that the bridge of the nose is positioned perpendicular to the table (Figure 5.17). Alternatively, a foam cushion may be used as a positioning tool. If maxillary and mandibular teeth are to be depicted in isolation, the jaws are pulled apart slightly by means of adhesive tape that is placed around the upper and lower incisors or by means

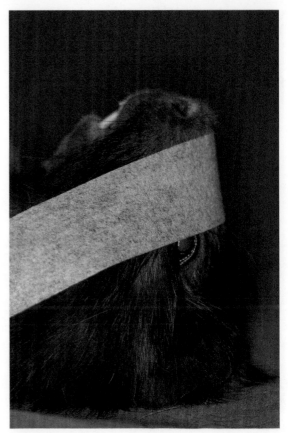

Figure 5.17 Positioning of a guinea pig for a rostrocaudal radiograph.

of gauze bandages hooked into the insicors. With these kinds of projections, a part of the tympanic bulla may also be depicted in isolation – depending on the angle of the head and the opening of the mouth (Figure 5.18).

If the maxillary occlusal plane is to be illustrated, the bridge of the nose must remain perpendicular to the table, while the lower jaw must get closer to the thorax. By contrast, if the mandibular occlusal plane is to be projected, the head is stretched to form a 45° angle and the mouth is kept open; the mandible must be directed perpendicularly upwards. Depending on the angle that is chosen, either the mandibular or the maxillary occlusal plane, or the length, slope or curvature of individual or various molars, or even a section of the temporomandibular joints will be depicted best. Different exposure times are used depending on whether there is a focus on the view of the temporomandibular joints, the row of teeth or the tympanic bulla.

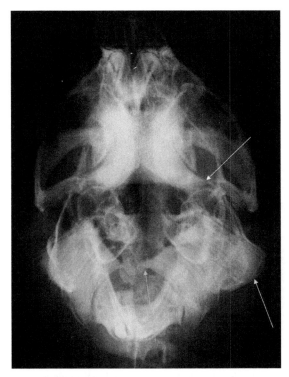

Figure 5.18 Malocclusion in a six-year-old guinea pig (open mouth rostrocaudal view), with buccal spurs as well as an intraoral elongation of all maxillary cheek teeth (more pronounced on the left than on the right; see white arrow), a lingual overgrowth of the first left mandibular cheek tooth (turquoise arrow) and a pronounced retrograde elongation of the last left molar (P4; yellow arrow). Despite some superimposition, the walls of the tympanic bulla appear normal.

Isolated views of the mandible in guinea pigs, chinchillas and degus according to Böhmer

For clarification of pathological changes of the mandible, the symphysis or the mandibular incisors and mandibular cheek teeth, the mandible of guinea pigs, chinchillas and degus can be depicted in isolation by means of a specific, species-specific kind of positioning (according to Böhmer, 2001a). In guinea pigs, chinchillas and degus, this projection technique is the ideal alternative to intraoral radiographs. It is not, however, suitable for rabbits because in these animals it is not possible to sufficiently isolate the mandible from the maxilla (there is a lot of complicating superimposition).

The patient is placed in ventral recumbency, with the front limbs extended toward the caudal end of the

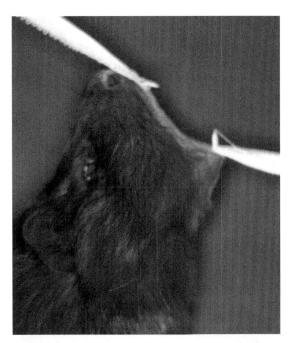

Figure 5.19 Positioning of a guinea pig for an isolated radiographic image of the mandible as described by Böhmer. The author acknowledges that hand-held positioning of conscious animals for radiography is against radiation safety regulations in the UK and thus advises that alternative positioning is used. This can be achieved by spreading of the jaws using a syringe body as shown in Figure 5.14.

animal and fixed to the thorax by an assistant on both sides. Alternatively, adhesive tape may be wrapped around the thorax and front limbs and then fixed on the table. The mouth is then opened as wide as possible; this can be achieved by placing two gauze bandages approximately 30 cm in length around the upper and lower incisors (Figure 5.19). At the same time the head is raised steeply off the table (approximately 45°) and positioned such that the central beam will be directed on to the middle intermandibular area cranially from the maxillary incisors and slightly caudally from the lower symphysis. In this way, both mandibles can be depicted largely in isolation without superimposition with the rostral part of the maxilla (Figure 5.20).

Starting from this kind of positioning, each individual mandibular incisor or cheek tooth can be projected in its entire length and thus be ideally evaluated if the head is rotated by approximately 45° to the right and left

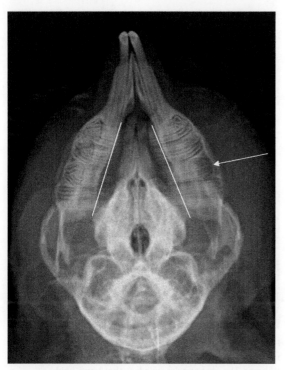

Figure 5.20 Right-sided abscess of the mandible in a three-year-old guinea pig (isolated view of the mandible as described by Böhmer), with subtle intraoral elongation of all cheek teeth (white lines), apical osteolysis of the second last molar (M2; white arrow) with a distinct soft tissue swelling.

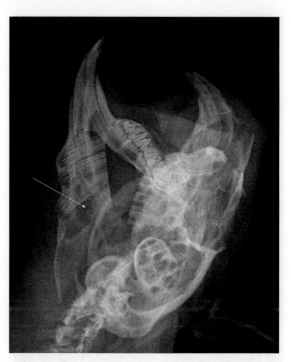

Figure 5.21 Abscess of the mandible in a five-year-old guinea pig (isolated view of the left mandibular dental arcade as described by Böhmer), 9 weeks post treatment, with an apicectomy of the last molar. The tooth socket appears normal, the cheek tooth has erupted toward the occlusal plane and is now occupying less than half of the tooth socket (white arrow).

(Figure 5.21). These kinds of projections according to Boehmer offer ideal views of the periodontum, split teeth, intraalveolar transverse fractures, partial or complete tooth loss and retrograde displacements of tooth apices or other changes in the apical area. It has to be kept in mind, however, that this oblique positioning technique will not yield a projection of the mandible closest to the X-ray table, but of the contralateral, upper section of the mandible (which is further away from the table). Hence with the patient in ventral recumbency, the skull must be rotated to the left in order to depict the right mandible, and vice versa (Figure 5.22).

Isolated views of the maxilla in guinea pigs and chinchillas according to Böhmer

In cases of suspected pathological changes of the maxillary cheek teeth, and in tooth-associated retrobulbar or intranasal abscessations, it can be impossible to identify exactly the tooth that is causing the infection by means of the classic radiographic projections that have previously been described. In addition, radiological findings may be very subtle in the early stages and may therefore be easily overlooked, particularly when considering the markedly curved molars of guinea pigs. In order to optimize diagnostics in this area, a specific projection technique has been developed by Boehmer. It allows for the maxillary molars of guinea pigs and chinchillas to be depicted largely without superimposition, in isolation (Böhmer, 2006). Depending on the positioning, not only can the apices of the affected teeth be evaluated well but also the tooth structures in their entire length. This radiographic method has proven to be very practical and informative for clarification of suspicious findings in the area of the maxilla, particularly in guinea pigs. Otherwise such information could only be obtained using intraoral radiography or costly methods like computed tomography.

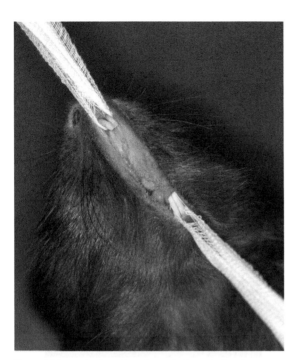

Figure 5.22 Positioning of a guinea pig for an isolated radiographic view of the left mandible as described by Böhmer (it shows the left mandible arch positioned furtherest from the table). The author acknowledges that hand-held positioning of conscious animals for radiography is against radiation safety regulations in the UK and thus advises that alternative positioning is used. This can be achieved by spreading of the jaws using a syringe body as shown in Figure 5.14.

The patient is positioned on the table in dorsal recumbency, and a relatively robust foam roller is placed under its neck such that the head (which is hanging on one side of the roller) is extended caudodorsally (Figure 5.23). A positioning tool with a diameter of approximately 4 to 5 cm can also be made by rolling up a few layers of cellulose and wrapping adhesive tape around them. If the apical parts of the posterior upper cheek teeth (M2/M3) are to be projected clearly, the patient's head is extended with a smaller angle (approximately 35°) (Figure 5.24). On the other hand, larger angles are chosen (approximately 45°) for isolated views of the apices of the two anterior cheek teeth (P4/M1) (Figure 5.25). The entire intra- and extraalveolar part of the maxillary cheek teeth can be projected in isolation by slightly rotating the skull to the left (for the left half of the upper jaw) and to the right (for the right half of the upper jaw) (Figure 5.26).

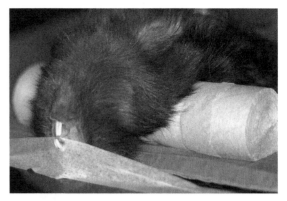

Figure 5.23 Positioning of a guinea pig for an isolated radiographic view of the maxilla as described by Böhmer.

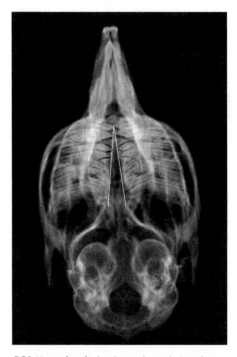

Figure 5.24 Normal occlusion in a guinea pig (specimen, isolated view of the maxilla as described by Böhmer). The apices of all cheek teeth are normal, but there is a subtle retrograde elongation of the last two molars (M3).

5.5 Interpretation of radiographs

Occasionally interpretation of radiographs in the various species of small pets can be rather difficult – particularly for less experienced practitioners. Primarily this is due to a lack of knowledge of the anatomy, which can be rather different in the various species, and of the pathological

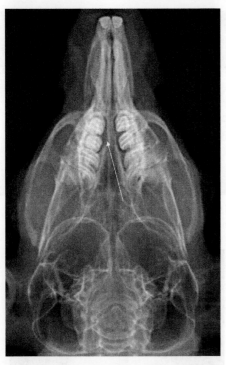

Figure 5.25 Isolated depiction of the maxilla as described by Böhmer in a seven-year-old chinchilla with mild clinical elongation of the upper cheek teeth, a subtle palato-interproximal osteolysis is visible between the apices of the first two maxillary cheek teeth (P4/M1; white arrow). There are no further pathological findings.

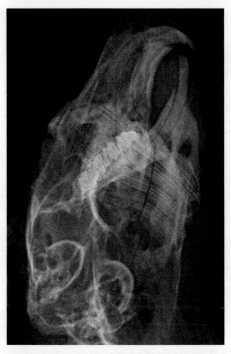

Figure 5.26 Normal occlusion in a three-year-old guinea pig. On an isolated view of the maxilla as described by Böhmer with slightly oblique positioning, the tooth structures of the last two maxillary molars (M3/M4) are clearly visible with no pathology.

findings related to the teeth and the jaws, which may vary greatly from species to species. Furthermore, the shape of the skull varies considerably within the species and possible superimpositions of various bony and dental structures may only be correctly interpreted with a profound anatomical knowledge (e.g. in guinea pigs, the zygomatic process superimposes on the occlusal plane of the mandibular cheek teeth in oblique projections of the head in a laterolateral view; see Figure 5.7). Therefore the following section will deal extensively with species-specific radiographic anatomy. In order to delve further into the subject, it can be very helpful to study macerated skulls closely from each species, with and without malocclusions, and to use them to clarify questionable radiographic findings, if necessary. Furthermore, radiographs of these specimens can be taken for comparison, if needed.

In order to interpret radiographs correctly and completely, care and patience are needed apart from a certain sense of a systematic approach (see below). Radiographs are diagnostically conclusive only in the context of careful clinical examinations. Otherwise intraoral buccal

overgrowths of maxillary molars may easily be confused with teeth having been displaced retrobulbarly or teeth with another growth defect. As for the latter, radiographs of the head in a dorsoventral view will clearly show dental tissue in the area of the orbit.

In healthy animals, the bones of the skull and the tooth substance are always well mineralized, although rabbits are said to have a physiological normal structure of the parietal bone that appears moth eaten (Harcourt-Brown, 2002a). Radiopacity of the skull and the teeth becomes considerably more inconsistent, however, in animals with a malocclusion or caries-like tooth lesions. This is due to poor or irregular calcification. In most of these cases the structure of the bones and teeth that can be seen on the radiographs is markedly different from normal. Individual cortical lines should usually be smooth and clearly detectable. On radiographs of the skull, they will appear as straight and continuous lines. In rabbits, the dominant structures visible on lateral views of the head are the mandibular and palatal bone plate, which are relatively large. In contrast, the maxillary plate is always a bit less distinct on radiographs of guinea pigs and chinchillas. In all species, the ventral margin of the mandible, the straight bony roof of the nose, which is thinner as a whole, will form other horizontal lines. Generally, there should be no bony asymmetries or pathological osseous formations involving the skull and jaws.

Healthy, aradicular hypsodont cheek teeth always appear a bit more radiopaque than the jawbone that surrounds them. Their dentin and crown cement is less radiopaque than their enamel, which clearly stands out and thus appears brighter on the radiograph. As a result, enamel folds of the cheek teeth can be identified relatively well in most cases as intradental, vertical, whitish lines. The lamina dura, which runs parallel to the tooth's longitudinal axis, also forms a fine line of marked radiopacity. The pulp cavity appears as a radiolucent, mostly conical, intradental structure that merges into an even more translucent area of bone at its apical end, the so-called dental sac with its germinal tissue (see Figure 3.11 in Chapter 3). The occlusal area of brachyodont teeth is covered by an enamel cap (which is more radiopaque and therefore clearly visible) only in very young individuals (see Figure 5.43 later).

When evaluating radiographs, the possibility of dental asymmetries must be taken into account. The number of teeth is checked, as well as their shape, position, structure and the reciprocal occlusion, with the corresponding occlusal planes. Evaluation of the parodontal area, which is relatively wide in rabbits and herbivorous rodents, and of the tooth's apex are also important. Periodontal diseases are relatively common but are also easily overlooked – not only during clinical examinations but also when evaluating radiographs. Typical findings in such cases are a progressive loss of the vertical alveolar bone and an expansion of the interdental spaces.

A radiographic examination of the tympanic bulla is also of great significance, as a chronic otitis can lead to pain-related anorexia (origin of the digastrics muscle at the paracondylar process). Gaps in the row of cheek teeth can be seen relatively often, particularly on radiographs of older omnivorous rodents like rats or hamsters. Individual molars may fall out due to chronic periodontitis with advancing age of the animals. Such changes may be a secondary finding but may also indicate a localized abscess.

If a chronic, tooth-associated abscess has progressed to an extent where the bone has eroded extensively due to infection and if the dental disease is too far advanced to reasonably hope for any therapeutic success, then there should be no hesitation in informing the owner in an appropriate way that euthanasia is the only alternative. In most cases the patients will be severely weakened as a result of their long-lasting disease and a majority of the affected animals will also suffer from severe disorders of the gastrointestinal tract. For this reason, it always makes sense to obtain radiographs of the abdomen when dealing with malocclusions.

Systematic interpretation of radiographs

Bone structure of the skull (disturbance of mineralization, increased bone density)

Bone structure of the mandibles (osteomyelitis, bone growth, osteolysis)

Asymmetry of the skull

Length of the maxilla and mandible and position of the two with respect to one another (brachygnathia, campylognathia)

Orientation of the lines representing the boundaries of the palatal bone and the mandibular bone with respect to one another (convergence, parallelism or divergence)

Occlusion of the incisors and cheek teeth (contact area, angle)

Reference lines (see Section 5.6)

Length of tooth structures– retrograde displacement (incisors and cheek teeth)

Incisors (shape of the occlusal edge, tooth surface, number, structure, curvature, apex)

Peg teeth (number, shape)

Alveolar bone in the area of the incisors (lysis, expansion of the periodontium)

Number of cheek teeth (hypo- or hyperdontia)

Cheek teeth (length, shape, curvature, position, structure, enamel folds, apex)

Occlusal surface of the cheek teeth (wave formations or step formations, uneven wear of individual teeth)

Displacement of individual teeth

Tooth substance (enamel hypoplasia, dentin hypoplasia, disturbance of mineralization, fracture, caries-like dissolutions)

Ventral boundary of the mandible (perforations, protrusions, bone growth, lyses)

Structure of the periodontal area (bone loss, expansion of interdental spaces)

Localization and radiopacity of the periapical germinative tissue

Temporomandibular joint

Tympanic bulla thickening of the wall, otitis)

5.6 Radiographic anatomy and reference lines according to Böhmer and Crossley

Even when following all general guidelines for examination and treatment of malocclusions, tooth and jaw disorders in lagomorphs and rodents still represent a formidable challenge for veterinarians. This is reflected in the large number of publications related to this topic that have been made in the last two decades. Most of these articles focus on the etiology of malocclusions as well as species-specific clinical and radiographic findings. In addition, they provide much advice on an adequate correction of the dentition (with and without extractions of teeth), although the extent of tooth shortening needed to re-establish normal occlusion is usually not clearly defined. However, the reference lines discussed below will help in determining this very precisely and will make treatment much easier, particularly for less experienced veterinarians.

Most specialized literature lacks information on the evaluation and classification of retrograde displacements of tooth apices, which are rather common in small mammals with elodont teeth. Pathological processes are usually described subjectively and defined very generally as being mild, moderate or severe. The extent of retrograde displacement may be evaluated differently by different persons, particularly depending on their experience. This, of course, will have an effect on the validity of their prognoses. An absence of objective guidelines for an evaluation also makes it difficult to document exactly the progressive changes over a longer period of time.

In order to facilitate proof of such retrograde displacements, a (dorsal) reference line that illustrates those kinds of changes very well for chinchillas was published by Crossley (1995b). It was followed by the description of a corresponding specific line for rabbits and guinea pigs (Böhmer, 2001a). As a result of this, further anatomical reference lines have been developed whose efficiency was reviewed in an evaluation of 528 head specimens (Table 5.1; Böhmer & Crossley, 2009, 2011).

These lines provide an objective and easily comprehensible means of staging retrograde displacements of cheek teeth in rabbits, guinea pigs and chinchillas. Furthermore, they provide a means of exactly localizing the normal occlusal surface for each individual patient. Hence it is now possible to precisely determine how much tooth substance needs to be removed during correction of the dentition in order to help re-establish normal occlusion (see Figures 5.36, 5.37 and 5.40a later). In addition, corrections can be reviewed objectively after surgery has been performed (see Figures 5.33b and 5.40b later).

These reference lines may also help explaining diagnoses to the pet's owner. Illustrative demonstrations will help nonprofessionals in understanding the therapeutic approach as well as the current prognosis. The lines will also make it easier to explain possible complications or treatments that may prove to be only short-term successful in individual cases.

5.6.1 Rabbit
Normal radiographic anatomy

In rabbits, the contact area between the maxillary and mandibular incisors appears chisel-shaped on radiographs of the head on a laterolateral view (Figure 5.27a). The pulp cavity can be seen in both the maxillary and the mandibular incisors, in the intraalveolar area and in the area close to the apex. The mandibular incisors are located shortly behind the upper ones, lying on the rudimentary peg teeth. The latter are relatively short and not very deeply anchored in the upper jaw; their occlusal plane is horizontal and blunt ended. The root area of the peg teeth is very variable, both in their length and curvature.

Table 5.1 Skull specimens examined for a review of the reference lines.

	Rabbit	Guinea pig	Chinchilla	Total
Radiographic examination				
Malocclusion	183	132	149	464
Healthy dentition	21	19	24	64
Total	204	151	173	528
Postmortem examination				
Specimens	52	41	131	224

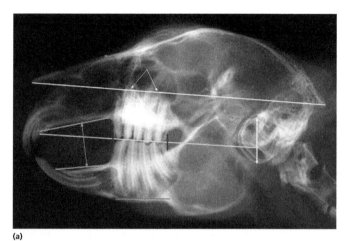

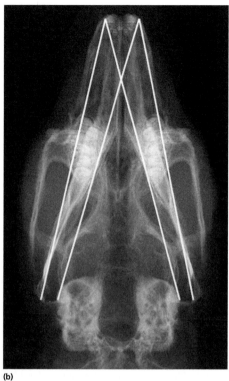

(a)   (b)

Figure 5.27 Anatomical reference lines for normal occlusion in a two-year-old rabbit in (a) a laterolateral view with a slight overgrowth of the mandibular incisors and (b) a dorsoventral view. The blue lines mark the medial mandibular cortical bone of the jaw (see also text).

The apices of the maxillary incisors lie approximately one-third to one-half of the length of the diastema and are located approximately 2–3 mm above the palatal bone plate, which appears as a straight, continuous line. The bone lamella is always a bit thicker in the area of the first maxillary cheek tooth. The apex of the mandibular incisor is close to the mesial plane of the first premolar and is located roughly halfway between the dorsal and ventral margin of the lower jaw. The radius of the curvature of the maxillary incisors is always significantly smaller than the radius of the mandibular ones.

The six maxillary and five mandibular cheek teeth form an occlusal plane that is largely horizontal. The chewing surface has a zigzag appearance on a laterolateral view that is typical for the occlusal surface of rabbits. This jagged structure can be depicted particularly well on laterolateral views of the head, with the mouth kept slightly open (e.g. by placing a thin layer of cellulose between the incisors). The last molar (M3) in both the upper and the lower jaw may sometimes be extremely small in comparison with the rest of the cheek teeth and may then be difficult to identify on radiographs. By contrast, the first mandibular cheek tooth (P3) very often has an extraordinarily robust tooth structure.

The germinal tissue (tooth sac), which can be seen particularly well in younger animals, is located at the apex of each individual mandibular and maxillary cheek tooth. It can be identified as a periapical radiolucency on the radiographs. The mandibular cheek teeth are clearly confined by a short, vertical and horizontal bone lamella (lamina dura) against the jawbone. The mandible itself has a well-mineralized bone structure and a smooth ventral margin. The caudal maxillary cheek teeth (P4–M3) apices are covered by a thin layer of bone tissue; here it is important to note that there must be no evidence of any retrograde displacement of the apices.

The structure of each individual cheek tooth can be seen particularly clearly on radiographs of each mandible (Harcourt-Brown, 2002a) (see Figure 3.11).

Each tooth's alveolus is surrounded by the lamina dura, which appears as a vertical radiopaque bone line mesially and distally; that same line runs horizontally below each of the mandibular cheek teeth. It consists of highly calcified tissue in which the periodontal fibers are firmly anchored. Between the lamina dura and the tooth there is the periodontal space. Each cheek tooth has a central, longitudinal, radiopaque line that is formed by the double-layered enamel fold and the cement in between. On both sides of that enamel fold, each tooth's pulp cavity can be seen intraalveolarly, close to the base of the tooth (dilophodonty). That structure appears as an elongated, radiolucent area on both sides of the fold, which becomes narrower close to the occlusal surface. At the apical end, the two halves form a single, wider pulp cavity, which is bounded by the lamina dura on the side of the bone. There are multiple parallel lines running in a vertical direction through each tooth and on the tooth's margins (except for the last molar); these represent the central enamel fold of each tooth as well as the corresponding vertical part of the lamina dura and the outer enamel lamellae. Those lines are much harder to identify – or are not recognizable at all – on radiographs of rabbits with a malocclusion of the cheek teeth, depending on the severity of the disorder.

Lateral views of the head show the palatal and mandibular plates, both of which are significantly radiopaque, converging slightly toward the rostral end. If they are parallel, then pathological tooth elongation is already present. In normal occlusion, the palatal bone merges almost directly into the oblique occlusal plane of the upper incisor. Within the maxilla, the bony portion of the nasolacrimal duct can often be seen as a fine, slightly more radiopaque double line that runs from the lacrimal bone straight past the anterior maxillary cheek tooth apex (P2) to the periapical area of the maxillary incisor. In rabbits, the parietal bone often has a moth eaten appearance, which is physiologically normal (Harcourt-Brown, 2002a); however, this peculiarity is not found in some of the wild animals.

In dorsoventral views of rabbit skulls, the maxillary and mandibular cheek teeth positioned vertically in the jaw superimpose almost completely (Figure 5.27b). While the palatal aspects of the maxillary cheek teeth form a single line (their inner edge), their buccal edges together form a slight arc outwards that is also visible on the radiograph. The periodontal space can be seen

particularly well in the first upper premolar (P2), which is slightly offset rostrally in relation to the lower cheek teeth. That tooth is surrounded by a relatively wide, radiolucent, oval halo whose periphery is formed by the lamina dura of the alveolar bone.

The maxillary and mandibular incisors are also poorly visible due to superimposition; the mandibular incisors are located between the maxillary ones, which are curved slightly buccally. The apical region of the maxillary incisors can sometimes be differentiated rather well, depending on the extent of the teeth's lateral curvature. The outer edge of the upper jaw's diastema, although fine and occasionally a bit blurred in rabbits, is also visible. It merges into the large base of the zygomatic process and the zygomatic arch at the level of the lacrimal process and the lacrimal bone, respectively.

A fine radiopaque double line running from the lateral to the rostromedial aspect may sometimes be seen just in front of the first upper premolar (P2); this is the bony portion of the nasolacrimal duct.

The zygomatic bone with the zygomatic process and the facial tuberosity which is located a bit further rostrally, are all readily visible on dorsoventral views. The lacrimal processus of the lacrimal bone, which is individually different, is located laterally from the second maxillary cheek tooth (P3). This bony protrusion becomes more prominent with advancing age of an individual animal, particularly in male rabbits. In young animals, the dominant feature in the anterior third of the zygomatic arch is a fine fissure that represents the boundary between the maxilla and the zygomatic bone. The temporomandibular joint, which is rather wide, is located caudomedially from the caudal part of the zygomatic arch.

Reference lines in normocclusion

In pet rabbits with normal occlusion, views of the skull in a laterolateral view (Figure 5.27a) should show no dental structure dorsally from a base reference line that runs from the proximal end of the nasal bone to the tip of the occipital protuberance. Another line runs – parallel to the above mentioned as a rule – from the rostral end of the hard palate, which is located immediately caudally to the peg teeth to the lower third of the tympanic bulla (yellow line). In order to exactly determine the caudal reference point, the height of the tympanic bulla is marked by a line that is divided into three sections of the same length. This reference line corresponds to the occlusal plane in most healthy pet rabbits. Although six maxillary cheek teeth occlude with five mandibular ones in the rabbit, the mandibular and the maxillary occlusal planes of the cheek teeth have approximately the same length. Using the reference lines it should be always kept in mind that exceptions to the rule are possible. Especially in larger breeds and rabbits that show a longer and lower skull (like most wild animals) the reference lines may not work. Therefore the whole skull anatomy always has to be taken into consideration while interpreting X-rays.

Furthermore, in normal occlusion the apical ends of the mandibular premolars and molars must not penetrate the ventral cortical bone of the lower jaw. The mandible should be evenly thick and regularly structured below the first three mandibular cheek teeth (blue line). Any change or remodeling of the ventral margin of the mandible located below the anterior cheek teeth, may indicate a retrograde displacement of the apical area of the teeth. In rabbits with a healthy dentition, the mandibular and palatal bone plates converge slightly toward the rostral end (green line), although the convergence can be distinctly different depending on the shape of the skull.

A number of relevant reference lines that help to differentiate normal occlusion from malocclusion can also be drawn in the dorsoventral skull view (Figure 5.27b). One pair of lines runs from the lateral boundary of the rostral aspect of the maxillary incisor to the medial edge of the mandibular ramus on the same side. Another pair of reference lines runs from the lateral wall of the tympanic bulla to the laterorostral edge of the opposite side's maxillary incisor. No dental structure should be visible outside of these lines, except for the outermost apical tips of the second and third upper cheek teeth (P3, P4), both of which are normally more curved. The two blue lines denote the medial boundary of the mandible. The cortical bone should be straight, smooth and regularly shaped in rabbits with a normal occlusion. The radiographic anatomy of the maxillary premolars can be seen without superimposing the mandible's structures in Figure 5.28.

Reference lines in malocclusion

Figure 5.29a and b demonstrates how the anatomical reference lines are used in practice. Both figures are radiographs of the head of a rabbit with advanced malocclusion. A clear retrograde displacement of the apices of several maxillary cheek teeth – denoted by white arrows – can be seen in the laterolateral view (Figure 5.29a).

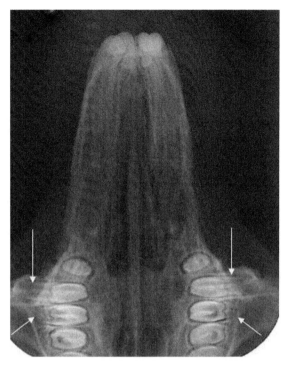

Figure 5.28 Intraoral view of the maxilla of a two-year-old rabbit with normal occlusion. The bodies of the second and third cheek tooth are curved slightly outwards (arrows).

Additional findings include a malocclusion of the maxillary incisor with a secondary perforation of the palatal bone by the apex of at least one maxillary incisor (green arrow). Furthermore, a significant loss of bone structure can be seen in the area of the mandibular incisor, which indicates a peridental (perialveolar) abscess of the jaw (blue arrows). The reference lines can be drawn even in laterolateral views with suboptimal positioning (slight obliquity); in such images the lines can be corrected accordingly and then used for a gross evaluation of the malocclusion. The second, yellow reference line, which has also been corrected slightly, shows rather clearly that the occlusal plane is almost normal in the rostral area, while the clinical crowns of the posterior maxillary cheek teeth are slightly elongated.

The radiograph of the skull in a dorsoventral view shows that there are clear pathological changes of the maxillary cheek teeth (Figure 5.29b). A retrograde displacement of the apices can be seen particularly on the right side. The zygomatic process has been perforated relatively extensively in the area of the facial tuberosity by the displaced apices of the maxillary cheek teeth

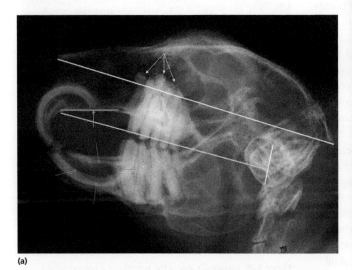

(a)

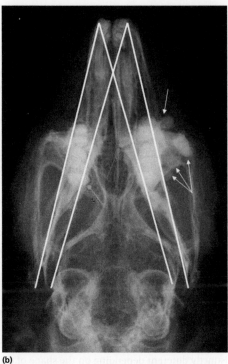

(b)

Figure 5.29 Anatomical reference lines for an advanced malocclusion in an eight-year-old rabbit. (a) In a laterolateral view, there is retrograde displacement as well as elongation of the maxillary cheek teeth and incisors, an intraoral elongation of the maxillary molars, a rostral abscess of the mandible (blue arrows) and an incisor malocclusion. (b) In a dorsoventral view, there is a retrograde displacement and elongation of the right maxillary cheek teeth, structural changes of the cheek teeth structure (on the right), a retrograde displacement of the first mandibular cheek tooth (P3; blue arrow) and a medial displacement of the second last left maxillary cheek tooth (M2; green arrow) (see also text).

(P2–M2) and the normal bone structure is significantly overshadowed by the latter. All maxillary cheek teeth on that side except for the last not only show lateral, intraalveolar tipping and curvature that is typical of rabbits with a dental disorder (a logical consequence of the radiological findings) but those teeth also appear more radiodense and have pathologically changes in the apical tooth structure. In addition, the second maxillary molar on the left side is displaced slightly medially (green arrow). On the right side, the apical area of the first mandibular cheek tooth (P3), which is displaced medially, can also be seen rather clearly (blue arrow).

The interpretation of those two radiographs shows that – just like in many other cases – further X-rays are necessary in order to comprehend the pathological changes more precisely and to assign them accordingly. At least two oblique projections (right and left oblique views) and an additional intraoral projection of the lower jaw would be necessary in that case in order to

verify conclusively whether the first mandibular cheek tooth (P3) is involved in the mandibular infection, which seems to originate from the incisor (uni- or bilateral?).

The reference lines in a laterolateral view as pictured in Figure 5.30a illustrate very clearly the pronounced retrograde displacement of the apices of various upper cheek teeth in another rabbit. In that case the middle maxillary cheek teeth are affected (P3–M2), with the alveaolar bulla of the second last cheek tooth exposed (white arrow). In addition, the bony portion of the nasolacrimal duct is pathologically dilated (red arrow) and the palatal bone plate is slightly deformed by a ventral protrusion as a result of a retrograde apex displacement of the maxillary incisors (green arrow). The occlusal plane of the cheek teeth is very uneven and stepped; moreover, different lengths of the mandibular and maxillary occlusal surfaces dominate. The shift of the occlusal plane resulting from this is marked by red lines. In addition, a more pronounced deviation of the second mandibular cheek

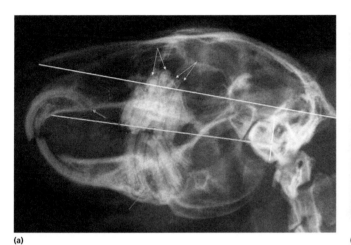
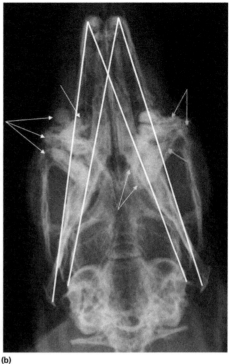

(a) (b)

Figure 5.30 Anatomical reference lines for an advanced malocclusion in a three-year-old rabbit. (a) In a laterolateral view, there is a retrograde displacement as well as an elongation of the middle maxillary cheek teeth (P3–M2) and incisors, a dilatation of the nasolacrimal duct (red double arrows), an intraoral elongation of the maxillary molars, a malocclusion of the mandibular incisors, a deviation of the second mandibular cheek tooth with an expansion of the distal and interproximal space and there are different lengths of the maxillary and mandibular occlusal surfaces (red lines). (b) In a dorsoventral view, there is a retrograde displacement and an elongation of the left maxillary cheek teeth (P2–M2) with a complete destruction of the facial tuberosity (white arrows), a corresponding change on the right side (P2–P4; green arrows), a retrograde displacement of the apices of the two anterior mandibular cheek teeth (P3/P4; yellow arrows) and an intraoral tooth spur (blue arrow) (see also text).

tooth (P4) together with a considerable expansion of the distal interdental area (blue arrows) can be identified, despite superimposition of the mandibles. Furthermore, there is a narrowing of the affected tooth structure.

The view in a dorsoventral projection (Figure 5.30b) indicates considerable destruction of the base of the zygomatic process (tuber faciale) as well as the lacrimal process. Responsible for this is a pronounced retrograde displacement of the elongated apices of five maxillary cheek teeth (P2–M2) on the left side (white arrows), whereas on the right side only the first three teeth (P2–P4) are affected (green arrows). The yellow arrows mark the medial displacement of the apices of the first and second mandibular cheek teeth (P3, P4) on the right side. When interpreting radiographs in a dorsoventral projection, attention must be paid to a distinction between an

intermandibulary retrograde displacement of the apices (yellow arrows) and an intraoral formation of tooth spurs (blue arrow). A thorough intraoral examination of the patient before the radiographic examination is performed is a crucial prerequisite for this. As in the preceding example, there is an indication for more radiographic images in this patient – bilateral oblique projections as well as an intraoral projection of the mandible – in order to differentiate the pathological changes more exactly.

5.6.2 Guinea pigs
Normal radiographic anatomy

In normal occlusion, the incisors are not in contact on a laterolateral view (Figure 5.31a). At rest – when the cheek teeth occlude – the mandibular incisors are located caudally to the upper ones. Just as in all rodents, the labial

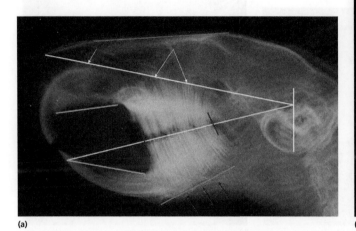

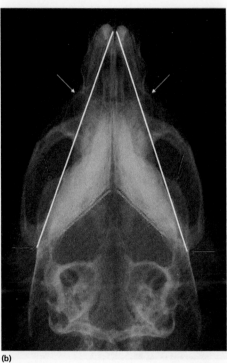

(a)

(b)

Figure 5.31 Anatomical reference lines for normal occlusion in a one-year-old guinea pig. (a) In a laterolateral view, there is a slight overgrowth of the mandibular as well as the maxillary incisors. (b) In a dorsoventral view, there is the masseteric ridge of the mandible (blue arrows), the medial border of the mandibular cortical bone (light blue line) and the apex of the first maxillary premolar (white arrow) (see also text).

surface of the maxillary incisors is covered with a smooth enamel layer that is clearly visible radiographically. In the intraalveolar area and the area near the apex of the maxillary and mandibular incisors, the pulp cavity can be seen – always more clearly in the maxilla than in the mandible. The root of the maxillary incisors ends just in front of the mesial surface of the first cheek tooth (P4) – a little further away from the palatal bone plate than in rabbits. The root apex of the mandibular incisor is located lingually from the row of lower cheek teeth, approximately on a level with the first molar (M1), and can therefore not be identified directly on lateral projections.

The maxillary and mandibular cheek teeth – four each – are relatively short and compact. The intradental enamel folds can be identified as multiple fine radiopaque lines of the individual teeth and the roots' germinal tissues are clearly visible as periapical translucencies. The ventral margin of the mandible is smooth in normocclusion. The cortical bone should not be perforated by retrograde elongation of the mandibular cheek teeth. The premolars

and molars, which are very curved intraalveolarly (buccally in the maxilla and lingually in the mandible, respectively), meet directly in the area of the occlusal plane (see Figure 3.20 in Chapter 3). Since the occlusal surface is normally tilted approximately 40°, it does not appear as a clear line on laterolateral radiographic projections. This is due to the medial edge of the maxillary occlusal plane superimposing the lateral edge of the mandibular occlusal plane. The occlusal surface is supposed to be consistently even, with a slight upward gradient from caudal to rostral correlating to the length of the cheek teeth. As a consequence, the palatal and mandibular bone plates converge rostrally – like in rabbits. Thereby the dorsal cortical bone plate of the mandible directly merges into the gnawing surface of the mandibular incisors. Contrary to this, many guinea pigs with a clinically normal occlusion exhibit a slight elongation of the mandibular incisors (as seen in the Figure 5.31a). In younger guinea pigs, a line resembling a fissure can be identified in the caudal part of the maxillary bone plate and should not to be misinterpreted as a fracture. It is the bony link between the incisive bone and the maxilla.

Radiographs of a dorsoventral skull view (Figure 5.31b) are usually of little validity when tooth elongation is not present as the curved cheek teeth superimpose extensively. The large zygomatic arch runs in a slight arc almost parallel to the row of mandibular cheek teeth that diverge widely caudally. The mandibular incisors are located – and are mostly clearly visible despite superimposition with the maxillary cheek teeth – in the rostromedial area parallel to each other. The maxillary incisors can be identified rostrally to the former and are curved more outwardly. Their apical portion is located near the mesial edge of the maxillary premolars (P4). The sled-shaped temporomandibular joints are visible caudomedial to the zygomatic arch.

Reference lines in normocclusion

Anatomical reference lines have also proven to be very helpful in guinea pigs. However, here too exceptions to the rule are possible if the skull anatomy of a single individuum deviates considerably from the norm. On radiographs of healthy dentition in a laterolateral view (Figure 5.31a), one of those lines runs from the rostral end of the nasal bone to the dorsal notch of the tympanic bulla, which is located at approximately three-quarters of the height of the tympanic bulla (white line). In young guinea pigs, the nasal bone forms an almost straight line with the dorsal skull, whereas in older guinea pigs the two meet at a slight angle creating a slight concavity where they meet (brown line in Figures 5.32a and 5.33a).

The outline of the occlusal plane, which is 40° oblique, can usually be drawn as a straight line. In order to determine the rostral reference point exactly, the mandibular bone plate is extended to the anterior edge of the mandibular incisors (green line) – a mark that would correspond with the normal physiological length of the mandibular incisors. That point, in other words the "normal" cusp of the mandibular incisor, is then connected with the notch of the tympanic bulla described above (yellow line). That second reference line marks the occlusal plane of the mandibular as well as the maxillary cheek teeth. In young guinea pigs with a perfectly normal occlusion, that line should touch the outermost tip of the chisel-shaped maxillary and mandibular incisors simultaneously when the jaws are closed. Hence the line marks the physiological length of the mandibular

and maxillary incisors – apart from the occlusal plane of the cheek teeth. However, this can rarely be seen in practice as most guinea pigs have a slight elongation of the extraalveolar crowns of the (upper and) lower incisors, which is often clinically not apparent.

In the periapical area of the mandibular cheek teeth, there are sac-like radiolucencies covered by thin cortical bone, which can usually be seen clearly on radiographs. If the ventral boundary of the mandible that is relatively smooth and uniformly thick (dark blue line) exhibits structural changes or is perforated, then a retrograde tooth elongation of the mandibular cheek teeth is present. In guinea pigs with a normal occlusion, the palatal and mandibular bone plates converge significantly rostrally (green lines) – much more pronounced than in rabbits. That convergence decreases when the clinical crowns of the cheek teeth become increasingly longer, and the lines will then become increasingly parallel or even start to diverge slightly. As is typical for rodents, the maxillary and mandibular occlusal surfaces of guinea pigs have the same length radiographically. In both cases it is made up of four cheek teeth (P4–M3) that – being antagonists – immediately occlude with each other at rest (red lines). Any radiographically visible change of length of those two occlusal planes, or even a shift with respect to one another, is a definite indication of malocclusion.

On dorsoventral skull radiographs (Figure 5.31b), the most informative reference line runs from the mesial border of the maxillary incisor to a caudolateral point on the ipsilateral mandible where the caudal boundary of the zygomatic arch crosses the mandible (red arrows). In guinea pigs without any significant retrograde tooth elongation only the radiolucent apical bulla of the first maxillary premolar (P4) extends lateral to that line (white arrows). More caudally the prominent nearly crescent shaped bone structure crossing this line (blue arrows) is the massetric ridge of the mandible where the deep part of the masseter muscle originates (see Figure 3.20 in Chapter 3). The blue lines mark the medial cortical borders of the mandibles.

Reference lines in malocclusion

Figure 5.32a shows the laterolateral view of the skull of an adult guinea pig (recognizable by the angle of the brown lines) with advanced malocclusion. The dorsal reference line clearly demonstrates a retrograde displacement of the reserve crown and apices of the last two upper cheek teeth (M2/M3; white arrows).

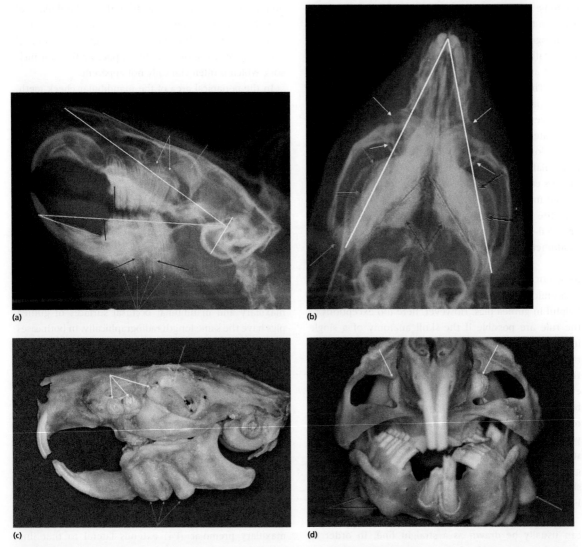

(a)

(b)

(c)

(d)

Figure 5.32 Anatomical reference lines for an advanced malocclusion in a four-year-old guinea pig. (a) In a laterolateral view, there is a retrograde displacement of the apices of the last two maxillary molars (M2/M3; white arrows), a radiodense bony structure in the area of the caudal orbit (green arrow), a malocclusion of the incisors with a significant elongation of the mandibular incisors, an elongation of the clinical crowns of all mandibular cheek teeth with a secondary prognathic jaw position (red lines) and a retrograde displacement as well as an elongation of all mandibular cheek teeth (unilateral; light blue arrows). The contralateral cortical bone is remodeled in an undulating way (dark blue arrows). (b) In a dorsoventral view, there is a retrograde displacement and an elongation of all mandibular and maxillary cheek teeth (more pronounced on the left than on the right; white and blue arrows) and the medial cortical bone of the mandible is visible (light blue lines) as well as a retrograde displacement of the apices of the last two maxillary cheek teeth (M3; red arrows). (c) The specimen gives a lateral view of the retrograde displacement as well as elongation of all maxillary and mandibular cheek teeth (white and light blue arrows), an increased bone density in the intraorbital area (green arrow) and an incisor malocclusion with rostral displacement of the mandible. (d) The rostrocaudal view of the specimen shows the retrograde displacement of the apex of the first maxillary cheek teeth on both sides (white arrows), retrograde elongation of the last right mandibular molar (light blue arrow) as well as the anterior right mandibular cheek teeth (dark blue arrows), an abnormal molar chewing surface with buccal spurs (on the left) and a vertical occlusal plane of the last molar (M3) and an incisor malocclusion with a thickening of the left mandibular incisor body (see also text).

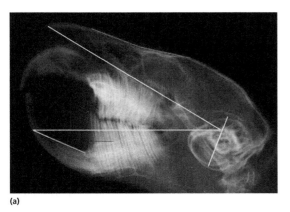 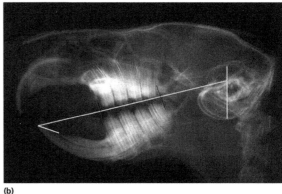

(a)   (b)

Figure 5.33 Anatomical reference lines for malocclusion in a one-and-a-half-year-old guinea pig. (a) In a laterolateral view an elongation of the clinical crown of both mandibular incisors and an elongation of cheek teeth with a rostral displacement of the lower jaw are visible (red arrows). (b) In a laterolateral view after correction of the occlusion, a re-establishment of intraoral normal occlusion is visible (see also text).

Dorsocaudally to that area, a radiodense bony structure is shown, which can also be identified on the macerated skull of the respective animal (see Figure 5.32c). The rostral point for the second reference line is determined by extending the mandibular bone plate cranially (determining the "normal" length and anterior tipping of the mandibular incisor). The reference point also marks the desired postoperative length of the lower incisors. When connected with the second reference point at the tympanic bulla, the line clearly shows an intraoral elongation of all lower cheek teeth (yellow line). Furthermore, the apices of some mandibular cheek teeth have unilaterally perforated the ventral mandibular cortical bone, thus exhibiting a distinct retrograde tooth elongation (light blue arrows in Figure 5.32a to d). The ventral boundary of the contralateral healthy cortical bone of the lower jaw, which has become slightly undulated in the area of the apices, is partly superimposed by these pathological changes (dark blue arrows in Figure 5.32a and d). In addition, a clear difference in length of the maxillary and mandibular arcades can be seen (red lines in Figure 5.32a) as well as a rostral displacement of the mandible. This is – particularly in the guinea pig – a reliable indication of a severely advanced stage of cheek teeth malocclusion.

On the dorsoventral view (Figure 5.32b) the references lines confirm the findings on the laterolateral view of a distinct and generalized retrograde displacement of the reserve crowns and apices of all mandibular and maxillary cheek teeth (more distinct on the left than

on the right). The apices of the elongated mandibular cheek teeth are located relatively far laterally from the reference line (light and dark blue arrows) and the maxilla shows similar changes. Not only the apex but also a part of the reserve crown of the maxillary premolar (P4) and the first molar (M1) is displaced beyond the reference line (white arrows) in this radiograph. The cortex is extensively perforated, particularly on the left side, a finding that can also be seen on the respective skull specimen (white arrows in Figure 5.32c and d). The light blue arrow in Figure 5.32d shows obvious retrograde tooth elongation and deviation of the fourth left mandibular cheek tooth (M3).

The second reference line which runs bilaterally along the medial cortical bone of each mandible on radiographs of the skull in a dorsoventral view (Figure 5.32b) shows some dental substance on both sides (red arrows). That finding indicates two possible changes: either a rostral displacement of the mandible, which is typical for guinea pigs with a cheek tooth malocclusion, or the retrograde displacements of the last two maxillary molar apices (M2/M3) – both or either.

Reference lines can be very helpful not only for the diagnosis but also for the treatment of malocclusions. For example, the second (yellow) line marking the physiological occlusal plane of incisors and cheek teeth on radiographs of the head in a laterolateral beam path makes it possible to evaluate objectively on postoperative radiographs whether the trimming of teeth was correct. The mandible is shifted rostrally in a species-specific way in guinea pigs with a tooth elongation. The extent of that rostral displacement of the mandible depends on the severity of the malocclusion (red arrows in Figure 5.33a). The yellow reference line shows that in this patient all mandibular cheek teeth as well as the incisors are too long and need shortening. The aim of the treatment is to create an occlusion that is as close as possible to the physiological situation (normocclusion). Thus after proper correction of the dentition, the mandibular and maxillary cheek teeth should be located exactly opposite one another and the correctly trimmed incisors should have no contact with one another (the tip of the mandibular incisor distal to the maxillary incisor). In the illustrated case all teeth were distinctly elongated intraorally without exhibiting any further significant changes in the apical area. Largely normal occlusion was successfully re-established by means of trimming the teeth (Figure 5.33b). The reference line shows that now the maxillary and mandibular cheek teeth, which are roughly the same length, are located immediately opposite one another again and also the

mandibular and maxillary occlusal planes are equal in length (red lines). When critically considered, the lower incisors are still a little too long (white line) and have blunt ends instead of the typical chisel-shaped tips.

5.6.3 Chinchillas
Normal radiographic anatomy

In the laterolateral view of the skull the incisors are not in contact at rest, whereas the four cheek teeth (Figure 5.34a). As in all rodents, the labial surface of the maxillary incisors is covered with a smooth enamel layer that is clearly visible radiographically. The pulp cavities of both the maxillary and the mandibular incisors are also clearly visible in the intraalveolar area as well as the area near the apices. The root apex of the maxillary incisor is located at roughly half or two-thirds of the length of the diastema, relatively close to the palatal bone plate. The mandibular incisor apex is located lingual to the first or second cheek tooth (P4/M1) and can be seen clearly despite superimposition of the cheek teeth.

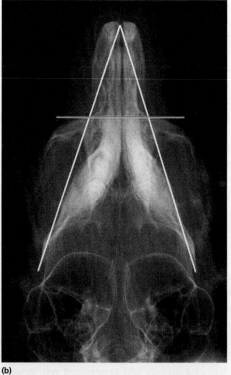

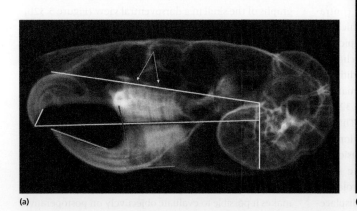

(a)   (b)

Figure 5.34 Anatomical reference lines for normal occlusion in a one-year-old chinchilla. (a) Radiographic examination in a laterolateral view. (b) Radiographic examination in a dorsoventral view (see also text).

The molars are relatively short and form a completely even, horizontally outlined occlusal surface. With perfect positioning of the head on a laterolateral radiograph, it can be identified as a clearly visible, absolutely straight, fine line (at rest). The apical germinal tissues appear as distinct periapical radiolucencies. The ventral cortical bone of the mandible is smooth and lacks protrusions. Especially in the chinchilla the laterolateral view is important to enable accurate evaluation of any retrograde elongation of the cheek teeth (see the reference lines), particularly if only subtle or no changes were noted during the intraoral examination.

On the dorsoventral skull view, a distinct rostrocaudal divergence of the maxillary and mandibular arcades can be seen (Figure 5.34b). The zygomatic arch is narrower than in rabbits and guinea pigs and is therefore usually less visible on radiographs. The periorbital and retroorbital areas of bone have smooth boundaries. The chinchilla has very large, multichambered tympanic bullae clearly visible on radiographs.

Reference lines in normocclusion

The most important reference line in the laterolateral skull view connects the dorsal margin of the upper incisor with the middle of the very large tympanic bulla. (rostrodorsal indentation) (Figure 5.34a). In healthy animals, the more radiolucent apices of the maxillary cheek teeth (P4–M3) should be located on a level with that line and no calcified dental tissue should be visible dorsally from that boundary. However, since most pet chinchillas exhibit a more or less pronounced retrograde displacement of the apices of the maxillary cheek teeth, it is very difficult to find animals without any abnormalities here.

The second reference line connects the tip of the upper incisors with a point that is located at three-quarters of the height of the tympanic bulla, measured from the rostrodorsal indentation toward the ventral end (yellow line). If the incisors are normal in length and occlusion, that line touches the tips of both the maxillary and the mandibular incisor rostrally, running distally parallel to the palatal bone plate and exactly on a level with the occlusal surfaces of the cheek teeth toward the bulla. The rostral point for this reference line will need to be estimated (in a similar manner as that described for guinea pigs above) if the incisors are severely elongated by extending a line rostrally along the mandibular bone plate (green line). On lateral images, the occlusal plane is usually clearly visible as a fine, black line (Figure 5.34a).

The third reference line (blue) starts at the most ventral edge of the mandibular incisor and continues caudally, running largely parallel to the occlusal plane of the cheek teeth, as far as the fourth molar (M3). It marks the outline of the mandibular cortical bone, which is located below the first three cheek teeth (P4–M2). That ventral border of the mandible should be smooth and even, without any narrowing of the cortical bone or distortions or perforations due to retrograde displaced apices of the mandibular cheek teeth.

In chinchillas, reference lines in a dorsoventral skull view (Figure 5.34b) are not as diagnostically conclusive as in guinea pigs with respect to an objective evaluation of a malocclusion, but they are still helpful. One reference line connects the mesial tip of each maxillary incisor with the caudal end of the ipsilateral mandible (white lines). In healthy animals it marks the lateral border of the caudal cheek teeth. Another reference line can be drawn in transversely where the line described above crosses the rostral end of the maxillary portion of the zygomatic process (green line). When the head is positioned correctly, this line indicates the rostral extent of the cheek teeth in a healthy chinchilla. Any calcified dental material rostral to this line is indicative of a malocclusion usually with retrograde elongation of (at least the first or more often all) maxillary cheek teeth.

Reference lines in malocclusion

Although an image of the skull in a laterolateral view (Figure 5.35) shows hardly any indication of an advanced malocclusion when asessing only the occlusal surface, the dorsal, white reference line contradicts this. It illustrates very clearly significant retrograde elongation of all maxillary cheek teeth together with dorsal displacement of the apices of the affected teeth (white arrows). The clinical crowns of the mandibular cheek teeth are also slightly elongated (dotted yellow line and yellow arrows) and will require the teeth to be trimmed. In order to correctly determine each of the rostral reference points for the yellow lines, the lengths of the maxillary and mandibular incisors are corrected (white lines in Figure 5.35), based on healthy dentition (Figure 5.34a). The increased divergent curvature of particularly the first (P4) and last (M3) maxillary cheek teeth, which cause the overall length of the chewing surface to increase, is also typical of an advanced malocclusion.

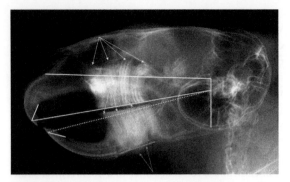

Figure 5.35 Anatomical reference lines for an early malocclusion in an eleven-year-old chinchilla. In a laterolateral view, there is a retrograde displacement and elongation of all maxillary cheek teeth, a subtle elongation of the clinical crowns of all mandibular cheek teeth (yellow arrows), a perforation of the ventral cortical bone of the jaw (M1/M2) and a slight overgrowth of the mandibular and maxillary incisors (see also text).

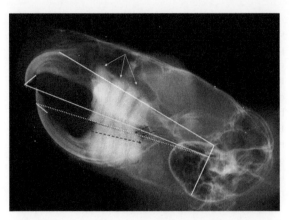

Figure 5.36 Anatomical reference lines for an advanced malocclusion in a five-year-old chinchilla. In a laterolateral view, there is a retrograde displacement and elongation of all maxillary cheek teeth (white arrows), a subtle elongation of the clinical crowns of all maxillary cheek teeth, a distal displacement of the mandible (red arrows) and elongation of the mandibular incisors (see also text).

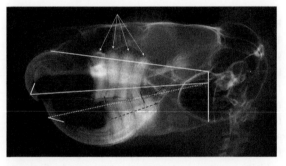

Figure 5.37 Anatomical reference lines for an advanced malocclusion in a five-year-old chinchilla. In a laterolateral view, there is a retrograde displacement of the apices of all maxillary cheek teeth (white arrows), an incisor malocclusion with an intraoral dental overgrowth, an elongation of the clinical crowns of all maxillary cheek teeth and a distal displacement of the mandible (red lines and arrows) (see also text).

Furthermore, the mandible's ventral cortical bone is perforated by the apices of the second and third cheek tooth (M1/M2) (blue arrows). Since the apical tooth changes in the maxilla and mandible are irreversible, recurrent malocclusions will occur at different time points, even after the best possible correction of the dentition with an approximation of intraoral normocclusion has been performed. Contrary to guinea pigs with a malocclusion whose mandibles shift rostrally with respect to the maxilla due to the elongation of all cheek teeth (Figure 5.33a), chinchillas with a malocclusion typically have their mandibles shifted caudally. That displacement can hardly be identified in Figure 5.35 as it is only very subtle. Most chinchillas with an incongruence of the jaws have significant problems chewing, with the degree of the mandibular shift correlated to the degree of intraoral tooth elongation. For example, the occlusal surfaces of the diseased animals may be shifted by half (red arrows in Figure 5.36) or even the entire width of a cheek tooth (red arrows in Figure 5.37).

In a dorsoventral skull view, pathological changes of the dental morphology (infection-related tooth resorptions) can be easily identified as certain irregularities within the dental structure. The blue arrows in Figures 5.38 and 5.39 indicate the elongated apices of the two posterior mandibular cheek teeth (M2/M3), with the apices having been displaced beyond the lateral margin of the mandibular cortical bone. Rostrally, calcified substances can be seen extending beyond the green

reference line on both sides indicating apical elongation and displacement of the two anterior maxillary cheek teeth (P4/M1; white arrows). Typically they elongate in an arc and penetrate the maxillary bone in this area, obstructing or obliterating the nasolacrimal duct (see Figure 5.40c and d).

When evaluating dorsoventral skull radiographs, it is important to make a distinction between intraorally elongated cheek teeth with corresponding buccal spurs (which can be seen in a clinical examination) and a

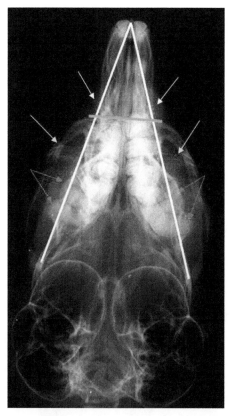

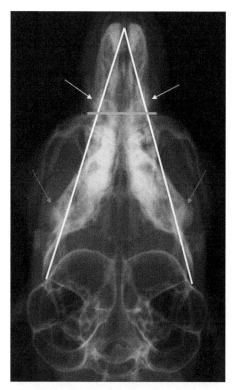

Figure 5.39 Anatomical reference lines for an advanced malocclusion in a five-year-old chinchilla. In a dorsoventral view, there is a retrograde apex displacement of the last mandibular molar (M3) as well as of the first maxillary cheek tooth (P4; white arrow) (see also text).

Figure 5.38 Anatomical reference lines for an advanced malocclusion in a three-year-old chinchilla. In a dorsoventral view, there is a retrograde displacement of the apices of the last two mandibular molars (M2/M3; blue arrows) as well as of the two anterior maxillary cheek teeth (P4; white arrows) and the lacrimal bone (yellow arrows) (see also text).

retrograde displacement of any apices. Crowns of cheek teeth that are elongated intraorally and growing buccally usually appear more radiolucent and more pointed when compared with a radiodense distorted retrogradely displaced apex of a molar closely surrounded by alveolar bone and soft tissue (blue arrows). The former must not be confused with the lacrimal bone, which is always located distally from the base of the zygomatic bone in chinchillas (yellow lines in Figure 5.38).

Just as in guinea pigs, a correction of the occlusion can be checked by means of certain reference lines. Figure 5.40a shows the laterloateral skull view of a chinchilla with marked intraoral and extraoral tooth elongation with an associated caudal displacement of the mandible and buccal tooth spurs (red arrows). The

two yellow reference lines show the normal occlusal lines for the maxillary and mandibular cheek teeth indicating how much tooth substance has to be removed during correction of the occlusion (the area between the lines). This is equal to almost a third of the entire length of the tooth structures in the area of the maxillary premolars. The reference lines drawn in after trimming the teeth (Figure 5.40b) show that, in this patient, the correction was suboptimal. The last mandibular cheek tooth (M3) is still a little too long intraorally (yellow arrow) and the mandibular incisor does not have a chisel-shaped tip. However, the occlusion as a whole is distinctly more normal; this can be clearly seen based on the position of the incisor tips, which are level just as a normal occlusion requires them to be.

The skull of the chinchilla that is depicted in Figure 5.40a and b could be examined more closely as the patient was later euthanized (Figure 5.40c and d). The

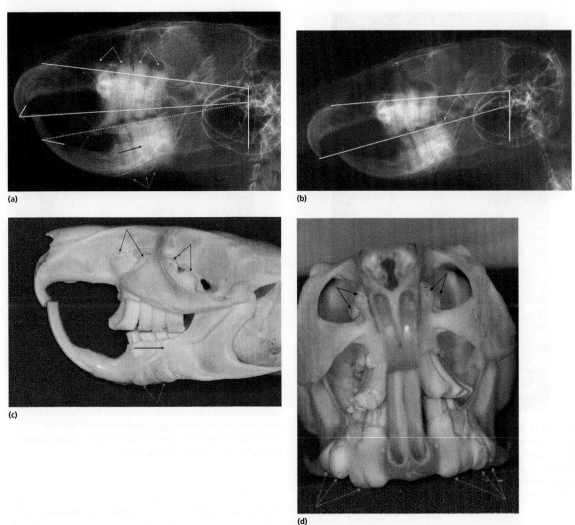

Figure 5.40 Anatomical reference lines for an advanced malocclusion in a six-year-old chinchilla. (a) In a laterolateral view, there is a retrograde displacement of the apices of all maxillary cheek teeth (white arrows), an incisor malocclusion with an intraoral dental overgrowth, an elongation of the clinical crowns of all maxillary cheek teeth with a large mesial overgrowth of the maxillary premolar (P4), a distal displacement of the mandible (red lines and arrows) and protrusions in the ventral cortex of the mandible (P4–M2; light blue arrows). (b) Immediately after correction of the dentition, largely normal intraoral occlusion is visible in a laterolateral view, however the last lower cheek tooth (M3) remains slightly elongated. (c) On a lateral view of the specimen, there is an advanced malocclusion with a severe intraoral as well as retrograde elongation of all maxillary cheek teeth, a distal displacement of the mandible, a distension of the ventral border of the mandible, an incisor malocclusion with an abnormal contact area of the incisors and extensive elongation of the clinical crown of the mandibular incisor. (d) On a rostrocaudal view of the specimen, there is an advanced malocclusion with a retrograde apex displacement of the anterior two maxillary cheek teeth (P4/M1; black arrows), a marked elongation and buccal deviation of the clinical crowns of all maxillary cheek teeth, a retrograde elongation of all mandibular cheek teeth with a resultant perforation of the ventral mandibular cortical bone (more pronounced on the right than on the left; light blue arrows) and multiple areas of osteomyelitis of the alveolar walls of the maxillary cheek teeth (more pronounced on the right than on the left) (see also text).

specimen shows a marked incisor malocclusion as well as a generalized intraoral tooth elongation. In addition, the apices of all maxillary cheek teeth are retrogradely displaced with penetration of the alveolar bone (black arrows). Such species-specific pathological bone changes could be extrapolated from the evaluation of the corresponding radiographs by means of the reference lines. There is a slight retrograde displacement of the mandibular cheek teeth as seen as distention of the mandibular cortex rather than actual penetration (blue arrows).

5.6.4 Degus
Normal radiographic anatomy

The laterolateral skull radiograph shows that the incisors of degus with a normal occlusion are not in contact – as in all rodents (Figure 5.41a). The apical area of the maxillary incisor is close to the apex of the first maxillary cheek tooth (P4), which is always slightly curved rostrally. The apex of the mandibular incisor, however, ends on a level with the last molar (M3) and cannot usually be seen clearly due to a superimposition with the apical sections of all four mandibular cheek teeth. Although the clinical crowns of the cheek teeth are almost vertical on intraoral examinations, the three maxillary molars (M1–M3) and the last mandibular cheek tooth (M3) are distinctly curved concavely in a caudal direction within the alveolus on lateral radiographs of the head. Just as in chinchillas, the occlusal plane is even and horizontal. Therefore it can be seen as a fine, black line on laterolateral views. The mandible is more arc-like than in guinea pigs and chinchillas and also has a smooth ventral border.

The dorsoventral skull view shows that the maxillary and mandibular incisor are superimposed due to the isognathic jaw relationship (Figure 5.41b). Each mandible diverges caudally. The mandibular incisor apices extend far distally and can be seen clearly in the mediocaudal area of each mandible, close to the temporomandibular joint. The clinical crowns of both mandibular incisors are located medially from the apices of the maxillary incisors. As in chinchillas, the multichambered tympanic bulla is relatively large.

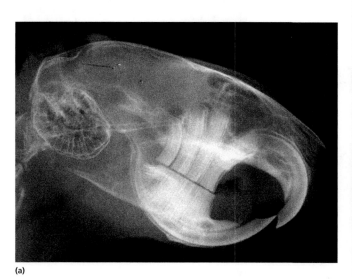

(a)

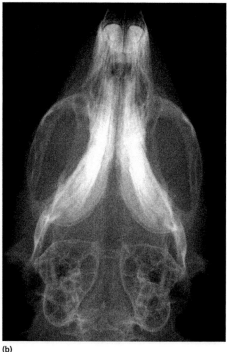

(b)

Figure 5.41 Normal occlusion in a two-year-old degu. (a) In a laterolateral view, there is a normal mesial deviation of the first maxillary cheek tooth. (b) In a dorsoventral view, the mandibular incisors are clearly visible as they extend far caudally.

5.6.5 Rats
Normal radiographic anatomy

In rats the incisors do not have contact, as is typical for rodents, unless there is a abnormal elongation (Figure 5.42a). However, most pet rats exhibit a slight overgrowth of the incisors, which is usually clinically irrelevant. The root of the maxillary incisor is located at roughly three-quarters of the length of the diastema, near the palatal bone plate. The mandibular incisor lies completely underneath the brachyodont, mostly three-rooted cheek teeth, with its apical area ending far behind the last molar (M3). In principle, the curvature of the rostral mandible corresponds with the radius of curvature of the mandibular incisor. In young animals, the occlusal surfaces of the cheek teeth are covered by a more radiodense enamel cap.

The dorsoventral skull radiograph shows that the rows of cheek teeth in the maxilla and mandible are still completely superimposed as a result of the isognathic jaw relationship despite the branches of the mandible diverging slightly caudally (Figure 5.42b). The apices of the maxillary incisors are located laterally from the crowns of the mandibular incisors and medially from the base of the zygomatic process. The caudal part of the mandible is a little wider than the maxilla; the apices of the mandibular incisors can be readily identified in the caudolateral area. The temporomandibular joints are distinctly shorter than in guinea pigs and chinchillas, and the tympanic bulla is relatively small.

5.6.6 Hamsters and mice
Normal radiographic anatomy

In hamsters and mice, the germinal root area of the maxillary incisor is located at half of the length and two-thirds of the length, respectively, of the diastema. The mandibular incisor ends on a level with or behind the last cheek tooth (M3) (Figure 5.43). On laterolateral skull radiographs, the delicate roots of the brachyodont molars as well as their more radiopaque enamel caps are clearly visible. The occlusal surfaces of the maxillary and mandibular incisors are not in contact unless there is a pathological elongation of teeth.

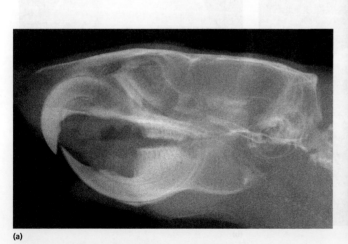

(a)

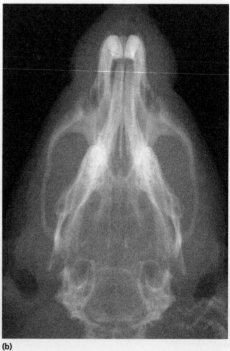

(b)

Figure 5.42 Normal occlusion in a six-month-old rat. (a) In a laterolateral view, there are radicular cheek teeth with enamel caps, with the apices of the long mandibular incisors being located far distally from the molars. (b) In a dorsoventral view, the apex of the mandibular incisors are located caudodistally from the rows of cheek teeth, which are clearly visible.

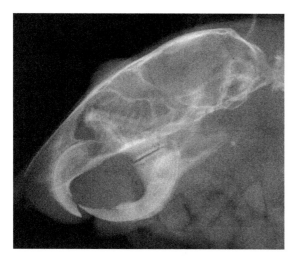

Figure 5.43 Normal occlusion in a six-month-old dwarf hamster. In a laterolateral view, there are radicular cheek teeth with enamel caps, the apex of the long mandibular incisors are located far distally from the molars and the cheek pouches are filled.

5.7 Intraoral radiography

Intraoral radiography is a method of examination that has long been established in human dentistry and is also commonly performed in veterinary medicine – particularly in dogs and cats. Individual teeth and their periapical area can be isolated without superimposition by using small, non-screen dental films or digital X-ray sensors – even in pets. For example, there is a publication describing the experimental performance of intraoral radiography in rats (Serota, Jeffcoat & Kaplan, 1981). Dental films are unique as they are very sensitive, allow a range of contrast and provide highly detailed images. This excellent fine-detailed image allows an precise interpretation to be made of even the most delicate bone and tooth structures.

As a result, intraoral radiographs are used more and more for the diagnosis of malocclusions in lagomorphs and rodents (Böhmer, 2001a). Although this technique takes more time and requires adequate processing, it does often provide the sort of information that could otherwise only be obtained by means of much more expensive methods (e.g. computed tomography); this is particularly the case for pathology in the rostral jaw area or the incisors. In some of those cases intraoral radiography cannot be beaten, especially in rabbits. The requirements for obtaining successful images for this specific technique are correct indication and adequate

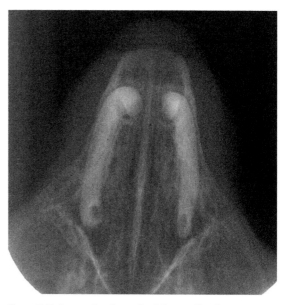

Figure 5.44 Intraoral radiograph of the maxilla of a one-year-old chipmunk, for a review of the retained fragments of teeth after a fracture of both maxillary incisors at the gingiva. The tooth structures and apices of both maxillary incisors do not show any pathology.

positioning of the patient as well as optimal film positioning and processing of the dental film.

5.7.1 Intraoral films

Flexible intraoral films are available in two different sizes that are relevant for our purposes:

Size 2: 31 mm × 41 mm (Kodak® DF 58; see Figure 5.47 later)

Size 0: 22 mm × 35 mm (Kodak® DF 54; see Figure 5.50 later)

D-(Ultra-Speed-)films and E-(Ekta-Speed-)films are available (product information). E-speed films can be exposed for a shorter time than D-speed films, but they have a lower resolution of the depicted objects. The larger-sized films are useful in rabbits whereas the smaller-sized films are suitable for intraoral radiography in guinea pigs, chinchillas and rats (Böhmer, 2007). The latter may even be used to image the incisors of small rodents when placed intraorally using just one corner (Figure 5.44).

Intraoral films are also available in a slightly more elongated shape with a bite-wing (28 mm × 55 mm). They can be helpful in imaging especially narrow and

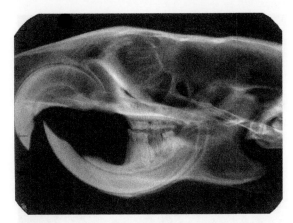

Figure 5.45 Radiograph of a one-and-a-half-year-old rat in a laterolateral view with a nonscreen occlusal film. The clinical crown of the second mandibular cheek tooth is missing (intraoral finding), there is loss of the second lower molar (M2), but all other cheek teeth and the incisors are without any pathology.

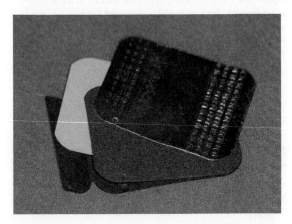

Figure 5.46 Opened package of a nonscreen dental film: metal foil with typical pattern, dental film lying between two paper strips and a embossed dot on all objects.

elongated oral cavities or retrograde overgrowth of extremely long incisors. Also available are so-called occlusal films (57 mm × 75 mm) that are big enough for the entire skull of small rodents to be imaged, with highly detail (Figure 5.45). In order to obtain overview images of the skull in two planes, the patient is placed directly on to the film and positioned accordingly.

Dental films can only be exposed from one side. Within their plastic coating, there is a fine metal foil that serves to reduce the amount of scattered radiation. Hence the films are placed into the oral cavity so that the front intraoral film faces toward the X-ray tube and the back side containing the foil faces away from the tube. Furthermore, ensure that the embossed dot (a small circle on the protective sleeve or a corresponding imprint) faces rostrally and toward the X-ray tube (Figure 5.46). This allows for correct orientation when viewing the film but also helps prevent damage to another area of the film that may be pieced during processing as this may otherwise create an artefact over a potential area of interest on the xray film.

A number of digital intraoral imaging plates that are suitably sized and similar in size to the classical intraoral dental films are now also available as an alternative to the "classic" dental film. The plate is exposed and then transferred to the computer and an image generated by means of special reading devices.

5.7.2 Positioning

Whenever the mandible of a rabbit is to be imaged with the incisors and cheek teeth in isolation, the patient is placed in dorsal recumbency and its neck is supported with a suitable foam roller. The film is then placed occlusally into the oral cavity such that the front side of the film, which is uniformly white, faces upwards.

For radiographic examinations of the maxilla, positioning of the dental film is performed with the patient in ventral recumbency. Before exposure, check that the film's two-toned back side, which has a small flap, faces toward the examination table. Otherwise the pattern of the metal foil, will be depicted on the image and would hamper interpretation of the findings.

In order to place the film as deeply into the oral cavity as possible, the tongue of the patient is grasped and pulled out of the mouth as far as possible, passing the incisors on one side. The jaws can be opened easily by simultaneously applying slight pressure on the mandible. It is then possible to introduce one corner of the dental film relatively deep into the area of the right cheek, and then slide the opposite side of the film just as deeply into the left cheek in a constant, flowing motion (Figures 5.47 and 5.48). The dental film can then be carefully introduced deeper and deeper into the oral cavity by means of repeated slight lateral movements, with the tongue remaining outstretched.

In the case of optimal positioning, only a small part of the film will remain extraorally. In rabbits weighing more than 1.2 kg, the dental film (Kodak® DF 58) can usually be successfully tucked behind the upper incisors,

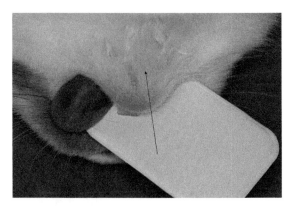

Figure 5.47 Positioning of the intraoral film in a rabbit; step 1: introducing a corner of the film into the right cheek.

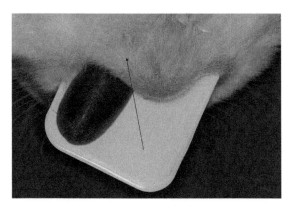

Figure 5.48 Positioning of the intraoral film in a rabbit; step 2: introducing the second corner of the film into the left cheek.

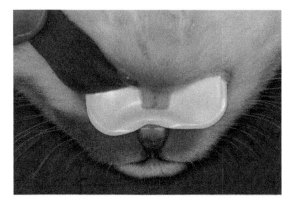

Figure 5.49 Final intraoral position of the dental film in a rabbit. The film (Kodak® D 58) is pushed behind the maxillary incisors in order to prevent any unintentional displacement.

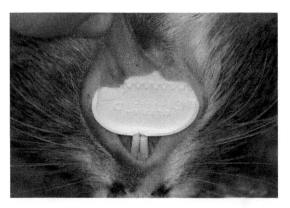

Figure 5.50 Final intraoral position of the dental film in a guinea pig. The film (Kodak® D 54) is pushed behind the upper incisors in order to prevent any unintentional displacement.

preventing any unwanted displacement (Figure 5.49). Correspondingly, smaller dental films (Kodak® DF 54) can also be placed behind the maxillary incisors of guinea pigs with a weight of more than approximately 600–800 g (Figure 5.50). The oral cavity of chinchillas is too small to allow that kind of optimal positioning of the film so here a small portion of the film will always remain extraoral. For intubated patients, the tube should be placed underneath the back side of the film to avoid superimposition on the image. In addition, the film package should not be bent during handling, as this may cause unwanted iatrogenic artefacts (black lines after processing of the film).

The intraoral film with the overlying part of the skull to be imaged are oriented as perpendicular as possible to the central beam by positioning the patient accordingly. An interpretation of findings concerning the mandible will be facilitated if the beam hits the cheek teeth as orthogradely as possible. To ensure this, support the nose by placing a small wedge of foam rubber or a few layers of cotton wool under the nose whilst the patient is in dorsal recumbency. This will allow the ventral border of the mandible to be oriented in a horizontal plane slanting slightly dorsally. However, if the focus is on the first mandibular cheek tooth (P3), which is slightly angled normally with respect to the remaining teeth of the mandible, then the head is positioned such that there is a 30° angle between the dorsal wall of the nose and the tabletop. The ventral cortical bone of the mandible will then represent a horizontal plane that may slightly slope upwards dorsally in some cases (Figure 5.51). For an equivalent orthograde view of the

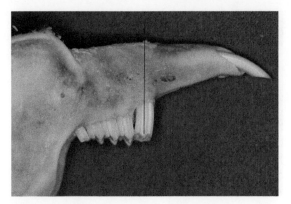

Figure 5.51 Positioning for an intraoral view of the first mandibular cheek tooth of a rabbit (specimen). The central beam runs parallel to the longitudinal axis of the first mandibular cheek tooth.

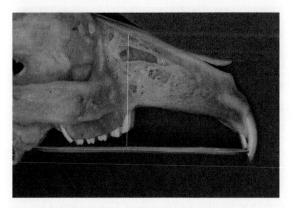

Figure 5.52 Positioning for an intraoral view of the first maxillary cheek tooth of a rabbit (specimen). The central beam runs parallel to the longitudinal axis of the first maxillary cheek tooth.

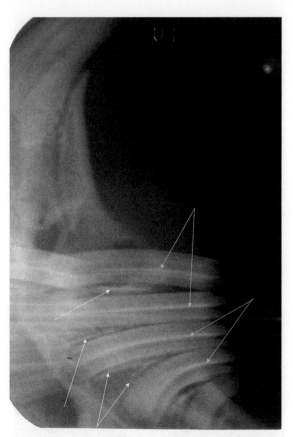

Figure 5.53 Intraoral, oblique radiograph of the mandible of a two-year-old rabbit: largely normal occlusion with a clearly visible, vertical lamina dura (white arrows) as well as an intradental enamel fold (turquoise arrows) of each individual cheek tooth, and a subtle expansion of the socket of the first mandibular cheek tooth (P3) as well as of the last two molars (M2/M3).

maxillary cheek teeth, the patient is placed in ventral recumbency and the rostral portion of the mandible is supported with a suitable wedge of foam rubber. The back of the nose will then slant ventrally by an angle of approximately 20° (Figure 5.52). The steeper the angle chosen, the better the distal molars will be imaged.

An oblique intraoral image can be obtained by slightly rotating the head by approximately 20° to the left or right. This will allow individual mandibular and maxillary cheek teeth to be shortened slightly on the image, but they will be visible in their entire length. With those kinds of images, particularly the periodontal and interproximal areas of the premolars and molars will be projected optimally and largely without superimposition (Figure 5.53).

5.7.3 Exposure values and focus-film distance

After positioning of the patient, the exposure field is collimated according to the film size. The central beam should ideally be centred at the level with the first cheek tooth (P3) in an intraoral exposure of the mandible. It is centred on the first maxillary cheek tooth (P2) for the maxilla.

Since intraoral radiography involves using films without an intensifying screen, a relatively high exposure (approximately 60 kV/32 mA or 75 kV/15 mA) is needed (Gorrel & Verhaert, 2006; Böhmer, 2007). The values depend on the size of the patient, the age of the X-ray tube, the choice of film and the film-focal distance. For healthy and safety reasons, these exposures are always taken with the patient under full anesthesia with its body and head secured using straps, adhesive tapes or rubber foam wedges. Most dental radiograph generators have default settings in fixed combinations, like kV values of 50–70 and mA values of 8–10. Electronic timers control the desired exposure time (Gorrel & Verhaert, 2006).

It is not essential to change the usual film-focal distance of more than 50 cm (standard height) for intraoral exposures and a specific dental X-ray unit is not specifically required either. A conventional (possibly digital) unit like the ones commonly used in veterinary practices is adequate provided the collimation can be adjusted. However, if a dental X-ray unit (a special wall-mounted device used in human dentistry) is available, it will significantly facilitate intraoral exposures as more elaborate positioning of patients becomes unnecessary. Instead of moving the animal, the arm can be moved together with the X-ray tube, which is then simply swiveled into position and lined up as vertically as possible to the film. More modern dental X-ray units are especially comfortable to handle as they have an X-ray head that can be tilted in every direction (ball joint revolvable by 360°). Furthermore, substantially smaller film-focus distances (approximately 10–20 cm) can be used with dental units than would be possible using conventional units, because the X-rays are focused directly on to the area to be depicted via a cylindrical tube. In this way, the scattered radiation is greatly decreased. For good images, the X-ray tube should principally always be placed as close as possible to the object to be imaged.

5.7.4 X-ray technique

If a rabbit's molar occlusal plane or the clinical crown of individual mandibular cheek teeth are to be imaged, the larger dental film (size 2) is carefully folded along its longitudinal axis and then inserted into the oral cavity parallel to the cheek teeth (Figure 5.54). Alternatively, the smaller dental films (size 0) can also be used. For this, the patient is placed in lateral recumbency (with the film positioned horizontally). For a horizontal orientation of the film, the tip of the animal's nose is supported with a small wedge of foam rubber. After choosing an appropriate collimation for the exposure field, the central beam should be directed at just about the level of the second mandibular cheek

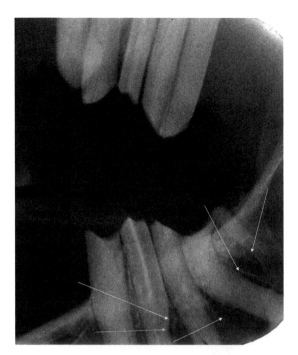

Figure 5.54 Sagittal intraoral view of a four-year-old rabbit with malocclusion: step formation, structural changes of all cheek teeth (predominantly a missing intradental enamel fold), an extensive loss of the lamina dura, an infection-related expansion of the tooth sockets in the area of the second (P4) as well as the fourth and fifth mandibular cheek teeth (M2/M3; white arrows), a basal narrowing of the second lower cheek tooth (P4; turquoise arrow) and a distinct distal deviation of the second last molar (M2).

tooth (P4). Indications for this technique are if carious changes are suspected or local demineralizations on the distal or interproximal surfaces of the mandibular cheek teeth, both of which are poorly visible on regular intraoral images.

In principle, intraoral radiographs of guinea pigs, chinchillas and degus can be taken following the same procedure as described above for rabbits. In these cases, smaller intraoral films (Kodak® DF 54) are used. For the maxilla, particularly the incisors but also all four cheek teeth may be depicted in isolation. Due to the strong curvature of the bodies of the molar teeth, the diagnostic conclusiveness of such kinds of exposures is often restricted in guinea pigs. However, they are usually very helpful if the apex of the molars is required to be imaged in finer detail (Figure 5.55).

For the mandible, the incisors as well as the rostromedial section of the mandible can be optimally examined

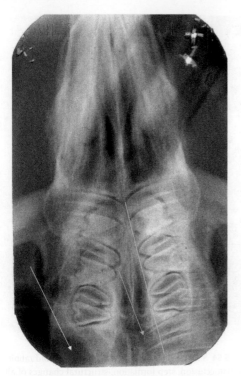

Figure 5.55 Intraoral radiograph of a four-year-old guinea pig taken 8 months after extraction of the last maxillary molar (M3; on the left). The area of the empty alveolus is without pathological findings (indifferent to stimuli; white arrow). Poor fixing and rinsing of the film is recognizable (black streaks), as is a subtle retrograde elongation of the last right molar (M3; turquoise arrow and line).

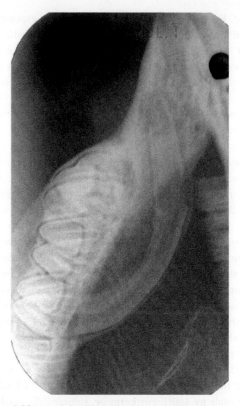

Figure 5.56 Intraoral radiograph of the mandible of a four-year-old guinea pig with slightly oblique positioning. The right incisor is missing (clinical finding). Visible are a residual intraalveolar tooth root with marked deformity of the tooth structure and an intramandibular expansion of the mandible. This is an indication for tooth extraction.

by means of intraoral radiography. In order to depict the incisors in their entire length, the patient is placed in dorsal recumbency and its neck is supported such that there is an approximate 30° angle between the back of the nose and the tabletop. However, this technique does not allow an interpretation of further distal findings because the mandibular molars cannot be included on those films due to the divergence of the mandibles caudally (by contrast, the maxillary cheek teeth can be depicted rather well). In order to clarify suspicious findings in the distal area of the mandible of guinea pigs and chinchillas, the better alternative is the special positioning technique for isolated projections of the mandible according to Böhmer, particularly if the focus is on pathological changes concerning the cheek teeth. By contrast, if the focus is on an isolated projection of the incisors, intraoral radiography provides a significantly better fine-detail reproduction and thus more information for those animals (Figure 5.56).

5.7.5 Film processing

For film processing, a darkroom or an automatic daylight developing system for intraoral films is needed. The saliva-proof slipcover is opened by pulling the triangular flap on the back side of the package before the dental film is uncovered and can be removed. It is wrapped in a two-layered protective paper and is additionally covered on one side by a thin metal foil (Figure 5.46). After the back side of the slipcover has been opened, a small mark can be felt in the left upper corner of the film; this is the spot where the clip is attached. The dental film can now be processed manually in the darkroom or by means of one of the special processing machines in normal lighting conditions.

Requirements for an intraoral radiographic examination

Standard X-ray unit or dental X-ray unit
Intraoral films of different sizes
Facilities to develop the film
Clips for use with manual wet processing
System for film filing eg. pockets or envelopes

For manual processing, three small containers (approximately 300–500 ml) made of plastic or ceramics are needed: one for the developer solution, one for the fixer and one for tap water. Having been freshly mixed, the developer solution and the fixer can be used for several weeks if stored appropriately and protected from light under a cover in the darkroom at 18–24 °C. The clip is held whilst the film is immersed in the developer solution, before being thoroughly rinsed and finally immersed in the fixer. After that, the film must be thoroughly rinsed again in running water until its surface does not feel slimy but smooth and clean.

The length of time required for manual developing and fixing, is dependent on the chemicals that are chosen (see the instructions for use). After the films have been thoroughly dried, the films can be stored in suitable transparent films (which are subdivided into several small pockets for films of different sizes). Extending the fixing time of the film will allow better preservation of the film during the storage period.

Processing can be simplified by using a so-called monobath. A single chemical is used for developing and fixing (duration of approximately 8 minutes). After that, the film must be rinsed or soaked in water for about 10 minutes. There are also dental film systems that contain chemicals for porcessing. After exposure, the films are kneaded appropriately in order to initiate the development process. Although those films provide viable images very quickly (within 15–60 seconds), they have low quality and can only be kept on file for a limited amount of time before deterioration.

Various errors may occur during film processing. If the processed film is too dark, it may be due to the exposure time having been too long or the kV value having been too high. The development time could also have been too long or too short. If there are hazy patches on a dark film, the lighting in the darkroom should be checked. On the other hand, if a dental film looks largely blurred or grey, it also indicates too high kV values. Dark patches on the surface are always caused by the developer, whereas white patches are due to the fixer solution. If there are grey casts on the intraoral films, it is time to replace the chemicals.

CHAPTER 6
Computed Tomography

Examination of the skull and teeth by means of computed tomography (CT) provides an alternative that may be better than radiography in certain circumstances, particularly if there are multiple findings in various jaw quadrants. CT can also be an additional diagnostic means for a closer evaluation of uncertain radiographic findings. One advantage is that the person examining the patient is not exposed to radiation, however all radiographs can also be taken without the need for manual positioning if the patient is under anesthesia and appropriate positioning tools are used. Another advantage of CT is the ability to image either the soft tissue or the dental and bony structures in finer detail, using different windows. CT is superior when diagnosing any kind of change in soft tissue, or when imaging the delicate intranasal structures or to clarify various neoplasia. Furthermore, it allows for a three-dimensional reconstruction of the entire skull or individual areas of the head, making it possible to assess suspicious findings in isolation and so evaluate them better (Figure 6.1).

The benefits of this CT though must not be overestimated. If the devices used are not of high performance or the sections made are more than a millimeter thick, then the diagnostic outcome of the images will not be significantly higher than with fully performed conventional radiographic techniques. Yet when using new, high-resolution devices and keeping sections less than a millimeter thick, this technique allows a image of the smallest changes in bone as well as dental structures. Even fine fistulous tracts can be depicted easily using high-performance devices. Hence hardly any pathology will be missed and many changes will be detected early

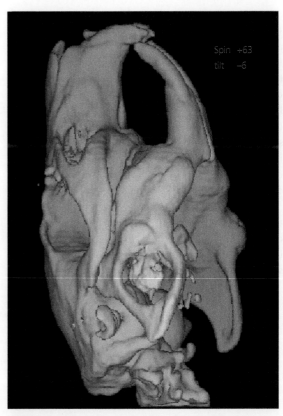

Figure 6.1 Three-dimensional computed tomographic reconstruction of the skull of a six-year-old guinea pig with an abscess of the mandible showing extensive osteolysis of the caudal right mandible. There is diffuse medial bone proliferation (partially ossified abscess capsule), retrograde apex displacement of the last right cheek tooth (M3) and retrograde elongation of the contralateral molar (M3; on the left), with a corresponding protrusion of the ventral cortical bone of the mandible.

on – even before they start to cause clinical symptoms. In addition, the time needed for examination is usually significantly shorter than for a full diagnostic radiographic set (Chesney, 1998; Crossley et al., 1998; Brenner et al., 2005; Capello, 2008; Mackey et al., 2008).

The best use of CT is to utilize it preoperatively and then monitor the further treatment by means of conventional radiography. This should be as focused as possible and therefore relatively cost-efficient; for example, intraoral images after an incisor extraction, verification of denti-noid formation or an infection spreading to adjacent structures. However, routine CT imaging of the teeth is currently still limited by the relatively high prices of CT diagnostics as well as the fact that this method can usually only be performed with a patient under anesthesia.

In calm animals, it may be possible to take a computed tomography of the head without sedation. The patient is confined within a relatively small paper box (with breathing holes), with the movement of the head additionally constrained somewhat by means of a few foam rubber wedges. The darkness inside of the box will calm the animals down quickly and then the box with the patient can be introduced into the CT tube. Images obtained in this way will certainly not be optimal (section thickness > 1 mm), but they are usually adequate for an overall impression, according to the author's own professional experience.

In order to avoid becoming entirely dependent on specialists or specialist hospitals for correct complete radiography of the teeth and skull, it is recommended to improve personal radiological knowledge and to use it in practice whenever time allows. Furthermore, it may occasionally be necessary to check the healing process radiographically during the postoperative stage of abscess treatments or tooth extractions or to find possible causes of delayed wound healing or other complications. This is best achieved by using inexpensive intraoral films or by choosing the specific kind of positioning that is suited for an individual case and a particular animal species (see Chapter 5).

CHAPTER 7
Anesthesia and Analgesia

7.1 Anesthesia

7.1.1 General remarks

When planning and performing anesthesia, take into account that the anesthetic risk is significantly higher for stressed animals and that exact control of the anesthesia usually poses a problem. A plane of surgical anesthesia can be achieved only with difficulty. The animals tend to react more defensively. Yet whenever concentration of anesthesia is only slightly increased, their breathing is extremely irregular and shallow. This means that the stressed patient's anesthesia is either too light or too deep. To avoid this, animals that are still agitated from their journey should not be anesthetized immediately but taken into a quiet environment where they can hide in a cage and have an opportunity to calm down. Two to three hours of resting time prior to anesthesia should be the minimum, the optimum being to plan anesthesia for the following day.

Rabbits in particular – depending on their individual character – tend to release an increased amount of catecholamines in situations where they are unfamiliar or uncomfortable (Henke & Reinert, 2006). This will raise their blood pressure and cause tachycardia as well as an irregular heartbeat. A sudden stress-related death may follow. When this happens the patients adopt lateral recumbency within a very short time and die while suffering mild cramps of the limbs. Resuscitation is always ineffectual. Frequent signs of a heightened level of stress are a swelling of the retrobulbar venous plexus due to an increased blood flow and the eyes being secondarily displaced from the orbit with a concomitant prolapse of the nictitating membrane (see Figure 4.12 in Chapter 4).

If anesthesia is planned in advance, stable patients are fed only water and hay *ad libitum* in the three to four hours before surgery; the hay should also be removed from the cage approximately 30 minutes before planned anesthesia (Baumgartner, 2010, personal communication). Longer preoperative fasting is not recommended, as this will have negative effects on the gastrointestinal tract (stasis) and could also quickly cause hypoglycemia as well as metabolic acidosis.

Patients with an anorexia-related, catabolic metabolism are first stabilized over the course of a few days before undergoing surgery under anesthesia: approximately 100 ml/kg BW/day of a mixture of glucose solution and electrolyte solution are given intravenously (i.v.) or subcutaneously (s.c.). As their gastrointestinal tract is mostly empty but bloated at the same time, they also receive assisted feeding: 30 ml/kg BW (body weight) of mashed pellets are syringe fed three times a day using an insulin syringe with a cut off end (ensuring there are no sharp edges) (see Figure 14.1 in Chapter 14). The slurry is made of pellets macerated in water with an addition of night feces of healthy animals or any suitable probiotic. In this way, the gastrointestinal tract is refilled, a dysbiosis is prevented and normal peristaltic action is re-established. Additionally, an antitympanic agent is administered, although its effect is questionable as bloating in pets is not caused by small-scale foam fermentation. Medication promoting peristaltic action can be used if necessary (metoclopramide 0.5 mg/kg KGW twice a day s.c. or per os (perorally or p.o.)). It will enhance emptying of the stomach, thus acting antiemetically and promoting peristaltic action. However, it does not have an effect on young animals (rabbits) and is reversed by atropine or opioids (Washabau & Hall, 1997).

Dentistry in Rabbits and Rodents, First Edition. Estella Böhmer.
© 2015 John Wiley & Sons, Ltd. Published 2015 by John Wiley & Sons, Ltd.

Additionally, sufficient analgesia must be provided in painful conditions (see Section 7.2).

The duration of preoperative assisted feeding is determined by the individual situation of the gastrointestinal tract as well as the general condition of the patient. One to two days of supported feeding will be enough for most animals. In exceptional cases, however, it may take up to a week before the gastrointestinal tract has returned to normal, and defecation is normal. Unless there is an emergency that requires intensive medical care, the animal's owner may well take over assisted feeding at home – after being shown practically and instructed accordingly.

In cases of severely cachectic or convalescing patients, where the primary aim is not just to refill and mobilize the gastrointestinal tract, special recovery foods (e.g. Critical Care® or Rodicare® for herbivores) are given. They have a higher energetic value and contain all essential vitamins, trace elements and minerals – apart from the necessary rough fibers. The powder is freshly blended with water and administered in a smaller dose (daily 50 ml/kg BW; see package). For the dental patient, the actual need for these preparations should be carefully balanced against the costs. Mostly the simple mashed pellets will be sufficient to return gastrointestinal passage to normal. It may often make more sense to spend the money on more elaborate radiographic diagnostics. Any given case should be assessed individually, and the situation discussed with the owner. In guinea pigs, additionally vitamin C (40–50 mg/kg BW) is substituted orally – or better still, administered subcutaneously in a dilution with the infusion solution – both before and after anesthesia. Generally, it must be kept in mind that patients will have a higher anesthetic risk after having suffered weight loss due to an extended period of anorexia, if that condition could not be remedied in the short term by means of assisted feeding.

7.1.2 Sedation

Various medications are available for the sedation of pets (see Table 7.1). Indications for sedation are when radiographs need to be obtained, intraoral examinations to be performed or peripheral venous catheters to be placed in a resistant patient. Sufficient analgesia must be provided during drain changes or straightforward wound debridement performed under sedation. For painful surgeries, a short anesthesia is the better choice.

7.1.3 Perioperative control of anesthesia

Immediately before inducing anesthesia, the patient is weighed. The scales must show the weight very precisely as even small deviations from the actual body mass (±5 g) can lead to a potentially fatal overdose of anesthetic agents, particularly in small rodents (Henke & Reinert, 2006). If a painful surgery is planned, the patient should receive a suitable analgesic (e.g. Carprofen i.m. (intramuscularly) or s.c.) at least 30 minutes prior to surgery. At the same time, an infusion solution (20–40 ml/kg BW) warmed to body temperature should be administered subcutaneously for perioperative stabilization of the circulation. For this, an electrolyte solution is mixed with a 5% glucose solution at a ratio of 3:1. Fluid replacement is necessary because of the marked diuretic effect of the medetomidine alone – provided that it is part of the anesthetic protocol (Henke & Reinert, 2006). Also needed is a suitable antibiotic, in order to ensure that a therapeutically meaningful concentration of active ingredients is already present in the tissue fluids during surgery.

It makes sense to use parasympatholytic drugs like atropine (0.1–0.5 mg/kg BW i.m.) to prevent vagal reflex bradycardia as well as increased salivation and bronchial secretion. Since up to 50% of all rabbits have atropinesterase, which quickly inactivates atropine, scientific literature often recommends higher dosages. Alternatively, further atropine must be added according to the effect obtained, or glycopyrrolate (0.1 mg/kg BW i.m.) can be used (Erhardt, Henke & Haberstroh, 2004). Unfortunately the latter is not available at the time of publication.

Following the pre-operative treatment, the patients are brought into a quiet, slightly darkened room to induce anesthesia. Alternatively, the cage may simply be covered with a towel. In the case of older patients or ones with a generally increased anesthetic risk, it is recommended to preoxygenate them first. To achieve this, the animal is supplied with pure oxygen for about five to seven minutes in a box that is more or less airtight (an aquarium with a lid, a sealable plastic box). Afterwards, the chosen anesthetic agent can be administered. The oxygen supply is maintained during the entire duration of the injectable anesthesia – especially in those patients at a high risk, and, if possible, in all patients. In order to provide that kind of supply, either an oxygen connection mounted on the wall in

Table 7.1 Drugs used for sedation and anesthesia of small pets.

Active agent	Class of drugs	Side effects	Rabbits	Guinea pigs	Chinchillas, degus	Rats	Mice, hamsters
Diazepam	Benzodiazepine	Low respiratory depression, almost no effect on cardiovascular system, antihypertensive in high doses	1–3 mg/kg s.c. (i.m. painful), i.v., i.p.	2.5–5 mg/kg s.c. (i.m. painful), i.p.	3–5 mg/kg s.c. (i.m. painful)	2.5–5 mg/kg s.c. (i.m. painful), i.p.	3–5 mg/kg s.c. (i.m. painful), i.p.
Midazolam	Benzodiazepine	–	1–2 mg/kg i.m., i.v., i.p.	2.5–5 mg/kg i.m., i.p.	1–2 mg/kg i.m.	2.5–5 mg/kg i.m., i.p.	5 mg/kg i.m., i.p.
Medetomidine	α2 agonist (1 ml = 1 mg; sedative with analgetic and relaxing effect; sedative effect up to 3 hours, analgetic effect up to approx. 40 minutes, to be used only in healthy animals as it causes cardiopulmonary depression)	Peripheral vasoconstriction, hypertonia, bradycardia, possibly respiratory depression and cardiac arrhythmias, increased diuresis (not in animals suffering from a heart or kidney disease); higher dosages do not enhance sedative effect but extend duration of effect	0.1–0.35 mg/kg i.m.	0.1–0.2 mg/kg i.m., s.c.	0.1–0.15 mg/kg i.m.	0.15 mg/kg i.m., s.c.	0.25 mg/kg i.m., s.c.
Butorphanol	Opioid	Relatively short duration of effect	0.1–0.5 (0.8) mg/kg s.c., i.m., i.v.	0.1–0.3 mg/kg i.v., i.m.	0.2 mg/kg s.c., i.m.	0.5–2.0 mg/kg i.m.	1.0–2.0 mg/kg i.m.
Propofol	Hypnotic (main field of application: induction or maintenance of anesthesia)	Quick uptake, short duration of effect because of fast degradation, respiratory depression in higher dosages or rapid injection	5–15 mg/kg i.v. strictly according to effect	3–10 mg/kg i.v. strictly according to effect	3–10 mg/kg i.v. strictly according to effect	3–10 mg/kg i.v. strictly according to effect	–

Adapted from Harcourt-Brown, 2002b; Erhardt et al., 2004; Morrisey & Carpenter, 2004; Henke & Reinert, 2006; Lichtenberger & Ko, 2007; Flecknell, 2009.

> Rabbits should be intubated, if possible, as many of them suffer from chronic respiratory diseases, and it also offers better opportunities in case of an emergency, e.g. a sudden respiratory arrest (see below) (Böhmer, Böttcher & Matis, 2002a).

> If no reflex can be triggered, the patient's anesthesia is too deep.

immediate proximity of the workplace (X-ray room, treatment station or operating theatre) is necessary or a transportable oxygen bottle. The oxygen can be introduced either via a suitable mask or a narrow-gauge plastic tube that is inserted intranasally.

In order to keep the body temperature constant, even for longer periods, the patient is placed on preheated cushions during transport, examination and surgery, and may additionally be covered with a blanket (e.g. a flokati rug) *ad libitum*. Any hypothermia will lead to a marked reduction in the metabolism, resulting in a prolonged anesthetic recovery and delayed convalescence (Henke & Reinert, 2006). Since it will always be more difficult to warm up hypothermic patients than to keep the body temperature within normal limits, temperature is carefully measured perioperatively as well as intra- and postoperatively. Small flexible thermometers with a permanent display are suitable for continuous monitoring.

For anesthesia monitoring, the respiratory rate and pulse rate are continuously monitored. A pulse oximeter, which can be connected via suitably sized pediatric probes (lower arm, toe, vulva, tongue), is particularly helpful here. The conjunctiva or the gingiva can be used for an assessment of the mucosal color. An

evaluation of the capillary refill time is usually assessed in the diastema – at least in larger pets. The depth of anesthesia is additionally checked by assessing the blink reflex and the corneal reflex as well as the toe pinch reflex (withdrawal reflex). The blink reflex is absent during surgical anesthesia whereas the corneal and the toe pinch reflex are still present at that stage, although the reflex response may be reduced somewhat.

7.1.4 Performing anesthesia

When treating patients with malocclusions and jaw abscesses (both lagomorphs and rodents), the fully reversable injectable anesthesia (the so-called triple anesthesia) has proven successful in everyday practice over the years. It has been shown to be especially reliable in all animal species and offers relatively high safety with the possibility of intraoperative or postoperative reversal of aneasthesia. This form of anesthesia is made up of three different components, which are drawn up in a mixing syringe in species-specific dosages (see Table 7.2). In rabbits, guinea pigs, chinchillas and rats, it is applied intramuscularly into the M. quadriceps (quick uptake) or intraperitoneally in smaller rodents like mice and hamsters. Subcutaneous administration is also possible, in principle, but not recommended as the surgery time is greatly increased. The animals will fall

Table 7.2 Triple anesthesia (adapted from Henke & Erhardt, 2004).

Anesthetic	Rabbits	Guinea pigs	Chinchillas, degus	Rats	Hamsters	Gerbils*	Mice
(mg/kg BW)	i.m., s.c.	i.m., s.c.	i.m., s.c.	i.m.	i.p., i.m.	s.c.	i.p., i.m.
Fentanyl	0.02	0.025	0.02	0.005	0.033	0.03	0.05
Midazolam	1.0	1.0	1.0	2.0	3.3	7.5	5.0
Medetomidine	0.2	0.2	0.05	0.15	0.33	0.15	0.5
Reversal							
Naloxone	0.03	0.03	0.05	0.12	0.8	0.5	1.2
Flumazenil	0.1	0.1	0.1	0.2	0.33	0.4	0.5
Atipamezole	1.0	1.0	0.5	0.75	1.7	0.375	2.5

In order to maintain anesthesia, one-third of the initial dosage may be added if necessary.

*In gerbils, increased states of excitation are possible.

Table 7.3 Vascular access in rabbits and rodents.

Species	Venous access
Rabbits	Vena auricularis lateralis, vena cephalica antebrachii, vena. saphena lateralis
Guinea pigs	Vena cephalica antebrachii (laterally in the lower arm), vena saphena lateralis
Chinchillas	Vena cephalica antebrachii, vena saphena lateralis and medialis
Degus	Vena coccygica, vena cephalica antebrachii, vena saphena lateralis and medialis
Rats	Vena coccygica, vena cephalica antebrachii, vena saphena medialis
Mice	Vena coccygica

into lateral recumbency approximately three to four minutes after injection of the anesthetic agent, depending on species and individual difference. At this point all patients should have had a peripheral venous catheter placed (see Table 7.3). It is possible in almost all pets, except in hamsters, which are too small and lack suitable peripheral veins. Blood vessels to be used are the tail vein in rats and mice, the lateral auricular vein in rabbits and the cephalic vein in guinea pigs.

Surgical anesthesia (see Table 7.4) is achieved after approximately 30 to 40 minutes, and radiography is now possible. Following radiography, required treatment can be performed, e.g. an uncomplicated correction of the occlusion or a simple tooth extraction. In cases of prolonged and painful manipulations, a suitable analgesic must be added intraoperatively because of the effect of the fentanyl lasting no longer than 30 minutes. Stable patients can also be administered a further third of the dose for inducing anesthesia (see details later for prolonged surgery).

To reverse the anesthesia, the individual components can be reversed by means of a mixing syringe with species-specific dosages of the antagonists. The recovery phase is relatively short (approximately 1 minute) if about one-third of the antagonist is administered intravenously. However, this should not be performed on a routine basis as it is accompanied by metabolic acidosis. The remaining amount is administered subcutaneously in case of a complete reversal. By contrast, the time that patients will take in returning to sternal recumbency is individually different after subcutaneous or intramuscular injections; it will usually vary between four to eight minutes.

During anesthesia, the patient's anesthetic plan can be lightened in critical situations, e.g. acute breathing problems or cardiovascular problems; this can be achieved by means of an intravenous reversal. The amount of drugs used for reversal depends on the individual reaction of the patient.

There is a variety of different anesthetic protocols representing possible alternatives to a triple anesthesia, but a discussion of other anesthetic protocols would go beyond the scope of this publication. There is no claim to comprehensiveness here in that respect.

When performing any prolonged surgery, e.g. a radical excision of a larger abscess in addition to a tooth extraction and correction of a malocclusion, injectable anesthesia is to be maintained accordingly. Such surgery, combined with immediate preoperative radiography, may well take one and a half to two hours. In order to continue from the primary injectable anesthesia, volatile anesthetics like isoflurane or desflurane are suitable. The anesthetic gases are introduced by means of an additional inhalation anesthesia or via the tracheal tube (in rabbits).

Alternatively, the stage of surgical anesthesia can also be prolonged by repeatedly administering small amounts of propofol (Diprivan) by means of a constant rate infusion (CRI) (0.5–1.5 mg/kg/min) (Baumgartner, 2010). This injection must be performed strictly intravenously. If a CRI cannot be performed temporarily, e.g. during radiography, the propofol can also be administered in increments of 0.1 ml each, using a full 1 ml insulin syringe. The amount of anesthetic to be administered always depends strictly on the individual patient's reaction (with

Table 7.4 Anesthesia stages in rabbits and rodents.

Stage	Term	Analgesia	Rabbits	Rodents
I	Analgesia	–	Disorientation, reduced motor function, no amnesia, raised heart rate and respiratory rate, failure of the righting reflex in the transition to the next stage	Disorientation, reduced motor function, no amnesia, raised heart rate and respiratory rate, failure of the righting reflex in the transition to the next stage
II	Excitation	–	State of excitation, significantly raised heart rate and respiratory rate, opisthotonus, nystagmus, nibbling, mydriasis (urination)	State of excitation, significantly raised heart rate and respiratory rate, flailing movements, trembling of the whiskers (urination)
III-1	Hypnosis	–	Relaxation, withdrawal reflex (WR) slightly +, blinking reflex ±, regular and deep breathing, respiratory and circulatory reactions to pain stimulus, failing swallowing reflex – intubation possible	Relaxation, WR slightly +, blinking reflex ±, regular and deep breathing, respiratory and circulatory reactions to pain stimulus, central position of eye
III-2	Surgical tolerance	+ (complete analgesia)	Slight WR can still be triggered, blinking reflex –, corneal reflex +, regular and deep breathing, stable heart rate, stable blood pressure, no reactions to pain stimuli, slight rotation of the bulb, slight prolapse of the nictitating membrane (slight drop in blood pressure toward the end)	Slight WR can still be triggered, blinking reflex –, corneal reflex +, regular and deep breathing, stable heart rate, stable blood pressure, no reactions to pain stimuli, slight exophthalmos (slight drop in blood pressure toward the end)
III-3	Depression	+	Abdominal, gasping respiration, drop in blood pressure, fast and shallow pulse, no WR, no corneal reflex, gazing in the distance ("fish eye"), mydriasis, prolapse of the nictitating membrane	Abdominal, gasping respiration, drop in blood pressure, fast and shallow pulse, no WR, no corneal reflex, severe exophthalmos
IV	Asphyxia	++	Complete loss of reflexes, agonal respiration, eyes fixed dead ahead with centrally positioned globe, dry cornea, dry mucous membranes	Complete loss of reflexes, agonal respiration, eyes fixed dead ahead with centrally positioned globe, dry cornea, dry mucous membranes

WR = withdrawal reflex.
Adapted from Henke, Haberstroh, Sager, Becker, Eberspächer, Bergadano, Zahner, M Arras[1] (2013), reproduced with permission of GV-SOLAS.

careful control of the anesthetic depth). Since propofol is merely a hypnotic agent ensure that sufficient analgesia is also administered (see Section 7.2).

Critically ill patients are merely sedated with a small amount of midazolam (see Table 7.1). An intravenous catheter can then be placed (rabbits, guinea pigs, chinchillas, degus, rats) and enough propofol administered strictly intravenously to induce a shallow anesthetic plane, allowing radiographic examination without resistance (Böhmer, Böttcher & Matis, 2002b). Rabbits can also be intubated using this anesthetic protocol. An anesthetic stage deep enough for radiography is maintained by repeatedly administering propofol (CRI or 0.1 ml steps strictly i.v.). Surgery, however, is performed under a light inhalation anesthesia with analgesia.

Intraoperatively, attention is paid to a sufficient (intravenous, if possible) volume replacement (approximately 4–5 ml/kg BW/h). As an alternative to plain electrolyte solutions, patients can be administered a

> Triple anesthesia results in a certain decreases in heart and respiratory rates so weak and unstable animals who are compromised cannot be administered the full dose. Here, half of the dose is usually sufficient (Erhardt et al., 2004).

[1]anaesthesie@gv-solas.de

mixture of 10 ml HAES with 10 ml glucose 5% and 30 ml electrolyte solution. The easiest way to infuse that mixture is by means of an infusion pump (Perfusor®; approximately 4–5 ml/kg BW/h), not only intraoperatively but also postoperatively if needed.

7.1.5 Anesthetic accidents

Pets are subject to anesthetic accidents relatively frequently – in comparison with dogs and cats. The respiratory depressive effect of the anesthetics causes different severe respiratory problems, e.g. a decrease of respiratory rate and/or a pathological breathing pattern. For this reason, monitoring the breathing pattern is one of the most important components of a careful anesthesia, apart from heart monitoring via an electrocardiogram (ECG). All rabbits weighing up to 600–700 g are intubated independent of the choice of injectable anesthetic, so that respiratory depression can be addressed quickly in case of an emergency using an ambu bag for direct artificial ventilation (Böhmer, Böttcher & Matis, 2002b).

Apart from conventional Magill tubes (2.0–3.5 mm in size), pediatric laryngeal masks have proven themselves in larger rabbits (>3 kg) (Figure 7.1). They can be attached easily, even by less experienced persons, and protect the trachea as well as the glottis because they do not cause mechanical irritations (Smith et al., 2004, Kazakos et al., 2007). Laryngeal masks are also suited for an emergency as they are applied blindly, i.e. without a laryngoscope. The inflated cuff causes the upper

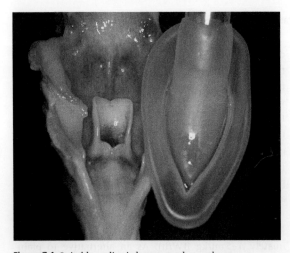

Figure 7.1 Suitable pediatric larynx mask on a larynx specimen of a rabbit.

section of the esophagus to be compressed concomitantly so that, at least in rabbits, there is no danger of pulmonary aspiration (especially since lagomorphs are unable to vomit). In addition, laryngeal masks seal up the area of the larynx and pharynx significantly better than normal tubes. This is also of great advantage during many intraoral procedures, like flushing, or in case of a discharging pus. Nowadays special supraglottic airway devices for rabbits are available (v-gel®). They can be easily inserted, but tend to dislocate during intraoral surgeries as an inflatable adjuster (such as that present in the v-gel® for cats) is missing.

In experimental surgery, a smaller, slightly modified prototype of laryngeal mask was developed for the use in laboratory animals (Imai, Eisele & Steffey, 2005). While the actual mask loosely encloses the larynx, an elongate, inflatable balloon lying in the upper section of the esophagus ensures that the anesthetic gases will only enter the trachea and gastric contents will not be aspirated.

If a conventional nose mask is used for artificial ventilation in an emergency, a large proportion of the air will get into the stomach (despite overflexion of the neck), worsening the initial respiratory situation significantly (elevated diaphragm). A gentle method of artificial ventilation is a repeated swinging of the patient. Whenever the head is inclined downwards, the intestinal loops exerts some pressure on the diaphragm, leading to expiration. As soon as the head is lifted back up again, the gastrointestinal tract draws the diaphragm back down, allowing the lungs to be refilled with air during inspiration.

In triple anesthesia, intravenous partial reversal can be performed at the same time as artificial ventilation in emergency cases, using approximately one-fifth to one-third of the initial dosage. In this way, the patient is reversed into a lesser plane of anesthesia, which often helps to prevent secondary cardiovascular failure (bradycardia, hypotonia, arrhythmia).

In rabbits, the following typical changes concerning the eye are indicators of critical anesthetic situations: mydriasis, exophthalmos and a prolapse of the nictitating membrane, resulting in a "fish eye". In case any of these findings are present, the current anesthetic situation should always be critically reviewed.

If no intravenous catheter is available for the use in a smaller patient, e.g. a hamster, the venous plexus cranial to the heart can be used as an alternative to peripheral

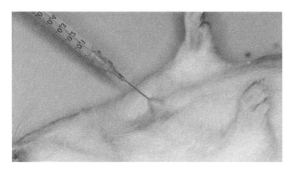

Figure 7.2 Aspiration of the venous plexus in a guinea pig, with area of needle insertion near the sternum.

intravenous drug administration. Thus, the emergency medication or antagonizing agent can be administered centrally into the circulatory system. This is done with the patient in dorsal recumbency; the thoracic inlet is pierced in the area of the venous pulse, craniolaterally from the tip of the sternum, in the direction of the contralateral stifle joint. A thin (blue) cannula is used for this, piercing approximately 5–10 mm deep at a relatively flat angle of approximately 20–45° (Figure 7.2). Afterwards the cannula is pulled back slowly while aspirating at the same time. As soon as blood can be drawn up into the syringe cone, the needle is fixed in that position, and the emergency medication that was drawn up is slowly administered intravenously. After removing the cannula, the piercing area is temporarily compressed a little. If the venipuncture is performed correctly, complications like hemorrhages or a cardiopuncture are extremely rare.

7.1.6 Postoperative care

Having partially or completely reversed the patient's anesthesia, it is moved to a quiet, ideally darkened room while constantly monitoring the body temperature, placed in sternal recumbency and still kept warm (heating cushion or heatable pad) until it is able to regulate body temperature autonomously. Caution should be exercised with infrared lamps as they can quickly lead to hyperthermia. If the animal is regaining consciousness very slowly, one-third of the already administered amount of antagonist can be added (intravenously or intramuscularly). In cases of delayed convalescence, additional help is provided by an increased oxygen feed (oxygen tent) as well as warm intravenous fluid substitutes. At the same time, analgesia should again be critically reviewed and improved if necessary, particularly in

cases of increased respiratory or heart rates (see Table 7.5). The first feed intake should ensue as soon as possible, and no later than two to three hours after the end of anesthesia. If the animals do not eat by themselves, syringe feed them in order to restart the gastrointestinal tract (see Section 7.1.1).

7.2 Analgesia

7.2.1 General remarks

When dealing with lagomorph and rodent patients, it can be very difficult to determine whether they are suffering pain because they are typical prey and flight animals and thus very much conditioned to disguise illnesses or pain. This is aggravated by the fact that in general they do not express pain by means of vocalization. Individual reactions to pain can be very different. In principle it must be assumed that – just like in humans – every surgical intervention entails pain requiring treatment, i.e. pain in animals is comparable with that in humans (Erhardt et al., 2004; Gorrel & Verhaert, 2006). Hence analgesics that are suited and appropriate to the situation should also be used perioperatively in pets. It should be added that pain leads to a general sympathetic activation, which always has negative effects on the circulatory system and the gastrointestinal tract.

A possible indicator of pain can be an animal that is generally quieter, or with reclusive behavior. Alternatively, it could be aggression toward a partner, changes in sleeping behavior or decreased grooming as well as pressing the head into a corner of the cage, hyperventilation (Lichtenberger & Ko, 2007) or an increased muscle tone, trembling, contortions whenever sensitive areas are touched, empty jaw movements or possibly bruxism (in rabbits). By contrast, if the muscles are relaxed and breathing is regular, it can be assumed that there is no pain.

In case of any prolonged pain in the oral area, the owner will notice a disturbance in feeding behavior. The animals will also start to eat selectively; i.e. they prefer soft food, change their chewing technique, or tend to grind the food on one side only, which would be the healthy side.

Pain therapy may temporarily enhance food intake of patients with a malocclusion, particularly in an early stage of the disorder. It is suggested that in the case of a retrograde displacement of the apices of the cheek teeth,

Table 7.5 Signs of pain in rabbits and rodents.

Rabbits	Rodents
Reluctance to move	Unkempt fur
Apathy	Chromodacryorrhoea due to reduced grooming
Sensitivity to touch	Bristled fur
Automutilation	Uneven gait
Inappetence or disturbed eating behavior	Apathy
Reduced bowel motility	Isolation from conspecifics
Aggression	Automutilation
Anxiousness	Inappetence
Increased muscle tone and trembling	Reduced bowel motility
Curved back	Diuresis
Bruxism and empty chewing movements	Long-term immune suppression due to increased cortisol and
Kicking the hind legs	catecholamine levels
Reduced grooming	Intraoperatively raised heart rate, increased blood pressure, possibly
Hyperventilation	cardiac arrhythmias, pale mucous membranes, raised breathing
Pressing the head into a corner	rate and shallow breathing
Diuresis	
Long-term immune suppression due to increased cortisol and catecholamine levels	
Intraoperatively raised heart rate, increased blood pressure, possibly cardiac arrhythmias, pale mucous membranes, raised breathing rate and shallow breathing	

Adapted from Bradley, 2001; Henke & Erhardt, 2001; Erhardt et al., 2004; Lichtenberger & Ko, 2007; Flecknell, 2009.

the nerve fibers in immediate proximity (branches of the nervus mandibularis and nervus maxillaris) are directly stimulated or even displaced (Figure 7.3). During feeding, the masticatory pressure causes an additional irritation of those sensory fibers, bringing about an sharp acute local, pain (Harcourt-Brown, 2002a). That pain can be controlled by means of administering an analgesic in cases with minor changes. In advanced stages, however, intraosseous change has become so dramatic that analgesics will have no effect or require very high dosages (see Figure 4.7 in Chapter 4). In the terminal stage of a malocclusion, a progressive loss of sensitivity will probably occur, so that at least pain medication will no longer be necessary for that reason (Harcourt-Brown, 2002a).

Furthermore, analgesics are used during more invasive, painful surgery of the teeth (tooth extractions) or the jaw (abscess excision). In such instances, a good analgesia should be given preoperatively – and intraoperatively in any case – in order to keep the patient from even becoming aware of the pain. This is easier than having to treat the pain postoperatively. Pre-emptive pain management involves administering analgesics

before the onset of the actual pain, thereby preventing a hyperalgesia due to an excessive central and peripheral pain sensitization (Henke & Erhardt, 2001; Erhardt et al., 2004; Gorell & Verhaert, 2006). It also allows the postoperative dose of analgesics to effectively be reduced. However, if the pain has already been established (acute or chronic pain), any analgesics that have not been administered until then will be significantly less effective, making a therapy of the postoperative pain much more difficult. The most convenient way to perform pre-emptive analgesia is to combine various analgesics, as this will allow smaller dosages (Lichtenberger & Ko, 2007). This can be done with a mixture of nonsteroidal anti-inflammatory drugs (NSAIDs), opioids or local anesthetics.

An analgesic that was administered preoperatively should also be consistently continued over the course of several days. Patients should remain free from pain for longer periods, and constantly at any rate. If certain pain stimuli cross the barrier time and again, there will still be a danger of hypersensitization (Erhardt et al., 2004). As soon as hyperalgesia develops, analgesics will no longer be sufficiently effective if administered in

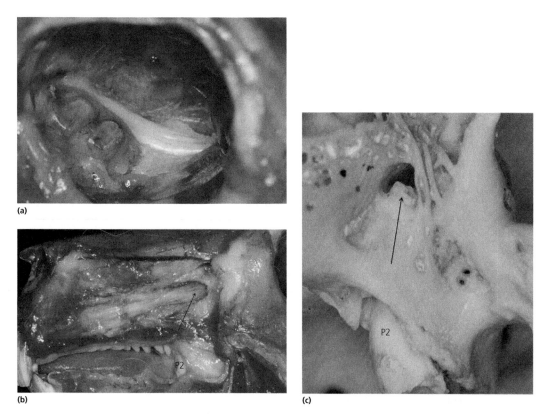

Figure 7.3 Maxillary nerve in a rabbit. (a) Intraorbital part of the maxillary nerve running medially to the apices of the caudal upper cheek teeth. (b) Maxillary nerve exiting the infraorbital foramen. (c) Narrowing of the infraorbital foramen as a consequence of retrograde tooth elongation (upper P2).

normal dosages. Pain management becomes difficult as tolerable increases of dose are usually not enough to sufficiently enhance the effectiveness of the analgesics. This can best be avoided by means of a constant rate of infusion (e.g. metamizole or buprenorphine) (see Sections 7.2.2 and 7.2.4).

The ideal analgesic for postoperative pain management should be potent and have a long-term effect, induce only minor side effects and act as a sedative. Nonsteroidal anti-inflammatories and the antipyretic metamizole come very close to these preconditions. All details concerning dosage and duration of effect of the respective analgesics are to be considered as mere guidelines (see Tables 7.6 to 7.12), with the most effective dose always having to be individually determined. There are huge differences between the species, and even within a species, so reactions will always be individually very different and depend on the situation (Henke & Erhardt, 2001; Lichtenberger & Ko, 2007). For example, it

depends on intensity, form and duration of the respective pain stimuli, as well as on age and general condition of the patient, and on whether other medication is administered (Otto, 2001).

7.2.2 Opioids

Opioids or opiate agonists such as morphine, fentanyl, alfentanil, etorphine, butorphanol and buprenorphine act in the centers of the central nervous system (Henke & Erhardt, 2001). They have a high analgesic potency, yet they cause a certain amount of cardiac and respiratory depression, especially in higher dosages. Hence they should not be used in patients with respiratory disorders. If administered for longer periods, opioids can also lead to a decreased peristalsis of the intestines and can have an immunosuppressive effect. Except for buprenorphine, they are predominantly used as analgesic components in various anesthetic protocols (Henke & Erhardt, 2001; Erhardt et al., 2004).

Table 7.6 Dosages for peri- and postoperative analgesia in rabbits.

	Class of drugs	Dose (mg/kg)	Way of administration	Dosage interval
Buprenorphine	Opioid	0.01–0.05	s.c., i.m., i.v.	30 min prior to the end of surgery and every 8–12 h after that
Metamizole	Antipyretic	20–50	Slowly i.v., i.m., s.c., p.o.(perorally), rectally	6 h
Carprofen	NSAID	4–5	i.m., s.c.	24 h
		1–2.2	p.o.	12 h
Butorphanol	Opioid	0.1–1–2	s.c., i.m., i.v.	4–6 h
		(0.1–0.5)	(i.v.)	
Meloxicam	NSAID	0.2	s.c.	24 h
		(0.6–1)	s.c. p.o.	

Adapted from Henke & Erhardt, 2001; Crossley & Aiken, 2004; Morrisey & Carpenter, 2004; Flecknell, 2009.

Table 7.7 Dosages for peri- and postoperative analgesia in guinea pigs.

	Class of drugs	Dose (mg/kg)	Way of administration	Dosage interval
Buprenorphine	Opioid	0.05–0.1	s.c., i.p. (intraperitoneally)	8 h
		0.05	s.c.	8–12 h
Metamizole	Antipyretic	80–100 (0.5–1–2 drops/animal)	p.o.	4–6 h
Carprofen	NSAID	4–5	s.c.	24 h
		1–2	p.o.	12–24 h
Butorphanol	Opioid	0.5–1–2	s.c.	4-6 h
Meloxicam	NSAID	0.2	s.c.	24 h

Adapted from Henke & Erhardt, 2001; Crossley & Aiken, 2004; Morrisey & Carpenter, 2004; Flecknell, 2009.

Table 7.8 Dosages for peri- and postoperative analgesia in rats.

	Class of drugs	Dose (mg/kg)	Way of administration	Dosage interval
Buprenorphine	Opioid	0.01–0.05–0.1	s.c.	8–12 h
		0.02–0.5	s.c., i.m., i.p.	6–12 h
Metamizole	Antipyretic	2 drops/animal	p.o.	6 h
Carprofen	NSAID	4–5	s.c.	24 h
		5–10	p.o.	
Butorphanol	Opioid	0.5–1–2	s.c.	4–6 h
Meloxicam	NSAID	0.2	s.c.	24 h
		(1)	s.c., p.o.	

Adapted from Henke & Erhardt, 2001: Crossley & Aiken, 2004: Morrisey & Carpenter, 2004: Flecknell, 2009.

However, pain management with opioids is always more effective when combined with NSAIDs. In principle they are not suited for pre- or postoperative analgesia (except for buprenorphine) as they only have a relatively short-term effect.

Butorphanol is an opiate agonist and an opiate antagonist at the same time (having an effect on K-opioid receptors). It acts more quickly than buprenorphine, but the duration of its analgesic effect is significantly shorter (two to four hours). Thus it must be administered

Table 7.9 Dosages for peri- and postoperative analgesia in chinchillas.

	Class of drugs	Dose (mg/kg)	Way of administration	Dosage interval
Buprenorphine	Opioid	0.05–0.1	s.c., i.p.	8 h
		0.05	s.c.	8–12 h
Metamizole	Antipyretic	80–100 (0.5–1–2 drops/animal)	p.o.	4–6 h
Carprofen	NSAID	4–5	s.c.	24 h
		5–10	p.o.	
Butorphanol	Opioid	0.5–1–2	s.c.	4–6 h
Meloxicam	NSAID	0.2	s.c.	24 h

Adapted from Henke & Erhardt, 2001; Crossley & Aiken, 2004; Morrisey & Carpenter, 2004; Flecknell, 2009.

Table 7.10 Dosages for peri- and postoperative analgesia in degus.

	Class of drugs	Dose (mg/kg)	Way of administration	Dosage interval
Buprenorphine	Opioid	0.05–0.1	s.c., i.p.	8 h
		0.05	s.c.	8–12 h
Metamizole	Antipyretic	80–100 (0.5–1–2 drops/animal)	p.o.	4–6 h
Carprofen	NSAID	4–5	s.c.	24 h
Butorphanol	Opioid	0.5–1–2	s.c.	4–6 h
Meloxicam	NSAID	0.2	s.c.	24 h
		(0.4)	s.c.	

Adapted from Henke & Erhardt, 2001; Crossley & Aiken, 2004; Morrisey & Carpenter, 2004; Flecknell, 2009.

Table 7.11 Dosages for peri- and postoperative analgesia in hamsters.

	Class of drugs	Dose (mg/kg)	Way of administration	Dosage interval
Metamizole	Antipyretic	80–100 (0.5–1–2 drops/animal)	p.o.	4–6 h
Carprofen	NSAID	4–5	s.c.	24 h
Butorphanol	Opioid	1–5	s.c.	4 h
Meloxicam	NSAID	0.2	s.c.	24 h
		(0.4)	s.c.	

Adapted from Henke & Erhardt, 2001; Crossley & Aiken, 2004; Morrisey & Carpenter, 2004; Flecknell, 2009.

Table 7.12 Dosages for peri- and postoperative analgesia in mice.

	Class of drugs	Dose (mg/kg)	Way of administration	Dosage interval
Buprenorphine	Opioid	0.02–0.5	s.q., i.m., i.p.	6–12 h
Metamizole	Antipyretic	80–100 (0.5–1–2 drops/animal)	p.o.	4–6 h
Carprofen	NSAID	4–5	s.c.	24 h
		5–10	p.o.	
Butorphanol	Opioid	0.5–1–2	s.c.	4–6 h
Meloxicam	NSAID	0.2	s.c.	24 h
		(5)	s.c., p.o.	

Adapted from Henke & Erhardt, 2001; Crossley & Aiken, 2004; Morrisey & Carpenter, 2004; Flecknell, 2009.

repeatedly within short periods of time postoperatively. In addition, it often does not have sufficient effect if administered on its own during more painful processes. Like all opioids, it should always be combined with an NSAID and/or metamizole.

A continuous intra- or postoperative analgesia can be achieved by means of a constant rate infusion of butorphanol: in rabbits 0.1–0.2 mg/kg i.v. as an initial dose, followed by 0.1–0.2 mg/kg/h (Lichtenberger & Ko, 2007). An infusion pump ensures that the substance is administered in the correct dosage.

Buprenorphine is the analgesic of choice in rabbits and rodents for short-term postoperative pain management (Henke & Erhardt, 2001; Erhardt et al., 2004; Flecknell, 2009). It is chiefly used for primary analgesia in a conscious animal. Administration is performed preferentially intravenously near the end of surgery. However, intramuscular and subcutaneous injections are also possible. Take note that the full analgesic effect will only be achieved after approximately 20 to 30 minutes. The duration of the analgesic effect will then be eight to twelve hours. Its very high analgesic potency should be mentioned; the effect of buprenorphine is approximately 20 times stronger than that of morphine and three times stronger than fentanyl. It is also analgesically more effective than butorphanol. However, buprenorphine should only be administered for the shortest possible time postoperatively as it has an immunosuppressive effect when administered for longer periods and can have negative effects on the gastrointestinal tract. In such cases, it is better to switch to nonsteroidal anti-inflammatories such as carprofen or meloxicam, especially considering that buprenorphine has no anti-inflammatory effect.

Buprenorphine is an opiate agonist/antagonist. It acts as an antagonist at the μ-opioid receptor, i.e. it keeps the agonists from binding to the μ-receptor by means of competitive inhibition, and then acts as an agonist itself. This can be used to counteract the respiratory depressive and sedative effect of the fentanyl, whereas the analgesic effect is largely retained thanks to its effect on the μ-receptors (Henke & Erhardt, 2001; Erhardt et al., 2004; Flecknell, 2009). Having said this, buprenorphine also has a slightly sedative effect, which can lead to somnolence and a secondary reduction of food intake (Erhardt et al., 2004). In addition, there have been reports of dysphagia and an uptake of foreign materials (allotriophagia).

The influence of buprenorphine on the circulatory system is rather small. The long and sustained duration of its effect is based on its very tight bind to the opiate receptor (very high affinity). Buprenorphine cannot be replaced by naloxone – a potential antagonist – by means of competitive inhibition (Henke & Erhardt, 2001; Erhardt et al., 2004).

> The effect of buprenorphine is almost impossible to reverse.

After a maximum effect has been reached, further dose escalation leads to a decrease of the analgesic effect, a phenomenon called the "ceiling effect" (Gaggermeier et al., 2001). If analgesia needs to be increased in individual cases, it is best achieved in combination with a nonopioid analgesic like metamizole.

Fentanyl can be given as a bolus for intraoperative analgesia during very painful surgery. The dosage is 0.01–0.02 mg/kg BW i.v. for rabbits and 0.05–0.1 mg/kg BW i.v. for rats, guinea pigs and mice. Since fentanyl causes bradycardia (apart from respiratory depression), this can be used in order to measure the efficiency of the pain relief. If fentanyl is administered intraoperatively, the patient should be intubated for safety reasons (Erhardt, 2010, personal communication).

A possibility of a continuous, intra- or postoperative analgesia is a constant rate infusion of fentanyl with 10–15 μg/kg/h i.v. (Lichtenberger & Ko, 2007). An infusion pump ensures that the substance is administered in the correct dosage.

Fentanyl is not suitable for a more long-term, systemic postoperative pain therapy as it has only a very short duration of effect of 20 to 30 minutes (Erhardt et al., 2004). By using fentanyl transdermal patches (12 μg/h plasters for up to 5 kg BW), however, a very consistent analgesia can be achieved. Those kinds of transdermal patches have proven to be very effective in therapies for dogs and cats for strong, enduring pains, although little experience has been gained regarding its use in rabbits or rodents. Problems may arise here, particularly when it comes to safely positioning the patches on the bare skin of the patients. In most cases a bandage is necessary, which also serves for protection of the patient.

In order to reverse the fentanyl, naloxone is used, which is a pure opiate antagonist (Henke & Erhardt, 2001; Erhardt et al., 2004). It counteracts both the analgesic and the respiratory depressive and sedative effects of the opiate agonist, which means it should be preferred over buprenorphine in principle (Henke & Erhardt, 2001). The pharmacological half-life of naloxone is 15 to 45 minutes, which means that the opiate receptors may be reoccupied by agonist molecules that are still present (rebound effect). In such cases, naloxone needs to be added at 0.003–0.03 mg/kg i.v., i.m. or s.c., prolonging its effect to one and a half to two hours. Since naloxone (contrary to buprenorphine) will completely reverse analgesia, it must carefully be ensured that the patient is provided with a sufficient amount of effective analgesic.

7.2.3 Nonsteroidal anti-inflammatories (NSAIDs)

Nonsteroidal anti-inflammatories (nonsteroidal anti-inflammatory drugs, NSAIDs) such as carprofen and meloxicam are most effective when administered prophylactically, in other words pre-emptively (Henke & Erhardt, 2001). The respective dosages can be found in Tables 7.6 to 7.12. Since the time to peak effect is almost 30 minutes, carprofen is injected approximately 10 to 15 minutes prior to the start of anesthesia (administration of anesthetics). Combined with opioids, it will thus take the full analgesic effect intraoperatively. NSAIDs are particularly suitable for the subsequent, more long-term postoperative analgesia, especially in the case of osseous or dental pain (Henke & Erhardt, 2001; Lichtenberger & Ko, 2007). They act peripherally and influence the inflammation process by inhibiting the formation of inflammatory substances like bradykinin and histamine, and at the same time intervene in prostaglandin synthesis as inhibitors of cyclooxygenase. The formation of prostaglandins, which are considered to be inflammation mediators, is inhibited. However, NSAIDs are also believed to have a central analgesic effect (Henke & Erhardt, 2001).

Thus NSAIDs not only have an analgesic but also an anti-inflammatory effect, the latter of which reduces swelling of wound areas. However, they are not effective against acute (sharp) intraoperative pain, which means that they are not suited for intraoperative analgesia (Henke, Erhardt & Tacke, 2008).

In summary, NSAIDs bring about a long-lasting postoperative analgesia and do not affect the central nervous system, the circulatory system or respiration. Potential side effects include the gastrointestinal tract as well as renal dysfunction; carprofen, however, only very rarely causes those kinds of problems even if administered to rabbits for several weeks (Henke & Erhardt, 2001; the author's personal experience). Having said this, it can only be used in patients that are well-hydrated and possessing a normal kidney function. Contraindications for the use of carprofen are hypovolemia, hypotension, ascites, shock, congestive heart failure, thrombocytopenia (blood coagulation defect), gastrointestinal disorders and ulcers, or trauma with significant loss of blood, kidney insufficiency and a prior administration of other NSAIDs (Henke & Erhardt, 2001; Lichtenberger & Ko, 2007). Since NSAIDs have a negative influence on bone healing, they should not be administered too long in cases of more severe jaw changes (Goodman et al., 2003).

7.2.4 Metamizole

The antipyretic metamizole has very good analgesic qualities, although its precise mechanism of action is not yet clear. It acts first and foremost centrally (centers in the brain stem), but also inhibits the peripheral stimulus transduction (Erhardt et al., 2004; Henke et al., 2008). In principle it is very well-suited for alleviating acute and chronic pain, both intra- and postoperatively. However, it has only a relatively short duration of effect of four to six hours. A great advantage is the fact that metamizole does not have a negative impact on the central nervous system, kidney function, respiration and the cardiovascular system (in stable circulatory conditions). Intraoperative analgesia can be continued postoperatively without any problems, even for longer periods. In this way, potential side effects involved in the use of NSAIDs can be avoided.

Agranulocytosis (which is feared in human medicine) has not yet been found in animals (Henke & Erhardt, 2001). Furthermore, metamizole has an antipyretic effect, as well as a small antiphlogistic effect and a spasmolytic effect on smooth muscle cells (gastrointestinal tract). Since it potentiates the effect of other analgesics, it works well intraoperatively when combined with opiates, allowing the latter to be used in smaller dosages (Erhardt et al., 2004; Lichtenberger & Ko, 2007; Clemm, 2008; Henke et al., 2008). Its biggest advantage is the fact that it has neither a respiratory depressive nor a sedative effect.

Whenever metamizole is administered intravenously as a bolus, it should be diluted 1:10 with physiological

NaCl solution and then be slowly injected over a period of approximately 3 minutes; otherwise there will be a danger of shock with a massive drop in blood pressure (decrease of vascular tone). A good alternative is a constant rate infusion containing 25 ml NaCl solution and 25ml of a metamizole preparation (500 mg/ml), with 1 ml of the infusion solution corresponding with 250 mg metamizole. This is equal to a dosage of 5–10 mg/kg BW/h or 0.025–0.05 ml/kg BW/h (Erhardt et al., 2004; Henke et al., 2008). Metamizole is suited not only for intraoperative but also for postoperative analgesia as it can be administered perorally in the form of drops, which means it can also be given by the owner. It does, however, have an unpleasant taste. Alternatively, rectal or intramuscular administration is possible.

Pain management with drugs (analgesia)

(based on Henke & Erhardt, 2001; Gorrel & Verhaert, 2006)

- Preoperative analgesia: 20–30 minutes before induction of anesthesia
  - NSAIDs
  - Metamizole (antipyretic)
  - Butorphanol (opioid)
  - Immediately preoperative local anesthesia (infiltration or nerve block)
- Intraoperative analgesia in the context of general anesthesia (opioids)
- Before the end of anesthesia: buprenorphine (opioid) or metamizole (antipyretic)
- Postoperative analgesia
  - Metamizole (antipyretic)
  - Buprenorphine (opioid)
  - NSAIDs (during the entire, painful healing process)

7.3 Local anesthesia and local analgesia

7.3.1 General remarks

Particularly when dealing with critical patients or in case of very painful surgery, additional local anesthesia is recommended as this allows the general anesthesia to be kept shallower; thus, the toxicity of the perioperative, systemic analgesics can be significantly reduced (multimodal analgesia or "balanced analgesia") (Henke & Erhardt, 2001; Eickhoff, 2005). The principle of regional and local anesthesia is a complete local block of sensory nerve pathways (sensory nerve block) by means of various local anesthetics (Gorrel & Verhaert, 2006; Lennox, 2008). In this way, referred pain is completely blocked. This leads to analgesia as well as anesthesia in the area of administration of the local anesthetic and the area of the nerve fibers located more centrally from that region.

Hence local anesthesia is an ideal method for an extremely effective, pre-emptive pain management. Central sensitization is avoided by simply keeping the stimulus that is induced by surgery from reaching the spinal cord or the supraspinal structures (Henke & Erhardt, 2001). These measures will allow for a significant reduction of the intensity of postoperative pain, although the pain itself will not be entirely avoided (Gorrel & Verhaert, 2006). In order to ensure that little pain is experienced during the recovery phase, additional analgesics will be necessary (in most cases buprenorphine, metamizole or NSAIDs).

Another advantage of local anesthesia are low costs and relative safety, as long as the local anesthetics are used correctly. Toxic side effects may arise if preparations are accidentally administered intravenously; these include centrally triggered cramps, tremor, myocardial depression, tachycardia, hypotonia, cardiac arrhythmias or extrasystoles (Henke & Erhardt, 2001; Gorrel & Verhaert, 2006). All this can be avoided by aspirating before injection of the local anesthetics. Another problem is excessive dosages of local anesthetics, which may not only lead to a systemic intoxication but also cause local damage to the tissue. In case of systemic complications, unwanted side effects such as cramps may be positively influenced by benzodiazepine or propofol, while cardiac problems may be helped with dopamine (Henke & Erhardt, 2001).

For local infiltrations of the skull or specific nerve blocks, amide-type local anesthetics such as lidocaine and bupivacaine have proven successful in veterinary medicine. They have a relatively long duration of effect and are tolerated well (Eickhoff, 2005; Gorrel & Verhaert, 2006; Lichtenberger & Ko, 2007). The potency of the various local anesthetics is measured with respect to procaine (ester type), with the potency of procaine defined as 1 (Henke & Erhardt, 2001).

Due to its long duration of effect, bupivacaine is the local anesthetic of choice. Its effect occurs after 15 to 20 minutes and lasts four to six hours. The maximum

Table 7.13 Local anesthetics.

Local anesthetic (potency)	Dosage without vasoconstrictor (with adrenaline)	Onset of action (lag time)	Duration of effect	Notes
Procaine (1)	6 mg/kg (8 mg/kg)	10–15 min	Short duration:30–60 min	Allergic reaction possible; use of a 1–2% solution for infiltration anesthesia or surface anesthesia
Lidocaine (2)	5 mg/kg (7 mg/kg)	Fast onset after 5–10 min	Longer duration:60–120 min	Most frequently used local anesthetic in veterinary medicine; use of a 0.5–2% solution for infiltration anesthesia, or 0.5–1.0 ml of a 2% solution for the peripheral nerve block
Mepivacaine (2.5)	5 mg/kg (7 mg/kg)	Fast onset after 5–10 min	Longer duration:90–180 min	Less tissue irritation than with lidocaine, locally not effective (surface anesthesia); use of a 1–2% solution for infiltration anesthesia
Bupivacaine (8)	2 mg/kg (3 mg/kg)	Very slow onset after 20–30 min	Long duration:240–360 min	Locally not effective (surface anesthesia); good effect with a 0.25% solution for infiltration anesthesia or 0.5% solution for the peripheral nerve block

dosage for infiltration anesthesia with bupivacaine 0.25% is 1–2 mg/kg BW (see Table 7.13).

Lidocaine has a quicker effect and is therefore better suited for intraoperative use (infiltration anesthesia or surface anesthesia). The maximum dosage for infiltration anesthesia with lidocaine 1–2% is 2–5 mg/kg BW (see Table 7.13).

The use of vasoconstrictors (adrenaline, L-noradrenaline) is supposed to reduce systemic absorption of the local anesthetic by means of vascular constriction, thereby reducing its systemic toxicity (Gorrel & Verhaert, 2006). Concomitantly, the onset of effect is accelerated and the duration of action extended two- to threefold. Adding them, however, also increases the risk of cardiac arrhythmias or ventricular fibrillations. Hence it is generally safer not to use vasoconstrictors in pets.

7.3.2 Infiltration anesthesia

When performing infiltration anesthesia, the local anesthetic is injected in the vicinity of the area of surgery in the form of small wheals or into the gingiva and the alveolus or the alveolar periosteum as a so-called intraligamentary local anesthesia (Henke & Erhardt, 2001; Gorrel & Verhaert, 2006). In order to avoid intravascular injections, always aspirate prior to injecting. In addition, a certain lag time (depending on the local anesthetic; see Table 7.13) must be awaited

before beginning surgery. When using local anesthetics, it should also be borne in mind that their effectiveness is markedly reduced in infected or inflamed tissue (slightly acidic conditions) as only a small portion of the anesthetic base is dissociated (Henke & Erhardt, 2001).

Intraligamentary local anesthesia has proven to be an excellent way of performing a planned tooth extraction without causing pain – both in the area of the incisors and in that of the cheek teeth (especially in rabbits and guinea pigs). For this, the local anesthetic is administered directly into the periodontal space; a special kind of metal syringe that allows control of the injection pressure and a very thin injection needle (30-gauge needle) is used (Fakler, 2003). The needle is pierced approximately 2–4 mm deep into the desmodontium before an amount of local anesthetic that has been precisely determined beforehand (by a mark on the metal syringe) is administered (approximately 0.1 ml/tooth). Since the alveolus of pet rabbits and rodents is relatively wide (compared with cats and dogs), for each tooth 0.2 ml of the local anesthetic may well be needed in a larger rabbit. The local anesthetic will diffuse as far as the apical area and will even enter the alveolar bone to some extent. When this happens, the vast number of small nerve endings in the periodontium is desensitized (Crossley & Aiken, 2004).

7.3.3 Conductive anesthesia (nerve block)

Conductive anesthesia interrupts stimulus conduction in individual nerves, thus achieving very effective pain suppression in their peripheral supply areas (anesthesia of the sensory fibers). For this, the entire nerve is surrounded as closely as possible with an injection of a small amount of suitable local anesthetic. Dosage, lag time and duration of effect of the local anesthetics can be found in Table 7.13.

A local block of various cranial nerves can be a relatively easy and specific method of anesthetizing one of the jaw quadrants (Henke & Erhardt, 2001; Gorrel & Verhaert, 2006; Lennox, 2008). Indications for this are extractions of single or various teeth and painful osseous abscess debridements. A very thin, short injection needle (22 to 30 gauge; 2.5 cm long) is used to inject a relatively small amount of the chosen local anesthetic in the vicinity where the nerve exits the foramen. After removing the needle, a finger is used to apply slight pressure to the injection site for about 20 to 30 seconds. This allows the local anesthetic to diffuse evenly in the nerve canal and around it. In addition, the formation of a local hematoma is avoided.

Generally, anatomical landmarks of pets are similar to those of dogs and cats when nerve pathways are concerned. Sensory innervation of the teeth is provided by branches of the trigeminal nerve lying in immediate proximity to the corresponding tooth roots. The maxillary nerve and its extensions (infraorbital and palatine nerves) innervate the maxilla as well as the maxillary cheek teeth and maxillary incisors, while the mandibular nerve innervates the mandibular teeth (Harcourt-Brown, 2002a).

During procedures of the cheek teeth, a caudal mandibular block can be used. For this, the alveolar nerve is anesthetized. It runs from the caudodorsal end along the medial aspect of the mandible, continuing mesially into the mandibular foramen. In guinea pigs and chinchillas, that small opening in the bone is located slightly caudally from the last molar (M3), at approximately half the width of the mandibular bone (see Figure 11.7 in Chapter 11). Its location in rabbits is almost identical, except that the opening is instead in the upper third of the mandible. It is relatively difficult to hit the nerve exactly; a delicate cannula is inserted toward the caudal inner surface of the mandible in a dorsorostral direction. The index finger of the other hand is positioned intraorally between the tongue and the mandible so that the tip of the finger can control and guide the needle. During this, the medial pterygoid muscle is punctured and the nerve is blocked locally. If the local anesthetic is deposited in the correct position, the entire mandible will be anesthetized.

However, if only the rostral area of the mandible is to be anesthetized, e.g. for an incisor extraction, then the mental nerve exiting the mental foramen is blocked locally in order to create a cranial mandibular block. In rabbits, the foramen is located in the upper third of the mandible, just rostral to the first mandibular cheek tooth (P3) (see Figure 9.3 in Chapter 9), whereas in guinea pigs, the opening is located halfway (see Figure 5.32d in Chapter 5). In contrast to this, the foramen of chinchillas is located relatively far dorsally, approximately 3–4 mm rostral to the premolar.

For surgery in the rostral area of the maxilla, for example an incisor extraction, the infraorbital nerve is anesthetized. In rabbits, the infraorbital foramen is located at midway and slightly rostral to an imaginary line running from the lacrimal process to the tuber faciale. Thus the nerve exits the maxilla in the immediate proximity of the apex of the first maxillary cheek tooth (P2) (see Figure 10.52 in Chapter 10). In guinea pigs and chinchillas, the nerve runs below the deep portion of the masseter muscle, continuing rostrally after exiting the infraorbital canal.

CHAPTER 8
Instruments for Examination and Treatment

8.1 Intraoral examination under anesthesia

Due to the poor view into the long, narrow oral cavity of lagomorphs and rodents, special instruments are necessary for intraoral examinations and procedures. In order to open the jaws and to clear away the hairy cheeks that protrude into the oral cavity, mouth gags and cheek dilators are used. These are available in different shapes and sizes: larger, more stable models for rabbits and guinea pigs as well as smaller, more delicate instruments for the small rodents.

There is a principal difference between models of mouth gags, ones with a quick-locking mechanism and ones with a turning mechanism. For welfare reasons, both kinds of instruments should generally only be used in anesthetized animals (see Figure 4.15 in Chapter 4). They serve to open the jaws, which is done in a careful way and by no means as far as the maximum limit; otherwise it may lead to overstretching of the masseter muscle as well as the temporomandibular joints. This gives the mouth gag with a turning mechanism a certain advantage because its blades can be extended slowly and in a controlled manner. In case of an emergency though, the instrument with a quick-locking mechanism provides greater safety as it can be opened and removed more quickly. If positioning of a gag is complicated by the presence of overlong incisors that also hamper the view into the oral cavity, the teeth could be shortened prior to placing the gag.

When opening the jaws in such a continuous fashion be wary of any possible drags (resistance to opening the jaw). For example, infections involving the last cheek teeth may spread to the respective temporomandibular joint and cause a "lockjaw" – particularly in rabbits and guinea pigs. In addition, a sudden lateral displacement of the mandibles whilst opening may be indicative of changes to the temporomandibular joint (Figure 8.1a and b).

The potential risks associated with using a mouth gag are mechanical damage to the incisors that occurs when jamming the gag, inversed positioning of the blades, a direct traumatization of the gingiva due to excessive pressure, an overextension of the temporomandibular joint, as well as the masticatory muscles, or even an iatrogenic fracture of the mandible occurring when opening the jaws extremely wide (beware! in case of jaw abscesses with an extensive osteomyelitis). Those complications can be avoided by carefully handling the instrument and ensuring sufficient depth of anesthesia. In order to protect the oral mucosa, additional small gauze cushions or sponge rubber cushions can be placed underneath the blades.

The blades of cheek dilators for rabbits are relatively wide, long and robust and the corresponding springs have a relatively high base tension. For guinea pigs and chinchillas, special instruments have been developed whose more elongate metal sides become narrower as they get closer to the tip. This allows them to be introduced deeper into the narrow oral cavity, enhancing the view of the caudal molars, which are relatively difficult to see. Furthermore, very fine and delicate cheek dilators are available whose small, short blades have an extraordinarily low base tension. These can also be used in rats, but they are still too large and bulky for smaller rodents like hamsters and mice. For the latter, fine anatomical forceps that are spread apart will help.

Dentistry in Rabbits and Rodents, First Edition. Estella Böhmer.
© 2015 John Wiley & Sons, Ltd. Published 2015 by John Wiley & Sons, Ltd.

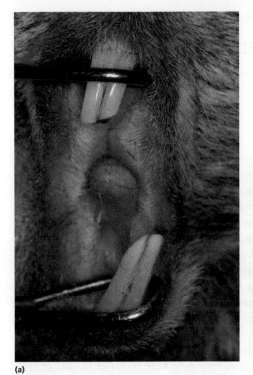

(a)

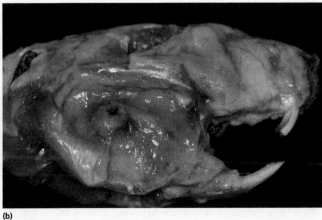

(b)

Figure 8.1 Abscess of the (right) mandible in a three-year-old guinea pig. (a) Lateral displacement of the jaws during opening of the mouth caused by spread of the infection concomitant with secondary pathological changes in the area of the right temporomandibular joint. (b) Specimen of the same animal with a view of the large area of abscess which is located below the masseter muscle with severe retrograde elongation of the last mandibular cheek tooth (M3) with lateral perforation of the mandible, spread of the infection to the nearby temporomandibular joint (partial lockjaw), incisor malocclusion and prognathic jaw position.

When introducing a cheek dilator, always ensure that it is placed below the mouth gag in order to avoid unwanted leverage effects occurring during procedures. (Figure 8.2). If no incisors are left due to tooth loss or extraction, two cheek dilators that are offset by 90 degrees with respect to their normal position are used to open the jaws. Whichever model has a higher spring tension is to be placed between the anterior part of the tongue and the rostral area of the hard palate.

A special mouth opener with a platform for rabbits is available at specialist retailers. The animals are fixed to the platform by means of two transverse poles, in ventral recumbency and with their heads raised; the degree of tilt can be adjusted. The poles are supposed to be just behind the maxillary and mandibular incisors and can be pushed apart by means of a turning mechanism. In order to avoid the patient becoming hypothermic, a heating pad should be placed on the lying surface of the device. When using that kind of restraining platform for a straightforward correction of a malocclusion, no assistant is needed in principle. Overflexion of the neck ensures that the respiratory passages are kept open. The disadvantage though is that kind of positioning poses an increased risk of pulmonary aspiration, particularly when using rotary instruments, because in such cases the cheek teeth will need to be repeatedly cooled down by means of waterlogged swabs. Correction of the maxillary cheek teeth in particular can be problematic in this position. Surgical treatment of jaw abscesses or the performance of an osteotomy may require repositioning of the patient on the operating table. Furthermore, the horizontal and vertical metal poles do sometimes restrict intraoral handling of instruments considerably. Generally, using classic cheek dilators and mouth gags gives more flexibility as the patient – lying on a suitable heating pad – can be easily shifted into the desired position. The animal's head can also be quickly lowered in case of an emergency (e.g. intraoral bleeding), thus keeping the respiratory passages free (Figure 8.3).

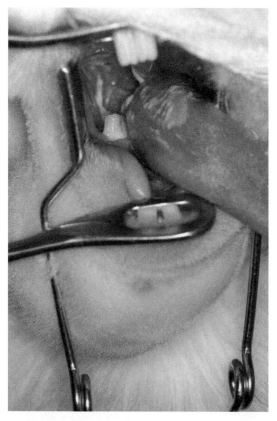

Figure 8.2 Abscess of the (right) mandible in an eight-year-old rabbit. Situation after opening of the mouth, apically ulcerated first mandibular cheek tooth (P3) with discharge of pus from the alveolus (on the right), cheek dilator positioned correctly below the mouth gag.

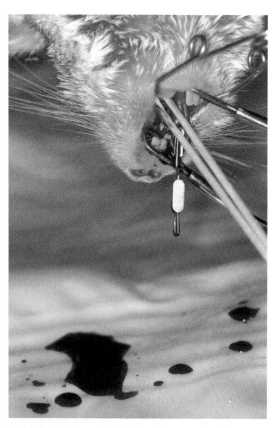

Figure 8.3 Situation after injuring the venous vessel in the jaw angle of a chinchilla. Mouth gag, cheek dilator and tongue-holding forceps are in position. For bleeding control, a cotton swab was introduced intraorally. The head is lowered to keep the respiratory pathways free.

In rabbits, guinea pigs and chinchillas, the view into the oral cavity is greatly impaired by the very thick tongue, which also bulges toward the palate (torus linguae). The intraoral view can be improved by grasping the tongue with two fingers and anatomical forceps or special kinds of tongue-grasping pincers, and then pulling it out of the mouth a bit. Alternatively, it can be pressed against the rostral floor of the oral cavity by means of an additional, vertically positioned cheek dilator (Figure 8.4).

For thorough examinations of the oral cavity, and in order to protect the soft tissue (tongue and cheek) during intraoral manipulations, a flat, concavely shaped metal or wooden spatula of a suitable size is needed. With this instrument, the tongue and cheek can be easily pushed aside (Figure 8.5). Firstly, an overview of the oral cavity is obtained. During this,

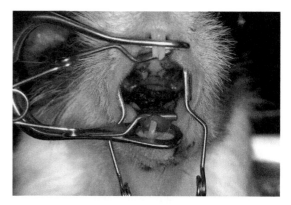

Figure 8.4 Examination of the oral cavity of a guinea pig, with mouth gag and cheek dilator in position; an additional cheek dilator is used to push the rostral area of the tongue down. Situation after extraction of the left mandibular incisor. Oral cavity is filled with food, wear of maxillary cheek teeth is slightly asymmetrical.

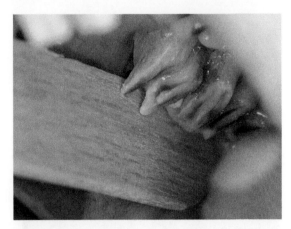

Figure 8.5 Malocclusion in an eight-year-old rabbit (right maxillary row of cheek teeth). A wooden tongue spatula was introduced in order to protect the soft tissue; preparation for burring of the buccal tooth spurs of the anterior two cheek teeth (P2/P3).

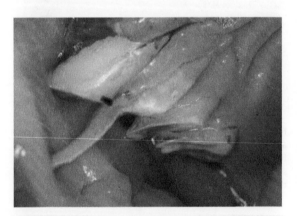

Figure 8.6 Malocclusion in a two-year-old rabbit (right maxillary row of cheek teeth). Intraoral view of four visible maxillary cheek teeth (P3–M2), pointed buccal spur of the third maxillary cheek tooth (P4) with a relatively small, secondary injury to soft tissue (ventrally from the tooth spur). The first maxillary cheek tooth (P2) is missing.

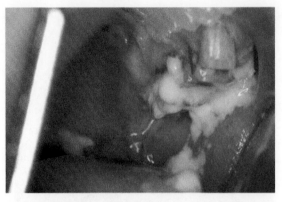

Figure 8.7 Retrobulbar abscess in a two-year-old rabbit (left maxillary row of cheek teeth). Discharge of pus from the alveolus of the fourth maxillary cheek tooth (M1) and displacement of the clinical crowns of all visible maxillary premolars (P2–P4).

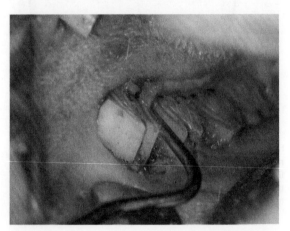

Figure 8.8 Early malocclusion in a one-year-old guinea pig (left mandibular row of cheek teeth). Enlarged and inflamed interproximal area between the first and second mandibular cheek tooth (P4/M1); removal of impacted foreign material (food fibers) with an explorer probe; early carious defects in the area of the lingual occlusal edge of the first three cheek teeth (P4–M2).

the lingual and buccal surfaces of each individual tooth are examined and the adjacent soft tissue (tongue, buccal mucosa) checked for injuries (Figure 8.6). Next, the entire occlusal surface as well as the gingiva and the interproximal areas of each tooth are examined. Attention should be paid to intraoral accumulations of pus or periodontal pus discharge (Figure 8.7). Lastly, the area behind the last cheek teeth, caudal of which the temporomandibular joints are located, is examined.

The sulcus of each individual tooth and the various interproximal areas are examined by means of a fine periodontal probe (Figure 8.8). At the same time, mobility of each tooth is assessed. Periodontal probes are available in different lengths and with pointed or slightly blunted ends. They are particularly suitable for a verification of plaque, calculus or food remains near the gingiva; all these must not be confused with discolorations caused by plant pigments. The latter are found particularly in wild animals or (domestic) rabbits that are left to graze and browse freely in the garden (see Figure 3.10 in Chapter 3). Periodontal probes will also be of use in examining tooth fractures or carious and resorptive tooth lesions more closely.

If no endoscope is at hand to optimally illuminate the intraoral area, a small mouth mirror can be used as an alternative for an examination of poorly visible parts of the dentition, although it will only be effectively used in rabbits. There is not enough space for mouth mirrors in the narrow oral cavities of guinea pigs and chinchillas, especially as the cheeks lie closely to the teeth when the jaws are open.

Optimal illumination of the oral cavity is essential for good intraoral examination. Special headlamps are particularly suited for this (apart from endoscopes). Inspection lamps could also be used in principle, but they require an assistant to be present unless one would want to work single-handedly. Since all pet patients are rather small and more subtle findings may therefore be overlooked magnifying loupes have proven successful for a complete examination. A headband can be used to attach the loupes to the head of the person performing the examination or they can be directly attached to a person's own pair of glasses. Particularly comfortable examinations can be made using stereo headband magnifiers with an integrated source of illumination, as the area of examination will be directly illuminated and magnified at the same time. However, their use is not easily learnt, as an acute three-dimensional vision is usually not achieved straight away.

If an animal's cheek bulges far into the oral cavity due to excessive swelling of soft tissue, e.g. a mandibular abscess or a phlegmonous lesion of the buccal mucosa, it can greatly impair intraoral examination and treatment. In such cases endoscopic intraoral examination

is of great benefit, particularly when examining the narrow, elongate oral cavities of guinea pigs and chinchillas. Suitable are rigid endoscopes (18 cm long) with a diameter of 2.7 mm, a straight or 30° optical system and a 3.5 mm protective sleeve (Capello, 2006; Hernandez-Divers, 2008). The integrated light source provides optimal illumination of the area of examination. The occlusal surface of the maxillary molars can be examined in closer detail by means of a 30° optical system. In order to examine the mandibular surface, the endoscope is turned by 180°.

A video camera connected to the endoscope can transfer the image to the monitor via an optical fiber cable (still frame or video recording). The data can then be saved to a suitable photo documentation system (harddisk, DVD, MOD) or printed out as a still frame. Alternatively, they can be transferred directly to the surgery's patient management system and assigned to the respective patient. With this kind of documentation, recent findings can be exactly registered and compared with earlier changes. This – along with an additional consideration of the corresponding radiographs – facilitates a more specific assessment of the individual prognosis.

As a general rule, even with the most meticulous clinical and intraoral examinations, no more than approximately 20% of all pathological changes in the skull can be found.

Thus all intraoral examinations should be followed by radiography as specific as possible. Otherwise important (intraosseous and intraalveolar) findings will be overlooked. As a consequence of that, the extent of malocclusion would be misjudged, resulting in an inappropriate

---

Instruments for intraoral examination and dental treatment

Otoscope with a metal or plastic funnel
Rigid endoscope with a monitor
Cheek dilator (various models, e.g. solid vs hollow wings or elongated models for small rodents)
Mouth gag (various models and different sizes)
Tongue/cheek spatula (metal or wooden)
Periodontal probe
Scaler
Special luxators for incisors and cheek teeth
18- to 25-gauge cannula (alternative to special luxators for incisor extractions)
30-gauge cannulae (local anesthesia)

(Continued)

Extraction forceps for cheek teeth
Special diamond rasp (various grits and shapes, smooth or hollow)
Anatomical forceps
Curette (fine models of different sizes)
Pean forceps
Special pincers for trimming of cheek teeth
Bone rongueur forceps (Luer forceps of different shapes and sizes)
Heidemann spatula
Explorer probe
Cotton swab (large and small)
Suitable source of illumination
Magnifying loupes
Headband loupes (binocular microscope)
Nasolacrimal cannula
Sterile pads with nutrition medium for sample-taking (aerobic, anaerobic bacteriological examination)
Dental unit (tabletop device)
Slow-rotating micromotor with a foot pedal (1000–20 000 rpm; rotation direction adjustable clockwise/counterclockwise)
Three-way syringe suitable for air and water – not indispensable
Straight handpiece without water cooling
Various diamond burs
Various diamond cutters (spherical, cylindrical and conical)
Special diamond cylinder with a suitable cap for protection of soft tissue
Cutting disc impregnated with diamond dust (with or without punch holes, cooling)

or incomplete treatment. As an additional consequence, the long-term prognoses will be wrong, as will be estimates of the costs of (mostly long-term) therapy.

8.2 Dental treatment

For professional corrective dentistry in small pets, suitable instruments are needed apart from a certain degree of professional knowledge and well-founded presurgical diagnostics. Iatrogenic damage to teeth and periodontium due to improper handling of instruments or the choice of unsuitable instruments cannot be underestimated. There have been many cases where malocclusions or even mandibular abscesses had to be ascribed to nonprofessional dental treatment or the choice of unsuitable instruments (Figure 8.9).

During the last few decades, various instruments of different shapes and sizes have been developed that are particularly suitable for examination and treatment of malocclusions in lagomorphs and rodents. Considering the patients' varying sizes and anatomical characteristics, they are essential for adequate corrective dentistry. Apart from "basic equipment," there is a range of rather specific non essential instruments (possibly for financial reasons or when the number of

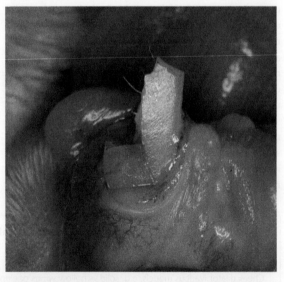

Figure 8.9 Chipped clinical crown of a rabbit's right mandibular incisor. Situation after incorrect clipping of the incisor with unsuitable forceps.

patients is small) but these tools make work so much easier that their acquisition should be contemplated in the future.

In order to perform adequate tooth trimming, a suitable dental unit with a slow-rotating micromotor that can be smoothly adjusted and operated by means of a foot pedal, as well as a straight handpiece are needed. The motor's rotation direction should be adjustable (clockwise/counterclockwise). In many devices, a maximum number of revolutions can be set exactly as desired by means of a small knob on the device. As an alternative to the usual dental tabletop devices, dental motors with a flexible shaft and a straight handpiece can also be used. The device can be attached to an infusion stand and thus be used in a rather comfortable way. Some dental devices are equipped with an additional three-way syringe for air and water. This is not indispensable, but is rather convenient. By means of the air jet, drill dust can be blown off the occlusal surface or food remains removed from periodontal pockets if necessary. Flushing intraorally usually cannot be performed in pet animals due to the risk of pulmonary aspiration, unless one uses a larynx mask that optimally seals the laryngeal area (see Figure 7.1 in Chapter 7). In order to avoid any overheating of the animals' teeth during burring, the dental tissue is continuously moistened with NaCl-soaked absorbent cotton swabs.

Instead of a special dental unit, a small multifunctional do-it-yourself power drill can also be used in exceptional cases, e.g. a Dremel®, although this device is absolutely not as ideal as proper equipment. Suitable devices have a relatively small, straight handpiece that is connected to the actual drill via a flexible, pliable shaft. That shaft can be attached to the table by means of a vertically adjustable tool stand. The velocity can be controlled via a foot pedal or varied using controls on the device. Such an alternative is absolutely recommended if an acquisition of a more expensive dental unit is not worthwhile for the moment due to low patient numbers. For professional burring of dental substances, various burs of different shapes and sizes, equipped with diamonds, are available, as are ceramic burs for a final smoothing of occlusal surfaces or sharp edges. The shank for the various attachments has a diameter of 3.2 mm, although thinner instruments can also be used if combined with special kinds of collets. One disadvantage is the fact that when using a do-it-yourself power drill, it is difficult to control the polishing head in a manner as steady as when using a dental unit.

Generally, the tooth substance is ground down by means of rotating instruments. It is important to choose a suitable abrasive bur. It can be made of various materials: stainless steel, hardmetal, tungsten carbide steel, corundum (a special form of aluminum oxide), silicium carbide or Arkansas stone. There are also various surface structures and shapes: spherical, wheel-shaped, cylindrical and conical burs. Ceramic burs differ with respect to their grit (green=coarse surface structure; white=fine surface structure). In addition, there is a multitude of different cutting heads equipped with diamonds. All burs can be attached to the straight handpiece by turn-locking, with the smooth shank of the instruments having a diameter of 2.35 mm in dental units.

Apart from diamond grinders, hardmetal cutters or fissure burs are sometimes recommended for use in tooth trimmings in pets, because they are able to remove comparatively high amounts of dental substance in a relatively short time (Gorrel & Verhaert, 2006). The surface of all cutters consists of sharp edges that remove the tooth substance as small strands. Hence they can only be used rotating in a certain direction (clockwise). A significant disadvantage of these instruments is the fact that chipping can occur during burring of teeth and that the cutting heads tend to slip off the tooth surfaces. As a result, there is an increased danger of injury to the soft tissue. The surface structures of certain cutters also produce vibrations that may possibly harm the periodontium and the apical area of the teeth (Gabriel, 2009).

The gentlest method of occlusal correction is by means of various diamond cutters or grinders that are available in different grits, shapes (sphere, cylinder, pointed cylinder, cone, roller, inverted cone, torpedo, flame) and lengths of shank (Figure 8.10). There are dull-edged or rounded tips of the instrument. The length and diameter of the abrasive bur also varies.

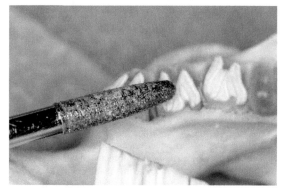

Figure 8.10 Situation during trimming of the cheek teeth of a guinea pig with a conical, diamond-impregnated bur (specimen, right mandibular row of cheek teeth); enlarged interproximal area between the first two cheek teeth (P4/M1) and fibrous material between the second and third cheek tooth (M1/M2).

Depending on shape and size of the chosen instrument, individual teeth may be trimmed in a specific approach or the entire occlusal surface remodeled in the desired way. Longer shanks will facilitate work in the narrow, hard-to-see oral cavities of guinea pigs and chinchillas.

The diamond cutting head of choice is gently positioned on the tooth or the occlusal surface with the hand simultaneously propped up on to the table or the patient to avoid wobbling and improve guidance of the instrument. This will ensure safe and specific control of the instrument. If one feels uneasy handling dental units or using rotating instruments, the method of correctly burring dental substance can be practised and learnt on skull specimens (Figure 8.11). Even experienced practitioners may be able to improve their technique in this way. In rabbits, tooth trimming is usually no problem as the intraoral view is good. For guinea

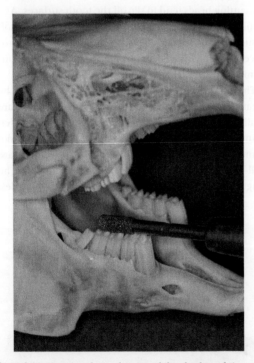

Figure 8.11 Situation during burring of the cheek teeth in a rabbit with a cylindrical, diamond-impregnated bur (specimen): normal occlusion. The first mandibular cheek tooth is normally thicker than the rest of the cheek teeth. Due to a lowering of the buccomesial alveolar wall, the clinical crown appears to be significantly higher than the rest of the cheek teeth (danger of overcorrection while removing dental substance); last molar (M3) tilted mesially (=physiological finding), clearly visible mental foramen.

pigs and chinchillas, using rotating abrasive burs for occlusal correction is significantly more difficult due to their elongated, narrow oral cavities. Generally speaking, any friction will generate a certain amount of heat – how much depends on the rotation velocity of the bur as well as the pressure exerted during cutting. Hence when removing tooth substance there is always a general risk of iatrogenic, thermal irritation of the pulp, particularly in the case of maximum shortening of teeth (near the gingiva). However, the risk of overheating will be relatively small if suitable diamond burs are used, as this will keep the amount of burring pressure acting on the tooth low (Crossley, 1996; Gabriel 2009). This is only true, however, as long as the surface of the cutting head is not coated with dental dust, which would greatly reduce its efficacy.

In order to keep the risk of thermal damage as low as possible, relatively low rotation velocities are used (15 000–30 000 rpm) and sufficient cooling of the dental tissue should be provided. The latter is achieved by repeatedly and thoroughly moistening the teeth with cool liquids using NaCl-soaked cotton swabs. Burring is always performed in the time in between, in short intervals (tooth contact lasting approximately 4 s). Thus the burring of the tooth substance is done step-by-step and carefully. Surplus water and burring dust is continuously removed using swabs or suctioning devices. If the dust is left in place, the tiny particles may cause irritation of the respiratory passages. In addition, the coarse surface of the burs will be covered with a mixture of saliva and dust if the latter is not removed. That would reduce the burring capacity and cause an increased heat generation during burring of the teeth. This is aggravated by the fact that in such cases one tends to automatically increase the pressure exerted on the tooth, further worsening the situation. More importantly, the burring dust hampers a continuous evaluation of the occlusal surface while work is in progress.

Should overheating of teeth occur due to inappropriate or excessive burring without adequate cooling, affected rabbits will exhibit sustained anorexia. It is caused by a rapidly developing, generalized pulpitis and a periodontitis, the latter of which will lead to an accumulation of pus in the tooth sockets of all teeth affected, after only a few days (Harcourt-Brown, 2002a). There is usually no hope of a successful therapy.

When using rotating instruments, there is also always a certain risk of iatrogenic injuries to soft tissues.

However, since the surface of diamond burs do not have particularly sharp edges, their use entails a lower overall risk of injuries than the use of hardmetal cutters. However, all patients with malocclusions have a certain degree of inflammable irritation of the oral mucosa, making them extremely sensitive to any kind of procedure. For example, inserting a suitable cheek dilator will still be enough to cause iatrogenic lacerations in many cases. Cheeks and tongue must therefore always be protected with a suitable metal or wooden spatula (see Figure 8.5). A discarded periosteal elevator will also be suited for this. Metal spatulas are available with either a straight or a concave working end. The concave metal surface helps to keep the tongue, which in rabbits can be very massive, in a simple and safe way. When using a straight spatula for this, the tongue tends to slip away from above or below the working end of that slender instrument, getting in the way in the treatment area and posing a risk of injury there.

Another advantage of diamond burs is the fact that in contrast to hardmetal cutters, they tend not to slip off the occlusal surface. They can also be used rotating clockwise or counterclockwise (Gabriel, 2009). This facilitates intraoral work as the direction of rotation is generally chosen as turning away from the soft tissues. On the other hand, an exclusive use of diamond burs requires a comparatively long time for removing larger

amounts of dental substance. This can be quite difficult when dealing with guinea pigs and chinchillas, as their cheek teeth often have to be shortened by up to 5 mm or one-third of the height of the entire tooth structure during occlusal correction (Figure 8.12a and b). Although the average pressure exerted on the tooth during burring with a diamond bur is low, the strain on the periodontal apparatus does accumulate over time. This is not to be underestimated when a (sub)clinical loosening of teeth is found – this is particularly true for chinchillas, whose teeth are often extensively resorbed intraalveolarly, causing them to sit in the tooth socket only very loosely (Figures 8.13a and 8.14).

In principle, incisors and cheek teeth of lagomorphs and rodents should be burred by means of rotating instruments. Specialist retailers offer special kinds of forceps that are suited for removing particularly long, thin and delicate tooth spurs relatively easily and in a way that protects the soft tissue (see Figure 4.18 in Chapter 4). Alternatively, fine Luer bone rongeur forceps can also be used for this. Afterwards the cheek tooth that has been pretreated in that way is further shortened by means of suitable rotating burs (Harcourt-Brown, 2002a). More compact tooth spurs of rabbits or partially tilted, overlong cheek teeth that exhibit a growth defect, however, should always be treated with suitable cutters. This is usually no problem as the intraoral

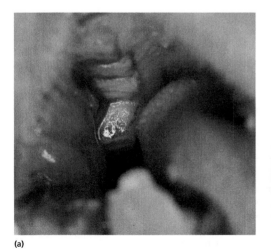

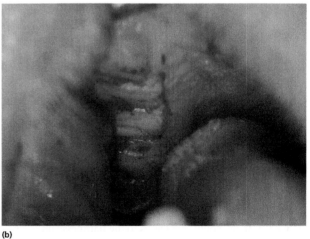

(a) (b)

Figure 8.12 Malocclusion in a six-year-old chinchilla (right maxillary row of cheek teeth). (a) Situation after trimming of the first three cheek teeth (P4–M2) with special forceps; the last molar's (M3) dental substance, which is still left to be removed, can be seen well. Since the anterior teeth are still slightly protruding over the gingival margin, they need to be reworked (trimmed) a bit with a diamond-impregnated bur. (b) Situation after trimming all cheek teeth (P4–M3) with special forceps; reworking of the occlusal surface with a rotating bur is necessary (slight shortening and smoothing).

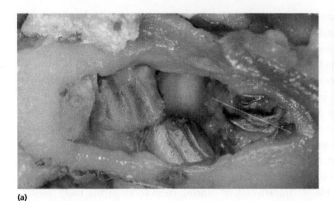

(a)

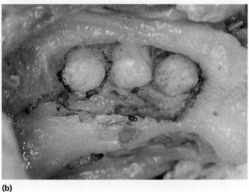

(b)

Figure 8.13 Look on the left (a) and right (b) maxilla of a postmortem specimen of a chinchilla with recurring malocclusion in an eight-year-old chinchilla. (a) Mobility of all teeth in the left maxillary row of cheek teeth as a result of a pronounced intraalveolar, odontoclastic tooth and bone resorption. No interproximal lamina bone is visible (or can be verified) and all tooth sockets have merged into a single, large bone cavity, which is distended when compared with a normal desmodontium. Impacted food particles have already been removed. There is a pronounced tooth displacement, an intraalveolar rotation of the last cheek tooth (M3; white line), recognizable by the longitudinal enamel pattern of the occlusal surface, and a generalized, inflammatory hyperplasia of the gingiva. (b) Situation of the right maxillary row of cheek teeth after tooth trimming with special forceps. The remaining tooth bodies have been dyed with ink and no fissures can be verified. There is a generalized loss of the alveolar bone, a pathological dilation of the desmodontium, an intraalveolar rotation of the tooth bodies, recognizable by the altered pattern of the occlusal surface, and a generalized, inflammatory hyperplasia of the gingiva.

access is good. When using forceps, molars that are too long should not be shortened in just one step ("clipped off") because otherwise the hypselodont, lophodont teeth tend to split. Intraalveolar tooth fissures or fractures as well as iatrogenic injuries to the pulp (exposed pulp with a secondary pulpitis) are frequent consequences of such actions (see Figure 8.9).

Exceptions are particularly soft, structurally changed cheek teeth of chinchillas that suffer from advanced malocclusion (Figures 8.13a and 8.14). Their molars can be easily shortened with special forceps designed for molars, as the entire hard substance of the teeth has become less resistant due to the pronounced dentin and enamel hypoplasia (Figure 8.13b). Afterwards the occlusal surface is reworked or flattened if need be, using rotating instruments. However, if the structure of enamel and dentin is unchanged, in other words it is hard and brittle, there is a danger of splitting teeth when using the forceps. In order to assess the quality of the tooth substance correctly, some experience and a good radiograph are needed. If any doubt remains as to the hardness and structure of a tooth, then that tooth is better burred with a cutter than worked on with forceps.

If the medical indication for tooth-clipping is correct (used basically in chinchillas) and cheek teeth are shortened in a professional, step-by-step fashion by means of

suitable forceps, the clipped tooth parts do not exhibit splits (Figure 8.15). Individual tooth prisms are also still connected with each other via the crown cement lying in between. It is important to correctly position the forceps on the molar as the entire width of the tooth body must be caught. Only optimally sharpened instruments should be used. Having said this, it is obsolete to simply "clip off" all overlong teeth randomly and uncritically. Areas where forceps must not be used include: the incisors of all animals (which is out of the question considering the shape of the tooth bodies) and all forms of malocclusion that are not associated with corresponding structural changes of the teeth, in other words hard and brittle teeth.

> Forceps must never be used for incisors of all animal species (which should be out of the question considering the shape of the tooth body) and in all types of malocclusion that are not associated with a corresponding structural change of the teeth, in other words in hard, brittle teeth.

Apart from diamond burs, there are also diamond hand files with different grits and a straight or concave

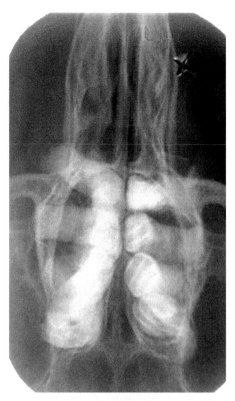

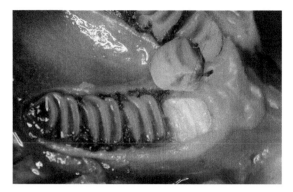

Figure 8.15 Malocclusion in a three-year-old chinchilla (specimen). Situation of the left maxillary row of cheek teeth after trimming of the first upper cheek tooth (P4) with suitable special forceps. Neither fragment nor occlusal surface are chipped. A slight gingival hyperplasia can be recognized.

Figure 8.14 Intraoral view of the maxilla of a six-year-old chinchilla with advanced malocclusion and severe dilation of all tooth sockets. There is a generalized loss of the lamina dura, severe buccal tooth displacement and a retrograde elongation of the tooth structures as a logical consequence of the apex displacements, and an intraalveolar rotation of several molars, recognizable by the altered pattern of the occlusal surface.

working surface. Those files can easily and effectively remove pointed sharp edges or particularly delicate buccal or lingual and palatal tooth spurs, especially in the area of the middle molars, all of which may have remained there after finishing shortening of the teeth. The concave shape of the working end helps to keep the file safely on the edge of the tooth while working on it, while accidental slipping off, which sometimes occurs when handling rotating instruments, is greatly reduced. This results in the risk of injury to the soft tissue being generally lower.

Hand files are not, however, suited for removal of tooth spurs in the last cheek teeth as the rostrocaudal working movements involve an excessive risk of injuring the blood vessel that runs along the jaw angle. Generally speaking, hand files can only be used for a relatively short period of time and without applying too much pressure, as otherwise excessive strain would be exerted on the periodontal apparatus. Besides, they are not suited for shortening the entire chewing surface of the cheek teeth because their effectiveness is far too low to be able to work efficiently while protecting the teeth.

The use of conventional, nondiamond hand files whose surface is made of multiple transversal grooves is obsolete. Handling them causes larger enamel and dentin lamellae to be torn off the occlusal surface. This leads to multiple coronal microfractures as well as an excessive strain on the periodontal apparatus due to strong shearing forces that can cause irreversible damage to the Sharpey fibers and ultimately a loosening of teeth.

The set of instruments used for the treatment of malocclusions is completed with disc-shaped burs that are used to shorten incisors (a cutting disc impregnated with diamond dust) and special kinds of luxators and forceps used to extract cheek teeth and incisors. Their use is explained in detail in the following chapters.

CHAPTER 9
Diseases of the Incisors

9.1 Primary incisor malocclusions

Primary incisor malocclusions occur independently from changes associated with the cheek teeth. They can be congenital or acquired (trauma, painful lesions of the gingiva, etc.) and have a traumatic or nontraumatic origin (Table 9.1). Omnivorous rodents often suffer from primary incisor malocclusions that are due to inappropriate husbandry, while rabbits and herbivorous rodents rarely exhibit that disorder.

9.1.1 Congenital malformations

Congenital malformations can affect the incisors themselves (dental malocclusion) or primarily affect the jaw (skeletal malocclusion) resulting in an incisor malocclusion. There have been few reports of congenital dental anomalies in lagomorphs and rodents, which are very rare. They include an inherited alteration of dental substance and dental structure (amelogenesis imperfecta) and an innate pathological radius of curvature of the incisors. Skeletal malformations such as inherited jaw and skull anomalies are much more frequent in rabbits. The most prevalent of these is a shortened maxilla in the form of the brachygnathia superior (see below).

By contrast, congenital malocclusions of the jaws are rare in herbivorous rodents. In examinations of 700 chinchillas, only one animal had a maxillary brachygnathia (Crossley, 2001a). There are no reports of malocclusions in omnivorous rodents, which is presumably because such animals generally would be unviable and thus unable to reproduce. Hence that disorder is self-limiting.

Brachygnathia superior in rabbits

In this congenital shortening of the maxilla, the curvature of the incisors is normal. It is an autosomal recessive hereditary defect where only the maxillary diastema or, additionally, the entire head can be shortened (Fox & Crary, 1971). Brachygnathia superior usually does not manifest itself before the age of approximately three weeks (Keil, 1966; Fox & Crary, 1971; Wiggs & Lobprise, 1995a). A typical early finding is abnormal contact of the upper with the lower incisors, and as a consequence the incisal edges have blunt occlusal surfaces and this is referred to as an "edge-to-edge bite" (Fox & Crary, 1971). Further development of changes in incisal occlusion is very variable (see below). If there are also pathological changes of the cheek teeth, for example an alteration to the occlusal angle or tooth elongations, these should be treated as early as possible. It is the only way – in combination with regular trimming of the incisors – to possibly recreate or preserve normal molar occlusion (Fox & Crary, 1971). Depending on the degree of maxillary brachygnathism and the relative mandibular prognathism as a result, different degrees of malocclusion develop, all of which lead to more serious complications within the first year of the animal's life (Gorrel & Verhaert, 2006). Often rabbits do not exhibit any symptoms during the initial stage of this malocclusion. The overlong incisors obstruct the narrow opening of the oral cavity resulting in rabbits only being able to ingest small food particles or hay stalks with their lips that are then ingested further with the aid of the tongue. The owners do not present their pets to veterinarians until the severely elongated incisors are clearly visible, or secondary injuries to soft tissue together with weight loss have occurred.

Dentistry in Rabbits and Rodents, First Edition. Estella Böhmer.
© 2015 John Wiley & Sons, Ltd. Published 2015 by John Wiley & Sons, Ltd.

Table 9.1 Etiology of incisor malocclusion.

Traumatic (primary)	Tooth fracture		
	Jaw fracture		
Atraumatic (primary or acquired)	Congenital	Tooth displacement	
		Jaw displacement	Campylognathia, brachygnathia
	Acquired	Purely feeding-related	Insufficient wear of incisors
		Calcium deficiency and vitamin D deficiency	Altered tooth structure and bone structure
		Result of an infectious irritation of the tooth apex	Inflammation in the periapical area
		Result of a mechanical irritation of the tooth apex	E.g. tooth intrusion due to chewing on cage bars
		Iatrogenic	Mechanical or thermal damage caused by incorrect tooth trimming
		Result of a gingivitis/periodontitis	Spreading infection, pain, lack of dental wear
		Result of a generalized malocclusion of cheek teeth	
		Neoplasia	

Maxillary brachygnathism primarily affects dwarf breeds with a weight of less than 1.5 kg as well as small lop-eared rabbits (Chai, 1970; Fox & Crary, 1971; Lindsey & Fox, 1994; Crossley & Aiken, 2004; Gorrel & Verhaert, 2006). This congenital defect has spread widely amongst rabbit populations due to the popularity of the 'cute', especially small rabbit breeds that have a short, round head (brachycephalia). As the discrepancy in length between the maxilla and mandible increases, the incisors cease to occlude at all and grow past each other.

The upper incisors are strongly curved and as they continue to grow, form an arc that curls into the oral cavity. This can lead to soft tissue injuries to the oral mucosa distal to the mandibular incisors or the lips (Figure 9.1). The maxillary incisors can also diverge while growing laterally past the lower lip, continuing dorsally in a relatively narrow arc. However, this occurs very rarely. In individual cases of extreme intraoral curvature of a tooth, injuries to the hard palate can also occur (Wiggs & Lobprise, 1995b). By contrast, elongated mandibular incisors have less acute curvature, causing them to continue growing rostrodorsally and past the maxillary incisors in a wide arc – much like elephant tusks. Both incisors either elongate running parallel to each other or they may diverge with respect to one another, caused by a slight intraalveolar rotation of the tooth. In many cases thick, matted tufts of hair interwoven with food debris accumulate around the base of the tooth, which can then lead to severe inflammation of the soft tissue (Figure 9.2).

A complication arising from primary congenital incisor malocclusion is secondary pathological changes

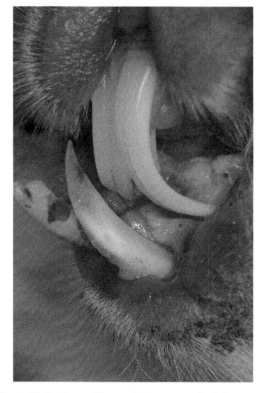

Figure 9.1 Brachygnathia superior in a one-and-a half–year-old rabbit with recurring incisor malocclusion: arc-like overgrowth of the left maxillary incisor with secondary gingival mucosal lesion, abnormal alignment and intraalveolar rotation of both lower incisors with discharge of pus from the left tooth socket (rostrally). There is an indication for preoperative intraoral radiographs as well as an extraction of all incisors.

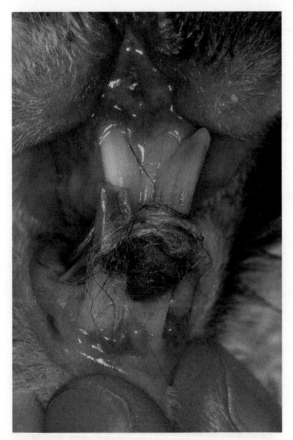

Figure 9.2 Brachygnathia superior in a three-year-old rabbit with recurring incisor malocclusion, matted hair in the area of the overlong mandibular incisors and overgrowth of the right maxillary incisor involving intrusion into the lower jaw and secondary mucosal lesions.

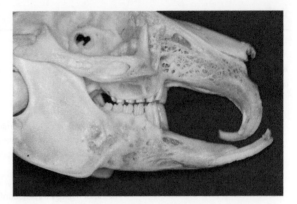

Figure 9.3 Brachygnathia superior in a two-year-old rabbit (specimen) with normal occlusion of the cheek teeth and severe enamel and dentin hypoplasia of the maxillary and mandibular incisors (transverse ridges).

The earlier maxillary brachygnathism is detected and managed by regular trimming of the incisors or extraction of incisors (see below) the better the long-term chance is of preserving normal occlusion in the cheek teeth. Therefore the long-time prognosis is good in these cases. Educating the owner also plays a crucial part in the management of the condition. Conversely, changes to cheek teeth will be more pronounced the later treatment is initiated and the less regularly trimming of incisors is performed.

Treatment
Generally, there are two possibilities of managing the incisor malocclusion: regular trimming of the incisors or extraction of all incisors as early as possible, with the latter being the preferred option.

There have been reports that it is possible to correct the incisor occlusion and obtain normal occlusion by early and frequent corrective shortening of the incisors (see Section 9.3), particularly in rabbits with milder forms of brachygnathism (Fox & Crary, 1971). However, there is a long-term risk of severe pathological alterations to the apical portion of the tooth due to changes in occlusal pressure of the incisors, which are transmitted via the longitudinal axis of the tooth to the apex. This simply shifts the problem from extra-alveolar to the apical part of the tooth. The changes in occlusal pressure (mostly increased) cause the maxillary incisor apices to get progressively closer to the palatal bone plate. At the same time, a pressure-related, mechanical irritation of the sensitive germinal

of cheek teeth that develops over time. The changes to the cheek teeth are caused by the constantly changing, abnormal incisor occlusal pressures as well as the changes in pressure of the molar occlusion. In addition, metabolic bone diseases and malnutrition play a certain part in the origin of the disorder. If the incisors simply elongate without contact one another and without causing trauma to the oral mucosa, the probability of secondary malocclusions of cheek teeth is reduced provided that the incisors are regularly shortened (Figure 9.3). However, if there is soft tissue trauma, the rabbit will be reluctant to chew properly due to pain resulting in less grinding and occlusal contact of the molars that tend to overgrow secondarily and a vicious cycle develops.

cells occurs, which may lead to those cells producing abnormal tooth material.

The time interval between corrective trimming depends on the degree of malocclusion, the structure of the teeth and their individual growth rates. In rabbits with otherwise healthy cheek teeth, the incisors need to be trimmed every four to six weeks throughout life – depending on whether the incisors are still partially in contact or out of contact all togeher (Wiggs & Lobprise, 1995c; Harcourt-Brown, 2002a; Crossley & Aiken, 2004). Many pet owners delay intervals between teeth trimming sessions – often for financial reasons – until ulcerations of the oral mucosa require an immediate response, or until the animal is hardly able to close its mouth correctly. As a result there are constantly varying axial loads on the incisors and cheek teeth, all with all negative consequences (Figure 9.1). If repeated radical trimming of incisors is performed in addition, the pulp cavity continues to shift more coronally. This results in less tooth substance being able to be removed after a while with an increased risk of iatrogenic pulp exposure. This will significantly reduce the optimal time interval between individual dental treatments. Given the potential complications of repeated tooth trimming, early extraction of all incisors seems to be the preferred treatment option both for the welfare of the patient and for a chance of preserving normal occlusion of the cheek teeth.

Complete removal of all incisors (see Section 9.4) in rabbits was first described by Brown in 1992, and then extended by Crossley by refining the operating technique and developing special luxators (Brown, 1992; Crossley, 1994). Since then, it has become a well-established and recommended method of treatment for rabbits with a congenital incisor malocclusion. If the tooth extraction is performed early enough, i.e. at an age of approximately six to nine months, the normal occlusion of the cheek teeth may be preserved for longer periods (Figure 9.3). The animals are able to eat normally after all incisors have been removed, but their food needs to be chopped up or grated before being offered. The food is prehended with the lips and then ground by the cheek teeth just as in healthy animals.

It must be pointed out, however, that an extraction of all incisors in the case of brachygnathism does not guarantee that a normal occlusion of the cheek teeth – if present – can actually be preserved in the long term. However, the chances of that happening are significantly higher than if repeated trimming of teeth were performed.

If rabbits are relatively young at the time of tooth extraction, the removal of all incisors is usually without any complications. It is a different situation in older animals with a hereditary brachygnathism whose incisors have already been trimmed several times. In these cases the tooth extraction is more difficult due to abnormalities of the intraalveolar shape of the teeth, and it is not uncommon to get postoperative complications. These are predominantly intraalveolar infections or partial necrosis of the alveolar bone. There is often delayed wound healing necessitating wound treatment. The owner should be informed of the risk prior to surgery, as this could significantly increase the costs of treatment. The risk of infections can be somewhat reduced by employing a sterile operation technique as well as antibiotics intra- and postoperatively. This re-inforces that the optimal time for tooth extraction should be as early as possible in animals with a congenital brachygnathism.

Campylognathia

Campylognathia is a special form of skeletal anomaly that also leads to a primary congenital incisor malocclusion (Keil, 1966). A lateral displacement and a concomitant twisting (distortion) of the rostral maxilla causes the incisors to lose contact with each other, and thus they fail to wear down correctly. This malformation occurs more frequently in rodents than in lagomorphs, but is very rare.

9.1.2 Trauma-related incisor malocclusion

A direct trauma for example a fall or a hit may result in loss of the clinical crown of one or several incisors that may result in a primary incisor malocclusion. In most cases the animals would have fallen down headfirst from a great height on to a hard surface, inflicting injury not only to their incisors but also to the rostral part of the jaw. Incisor traumas occur relatively frequently in herbivorous pet rodents (Crossley & Aiken, 2004). In rabbits, guinea pigs, chinchillas and degus, all of which have a bony link between the two mandibles, loosening (fracture) of the symphysis may occur in addition. In order to proceed further, it is crucial to distinguish between an incisor fracture with or without pulp exposure (see Section 13.2 in Chapter 13, symphysiolysis, and Section 9.3, vital amputation).

Associated injuries, such as jaw fractures, separation of the symphysis of the mandibles or lesions involving the bony alveolus, need to be identified by radiography prior to treatment. Suitable radiographs include intra-oral exposures or an isolated view of the mandible in guinea pigs and chinchillas.

Any affected tooth will regrow without any complications if the germinal cells in the tooth apex are still vital. This is the reason why an incisor that is completely knocked-out can regrow provided the dental sac is still present. If, however, the germinal tissue has been partially or completely destroyed due to the force exerted on the tooth, the incisor will not regrow at all or will be severely altered structurally. In such cases, or if primarily there is a suspected additional intraalveolar injury, radiographic diagnostics are performed. Intraoral views are suited for this in rabbits, whereas in guinea pigs and chinchillas special projections are best for an isolated view of the mandible as described by Böhmer (see Section 5.4.2 in Chapter 5).

Treatment

If an incisor is fractured its counterpart is no longer able to occlude and therefore will not be abraded and continue to grow more quickly than normally – meaning tooth eruption is increased temporarily. Hence temporary corrective trimming of that tooth is necessary until the injured antagonist is able to resume normal abrasion. To avoid the need of repeated trimmings, both incisal antagonists (or even all four incisors) are trimmed to identical lengths immediately after the trauma, using a diamond-impregnated cutting disc. The length is determined by the remaining length of the fractured tooth. If the tooth fragments are of reasonable length, a chisel-shaped occlusal edge should be created in addition. If, however, the fracture is close to the gingiva, the incisors are burred bluntly with any sharp edges being thoroughly smoothed to avoid the risk of additional soft tissue injuries (tongue). Following this treatment, the incisors regrow at equal rates until they naturally meet again in normal occlusion (Figure 9.4a to c). The patient must be offered particularly fine hay and fresh food that has been chopped up to enable the food to be taken with the lips until the incisors have grown to their normal lengths (after approximately 3–6 weeks).

Fractured incisors without pulp exposure, are smoothed and any sharp edges rounded with a diamond coated bur or the cutting disc to avoid further soft tissue injuries. Since it must be assumed that the trauma (pathological tooth intrusion and intraalveolar jamming/tilting) has also damaged the germinal dental tissue as well as the periodontium, the affected incisor is

trimmed a bit more in order to temporarily immobilize it. The respective antagonist is also trimmed slightly to allow the injured tooth to temporarily regrow unopposed. If a fractured incisor does not regrow properly, a specific radiographic examination is performed in order to determine further treatment required.

In the case of tooth fractures close to the gingiva with pulp exposure, there is an extremely high risk of an infected pulpitis, which can advance to a pulp necrosis and ultimately lead to the formation of an apical abscess. In order to prevent an infection, the tooth is treated endodontically. A cavity preparation with a partial pulpectomy is performed and then direct pulp capping is carried out with calcium hydroxide cement (Crossley & Aiken, 2004; Wiggs & Lobprise, 1995c). After pulp treatment, sharp edges are removed as well and the antagonist is trimmed accordingly. Adequate postoperative analgesia must be ensured as this is a painful procedure. This approach though is usually sufficient to preserve the incisor in a fully functional and healthy state. The patient should be monitored at regular intervals as often as possible over a period of several weeks until normal incisor length occlusion has been re-established.

9.1.3 Acquired, non-trauma-related incisor malocclusion

Pathological changes of the incisors can also be the result of an irritation to any part of the tooth structure or merely to the apex. This includes mechanical, infectious or thermal injury. If such a stimulus reaches the germinal tissue, it can either lead to an abnormal tooth eruption or be detrimental to the form and quality of the newly-formed tooth substance (Figure 9.5). However, gingivitis may also be a pain-related cause of decreased dental wear, resulting in a malocclusion, e.g. following the use of mouth gags without anesthesia.

The principle of the aradicular hypselodont teeth of rabbits represents a balance that is both constant and extremely susceptible to disturbances; it balances the continuous, appositional growth of the teeth and the simultaneous wear of the tooth substance due to constant abrasion during feeding. In principle, any situation that can lead to an imbalance of the two factors inevitably results in a malocclusion of the incisors.

That delicate balance of continuing tooth growth is most often disturbed by errors in feeding (Crossley, 1995b). Under normal conditions, e.g. whilst browsing on a meadow, the incisors chop up the food into smaller

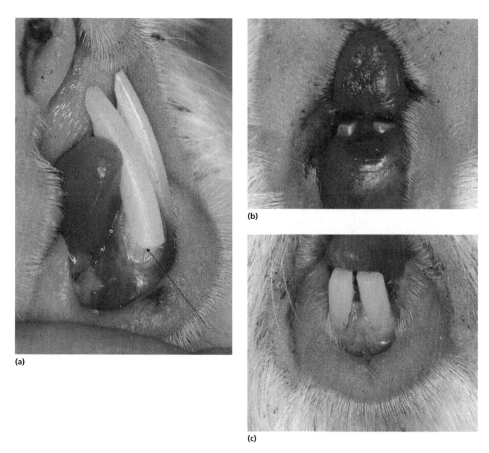

Figure 9.4 Fall-related injury of the incisor of a one-year-old guinea pig. (a) Fracture of the right lower incisor near the gingiva. (b) After maximum shortening of the mandibular incisors; blunt biting edge with rounded occlusal surface. (c) Three weeks following maximum shortening of incisors; incisors regrow evenly.

pieces by making lateral movements, causing wear of the incisors. Therefore daily feeding of a suitably structured, long-stranded, abrasive food, is crucial for keeping the incisors healthy. It would be best to let the animals browse on a meadow on a daily basis and offer hay *ad libitum* at the same time.

If, however, rabbits that are kept in cages or left to roam freely inside a house have access to customary mixed foods throughout the day, they will – apart from some hay – preferentially eat those mixtures (good acceptance). This results in neither the incisors nor the cheek teeth being sufficiently worn down. Although special food mixtures do contain longer fiber elements that are suited for incisor abrasion in principle, small pellets taste better and are taken up preferentially. This selective feeding behavior results in dental abrasion being insufficient as long as feeding dishes are refilled daily. In principle, pellets that are large enough to pre-

vent being easily taken up with the lips are more beneficial for incisor abrasion. In this way the animal is forced to use their incisors, which leads to a certain amount of dental abrasion. This is not however a substitute for natural browsing on a meadow.

Furthermore, a primary calcium deficiency or vitamin D deficiency may play a part in the etiology of incisor malocclusions (Harcourt-Brown & Baker, 2001). An undersupply of those two minerals which are required for the production of new, hard tooth substance results in enamel and dentin that is less resistent. An indication of this kind of temporary malnutrition may be visible horizontal lines (grooves) in the enamel of the incisors (and also the cheek teeth) (Harcourt-Brown, 1996, 1997) (see Figure 2.15 in Chapter 2).

The elodont incisors of rodents are subject to particularly strong occlusal pressures because they act as true gnawing teeth. For this reason, a stable equilibrium

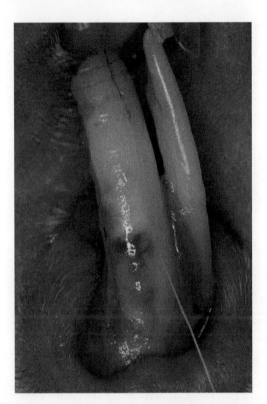

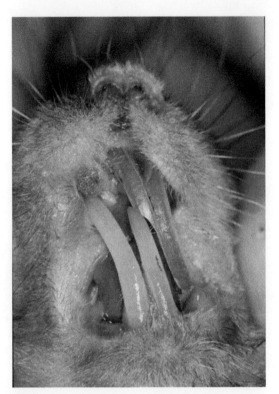

Figure 9.5 Recurring, primary incisor malocclusion in a three-year-old guinea pig: chronically thickened lower incisor with longitudinal splitting of the tooth body. There is an indication for intraoral radiographs as well as subsequent tooth extraction as no physiological abrasion is possible (alternative: isolated radiographic view of the lower jaw according to Böhmer).

Figure 9.6 Pronounced incisor malocclusion in a two-year-old rat with severe mandibular as well as maxillary incisor overgrowth, secondary mucosal lesions and soft tissue swelling in the area of the right upper jaw (lip), abnormal enamel pigmentation of the mandibular incisors.

between growth and wear of the incisor is of crucial importance (O'Malley, 2008). The exact regulation mechanism for this complex interaction is still widely unknown.

Possible causes leading to an incisor malocclusion are acquired tooth displacements, insufficient dental wear due to poor husbandry, traumatic lesions (fall-related tooth fractures or tooth intrusion), an apical infection or structural changes of the tooth substance such as enamel and dentin hypoplasia or a thickening of the tooth. Another cause of malocclusion can be an abnormal chewing behavior associated with abnormal wear, e.g. caused by constant chewing on the cage bars (Wiggs & Lobprise, 1995b; Crossley & Aiken, 2004). Hormones and minerals also have an influence on tooth growth. For example, horizontal enamel grooves and dentin grooves have been experimentally induced in the incisors of rats as a consequence of a hypophysec-

tomy (Schour & Van Dyke, 1932; Becks et al., 1946; Baum et al., 1954) and an undersupply of magnesium (Kusner, Michaeli & Weinreb, 1973; Weinreb, Kusner & Michaeli, 1973).

The most frequent cause of primary malocclusions of incisors in omnivorous rodents (rats, mice, hamsters) is insufficient dental wear due to a lack of surfaces for gnawing provided by the owner (Manville, 1954; Crossley & Aiken, 2004). The elongated incisors cause injuries to soft tissue and problems with feeding and ultimately anorexia. The animals continuously lose weight and exhibit hypersalivation due to the painful mucosal injuries (Figure 9.6). As a result of reduced grooming, many rats develop chromodacryorrhoea ("red eyes") and the eyelids of mice and hamsters also stick together (Wiggs & Lobprise, 1995b).

In small rodents, the incisors do not just grow out of the alveolus forming a simple arcc, but also form a spiral

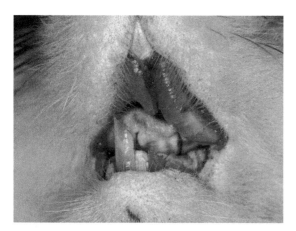

Figure 9.7 Severe incisor malocclusion in a dormouse (postmortem specimen) with marked thickening of the left maxillary incisor and pronounced buccal displacement of the tooth body, abnormal enamel pigmentation of the right mandibular incisor and pathological, oblique occlusal plane of both lower incisors.

(Schour & Massler, 1962; Keil, 1966; Thenius, 1989). As a result tooth elongation always involves a lateral deviation and a concomitant spiral deformation of the tooth. The temporomandibular joint is firmly restricted and does not allow lateral movements in the gnawing position; thus a slight lateral displacement of any individual incisor or a lateral increase of its occlusal surface may already be enough to cause insufficient dental wear of that incisor by the opposing tooth (Miles & Crigson, 2003). Without that functional abrasion, the tooth becomes longer on one side, starts to twist more laterally due to the abnormal pressure and ultimately grows in length unopposed by any kind of tooth contact (Figure 9.7). Depending on the individual curvature of the tooth and the deviation of the elongated incisor, there are often superficial ulcerations or deeper injuries of the lips or the gingiva of the opposing tooth. Only very rarely will the elongated incisors of small rodents simply grow past each other without any kind of contact.

In herbivorous rodents (guinea pigs, chinchillas and degus) poor husbandary resulting in insufficient dental wear is not as important. The animals are not dependent on wearing down their incisors by regularly gnawing on things. In these species it is more important that both the incisors and the cheek teeth are worn down sufficiently by feeding on a suitable fibrous food (coattrision of the incisors during grinding movements).

Purulent incisor infections are relatively frequent, both in omnivorous and in herbivorous rodents. The infection

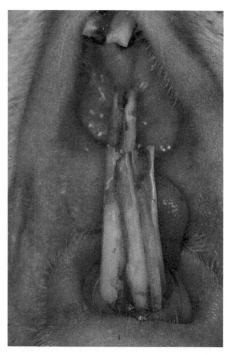

Figure 9.8 Primary incisor malocclusion in a two-year-old guinea pig. The left incisor is thickened and split longitudinally; additional narrow rostral dentin column, enamel and dentin hypoplasia of both mandibular incisors, abnormal length of their visible crowns and pathological occlusal planes on both sides.

most commonly leads to a slight deviation of the tooth with respect to the neighboring tooth, as well as structural changes of the tooth substance in the form of transverse grooves, longitudinal splits, color changes, enamel and dentin hypoplasia, etc. (Figure 9.8). In addition there is increased pain during palpatation of the rostroventral mandibule or in the case of the maxillary incisors, the palatal bone plate. An axial compressive load on the affected tooth and a lateral shear movement are also uncomfortable. Due to the pain, the tooth is no longer worn down correctly, which secondarily leads to overgrowth and the formation of an abnormal occlusal plane. The tooth becomes more mobile as the periodontal ligament enlarges, and often there is a purulent discharge from the alveolus.

Chronic infections of the incisors can be clinically asymptomatic for a long time in guinea pigs and chinchillas. Over time, however, the continuous irritation to the germinal cells will cause the new formation of normal tooth substance to halt, and then only abnormal dental tissue is formed (Figure 9.8). This can also be caused by a mechanical irritation of the apex (abnormal occlusal pressure).

These acquired changes of tooth substance are relatively common in herbivorous rodents, whereas no reports have been found about congenital dysplasias. The incisors become lighter in color (missing enamel or badly mineralized enamel) and more brittle (enamel and dentin hypoplasia). Often they show a enlarged thickening or a longitudinal splitting of the entire tooth structure (Figure 9.5). Dental wear is secondarily altered.

Treatment

Insufficient wear of incisors in small rodents with brachyodont teeth can usually be treated by a single treatment of trimming the incisors (see Section 9.3) and then improving the husbandary (more gnawing possibilities) (Figure 9.6).

If individual incisors are significantly longer than their counterpart, they will hamper the eruption of the latter. In many cases there is no antagonist at all (Figure 9.9) and just a pronounced, painful soft tissue lesion at the site of an empty alveolus. In order to allow new normal tooth growth, the elongated incisor is trimmed down to the gum margin, which in principle will allow the opposite tooth to regrow undisturbed. This, however, requires a functional incisor to be present. This can be confirmed by means of an intraoral radiograph (see Figure 5.44 in Chapter 5). The incisors will then mostly meet again in the normal occlusal plane after two to three weeks. While a subsequent correction may be necessary in some cases, in general the prognosis is good.

In the case of more severe tooth deformations or apical infections, however, a tooth extraction is indicated (see Section 9.4) (Figure 9.10). The apices of the mandibular incisors of omnivorous rodents are located far behind the last molar. Thus the entire ventral mandibular area almost entirely consists of the tooth bodies of the incisors, which are covered with correspondingly thin bone lamellae (see Figures 5.42a and 5.45 in Chapter 5). Particular care needs to be taken when extracting these teeth, to avoid iatrogenic jaw fracture or trauma to the apices of the molars, which lie in close proximity. The luxators that were developed for rabbits are too large to be used in most small rodents (the exception being larger rats). Therefore suitably-sized cannulae that have been bent accordingly are preferentially used for mobilizations of these teeth. An

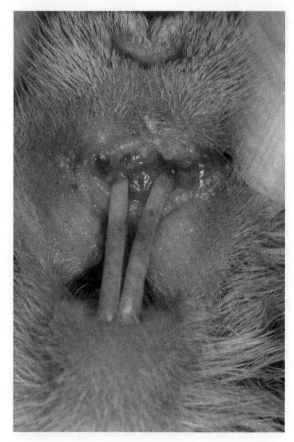

Figure 9.9 Incisor malocclusion in a nine-month-old mouse with marked intraoral elongation of both lower incisors and a secondary maxillary mucosal lesion. There is an indication for a radiographic examination of both maxillary incisors and a substantial shortening of the incisors.

extraction of an incisor can be facilitated by a ventral osteotomy of the tooth socket (Figure 9.10). At the same time, this allows follow-up aftercare of the mandible which may be infected. Postoperatively, the remaining incisor is usually able to sufficiently abrade both antagonists in the long term. Otherwise repeated tooth trimming sessions are going to be necessary.

If there are changes to the tooth structure in herbivorous rodents, then there is an indication to carefully examine and evaluate the intra-alveolar section of the affected incisor radiographically. In most cases a peri- or intradental infection is present, necessitating tooth extraction (see Figure 9.56a later). If, however, the intraalveolar section of the tooth is normal, no treatment is needed. Occasionally the structure of the tooth may

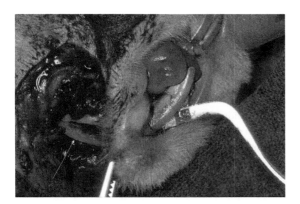

Figure 9.10 Abscess of the (right) mandible in a one-year-old rat, intraoperative view : extraction of the apically ulcerated right lower incisor. The tooth socket is partially dissolved ventrolaterally due to inflammation (white arrow), localization corresponding with an osteotomy and mobilization of the incisor by means of a small Heidemann spatula.

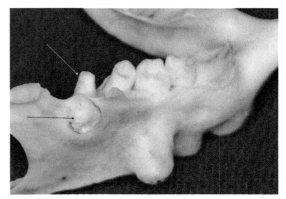

Figure 9.11 Malocclusion in a four-year-old degu (specimen, right mandible) with severe retrograde displacement of the incisor apex with medial (white arrow) and lateral perforation (black arrow) of the mandible in the immediate proximity of the temporomandibular joint, mesial spur on the first cheek tooth (P4; turquoise arrow) and lateral and ventral prominence of the cortical bone of the lower jaw as a result of a retrograde elongation of the first to third cheek teeth (P4–M2; red arrows).

return to normal without any further treatment. For example, there is a chance that at some point, a vertically fractured mandibular incisor of a guinea pig may regrow as a normal tooth. A possible explanation for this is that the germinal cells have not been irreversibly damaged as a result of a singular trauma or unknown specific incident. This indicates that there is only temporary disruption to the normal formation of the tooth that returns to normal as soon as the germinal cells have had time to regenerate (usually within a few weeks).

In cases of chronic duration of split teeth or thickening of tooth substance tooth extraction is indicated earlier on. Experience shows that incisors that have undergone those kinds of changes are unable to regenerate as there has been irreversible damage or irritation of the germinal cells. Because of its abnormal size and thickness, the affected incisor cannot be sufficiently worn down by the opposing tooth (Figures 9.8 and 9.5). This leads to a severe incisor malocclusion requiring constant tooth trimming. A secondary complication from abnormal incisor wear is abnormal wear of the cheek teeth. This is mostly due to an asymmetrical grinding action of the molars (due to incisor asymmetry) or because of pain associated with apical inflammation of the cheek teeth (see Figure 9.35c later). In addition, apical infections may easily extend from the incisors to the molars, or vice versa. This applies not only to the teeth of guinea pigs but also to the molars of chinchillas and degus as well as small rodents (see Figure 9.26 later).

9.1.4 Pseudo-odontomas

A pseudo-odontoma is a dysplastic malformation of tooth substance where odontogenic tissue is continuously deposited in the periapical area of elodont teeth, causing remodeling of the alveolar bone. The maxillary incisors are predominately affected and this has been reported in squirrels, prairie dogs as well as small laboratory rodents or pet rodents (Wagner, Garmann & Collins, 1999; Phalen, Antinop & Fricke, 2000; Ida-Yonemochi et al., 2002; Miles & Crigson, 2003; Crossley & Aiken, 2004; Ohshima et al., 2005; Boy & Steenkamp, 2006; Jekl et al., 2008b). Most publications relate to prairie dogs but the formation of a pseudo-odontoma may occur in all pet species with elodont incisors – for example in rabbits and more frequently than expected in degus (Jekl et al., 2008b) (Figure 9.11 and see Figures 9.13 and 9.17 later). Since many affected animals do not exhibit clinical symptoms in the early stages of the disease, adequate radiographs are necessary for an early detection of changes.

It is mostly a bilateral, primarily benign tumor-like lesion whose pathogenesis has not been clarified (Ohshima et al., 2005). It is supposed, however, that apart from many other factors, chronic apical infections or simply aging processes are the main factors to have an influence on the origin of pseudo-odontomas. Another influence proposed is possible damage of the germinal tissue due to a pronounced retrograde displacement of the apices. Similar apical dysplasias have been provoked experimentally in rats via a hypovitaminosis A (Burn, Orten & Smith, 1941). Viral infections are discussed as another possible cause (Baer & Kilham, 1974). For example, hamsters developed odontomas after having been infected with a specific mouse virus (MVM, minute virus of mice). An osteopetrosis may also be a possible cause (Boy & Steenkamp, 2006). For example, osteopetrotic mice have been shown to mainly exhibit a reduced bone resorption during tooth growth. Hence in those animals, the odontomas were more like a crowding together of odontogenic tissue than a true, excessive proliferation.

In larger rodents, especially prairie dogs, the most important factors responsible for the formation of typical pseudo-odontomas or elodontomas seem to be recurrent injuries or irritations of the incisors, such as tooth fractures that lead to an injury to the surrounding jawbone and the apex (Phalen, Antino & Fricke, 2000). The animals will often keep chewing on the cage bar and one preliminary report states that there is usually a history of a fall from a great height. The traumatic intrusion of the incisors and the apical infections and irritations lead to a damaged germinal, odontogenic tissue. Tooth eruption is further hampered by the chewing on the cage bars, due to the increased axial load of the teeth.

Depending on the type and duration of the trauma, different pathological changes are found in squirrels (Boy & Steenkamp, 2006). In case of a mild, chronic irritation of the germinal cells, there will merely be an irregular formation of enamel and dentin in the area of the labial tooth surface. At first glance, the teeth seem to have hardly changed. Larger, more odontoma-like proliferations are predominantly formed after more severe traumas, such as a fall. The injury causes stem cells and daughter cells to be torn out of their complex and start to form multiple odontogenic islands. Each of those islands will independently continuously form different types of dental hard tissue, and as a result will give rise to so-called hamartomatous masses, which spread uncontrolled in the apical direction (Ida-Yonemochi et al., 2002). This also explains why no normal pulp cavity can be found in teeth that are severely affected (Boy & Steenkamp, 2006).

Odontomas are often called odontogenic hamartomas, particularly in English scientific literature. As odontogenesis occurs throughout life, stem cells in the apical area of hypsodont teeth constantly divide. Those cells, which are constantly renewed, form the ameloblasts, odontoblasts and cementoblasts that are necessary for the formation of teeth (Ohshima et al., 2005). In the case of a hamartoma, abnormal odontogenesis occurs involving the formation of a localized, unorganized, benign excessive tissue – a type of tissue that usually occurs in that localization. Hence odontomas are odontogenic hamartomas. Those benign, tumor-like tooth proliferations can also be called elodontomas as they exclusively affect continuously erupting (elodont) teeth (Boy & Steenkamp, 2006).

Experience has shown that – apart from microtraumas and any hindrances of the tooth eruption – a vitamin A deficiency is a factor in the origin of odontomas (Crossley & Aiken, 2004). If the dental dysplasia is detected before the apical tooth area is more severely deformed and bulbous new formations occur, the situation can often be improved by the following protocol: incisor trimming, enhanced dental wear due to more gnawing possibilities and an adequate supply of vitamin A provided by young grass. On the other hand, however, an oversupply of vitamin A may accelerate apical tooth growth to such an extent that the pseudo-odontoma becomes rapidly larger (Crossley & Aiken, 2004). Hence it should merely be ensured that there is a sufficient supply of natural vitamin A; by no means should it be parenterally substituted.

If the intraalveolar tooth substance has become more markedly folded or if a larger, dense dental mass can be found apically, then the continuous tooth eruption is hampered; ultimately eruption will stop. Since new dental tissue is still being formed apically, the pseudo-odontoma expands internally around the apex growing slowly (Crossley & Aiken, 2004). These proliferations, which are constantly getting larger, are unlikely to cause further complications in the mandible unless they involve the temporomandibular joint, however in the maxilla, they can cause obstruction of the nasal cavity. As these pets are obligate nasal breathers, affected animals exhibit severe respiratory problems, which may even lead to death by asphyxiation (Figures 9.12 and 9.13).

Unless the intranasal, dysplastic dental mass is too large, it can be removed along with the affected incisor

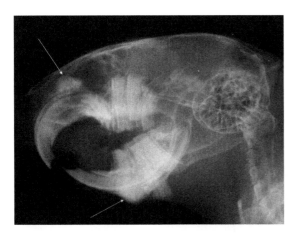

Figure 9.12 Severe malocclusion of the cheek teeth in a five-year-old degu (laterolateral view) with radiopaque swelling dorsal from the maxillary incisor (elodontoma; white arrow), clearly visible step mouth, pronounced retrograde displacement of all apices of the mandibular cheek teeth with perforation of the ventral cortical bone of the lower jaw (M1), slight intraoral overgrowth of the incisors and odontoma-like reconstruction of the apex of the first mandibular cheek tooth (P4; turquoise arrow).

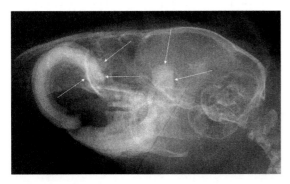

Figure 9.13 Severe incisor malocclusion in a dormouse (laterolateral view) with odontoma formation in the area of the apices of the maxillary and mandibular incisors (white arrows).

via an extraoral, lateral approach (incisor extraction). In the case of larger apical formations that are associated with an inflammatory resorption of intranasal structures (conchae), a rhinotomy or a permanent rhinostomy is performed. Alternatively, a transpalatal approach can be used, which is recommended especially for the removal of intraalveolarly fractured incisors (after an extraction attempt) (Wagner, Garman & Collins,1999). The palatal bone is opened above the apex and the overlying mucosa

is stitched up again after the dental tissue has been removed. Possible complications include the formation of an oronasal fistula.

9.2 Secondary incisor malocclusions

The most frequent disorder affecting the incisors of rabbits as well as herbivorous rodents is an acquired secondary incisor malocclusion, which usually arises as part of a mostly generalized problem of the cheek teeth. A primary incisor malocclusion usually occurs during the first year of age but secondary incisor malocclusions don't usually present before the second year of age. Quite often, however, much younger rabbits are also affected. As cheek teeth elongation advances, the jaws are pushed apart leading to secondary elongation of the incisors. Very slowly, the incisors change in structure, length and shape in a rapidly advancing process that even the animal's owner can easily recognize.

Often the incisors have different lengths and are abnormally curved, structurally altered, deformed or pathologically fractured. In addition, they often have transverse grooves or discolorations of the teeth, both of which indicate an apical irritation (see Figure 9.27 later). Furthermore, there is abnormal occlusion of the incisors and the occlusal surfaces change (they are no longer chisel-shaped). All these changes may indicate an early or advanced primary cheek tooth problem which needs to be addressed by means of a thorough clinical as well as radiographic examination. Merely trimming the incisors will not solve the problem, even though the patient may not be exhibiting any other clinical symptoms that might indicate a molar malocclusion. The sooner the affected cheek teeth are treated, the better the disease can be managed and further treatments delayed. Creating awareness amongst owners that changes to incisors may only be a small symptom of a further underlying problem is essential.

With primary or secondary malocclusion the elongated incisors that immediately contact each other cause a persistent raised, axial load on the apices resulting in a mechanical irritation of the germinal tissue. The clinical signs of this are transverse grooves in the newly-erupting tooth substance. In the case of sustained abnormally high pressure, there will inevitably be a progressive retrograde displacement of the tooth apices that will often be associated with a more pronounced intraalveolar curvature of the teeth in the maxillary area. In the mandible, the apex of the affected incisor visibly migrates to the mesial wall of the first cheek tooth. In the maxilla, the apex becomes progressively closer to the palatal bone plate, which in an extreme case may even be perforated (see Figure 5.29a in Chapter 5). This is very painful during intraoral palpation of the area. An abscess may also develop in that area, but that may be difficult to detect clinically as it continues to be covered by the hard palatal mucosa (Figure 9.14). Changes of this kind are often not detected clinically until the infection has perforated into the oral cavity or the nose, e.g. in a unilateral, chronically purulent rhinitis.

In the mandible where the mandibular incisors are less curved, part of the abnormally increased occlusal pressure is not transferred directly on to the tooth base, but is instead conveyed on to the actual mandible via the ventral alveolar wall. As a result there is remodeling of the alveolar bone causing the incisor to be displaced more ventrally to the ventral mandibular cortex (Figure 9.15). The tooth apex is simultaneously displaced toward the mesial wall of the first mandibular cheek tooth, which allows direct transfer of infection from the incisor to the cheek tooth. The occlusal surface of the mandibular incisor also changes secondary to the changes of the tooth in its socket. Often the incisors will cease to occlude with one another, further worsening the situation.

Often the retrograde displacement of the incisors in the maxilla also causes partial or complete obstruction of the nasolacrimal duct, which runs immediately medioventrally to the tooth apex (Figure 9.16). The duct is anatomically very narrow at that particular point and there is also an abrupt change in its direction here. A periapical remodeling of bone and tooth is responsible

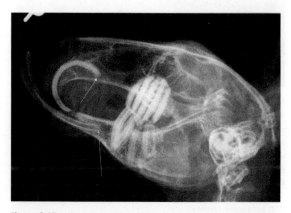

Figure 9.15 Advanced malocclusion of incisors as well as cheek teeth in a six-year-old rabbit (laterolateral view): structural change and pathological shape of the tooth structures as well as severe elongation of all incisors, retrograde displacement of the maxillary incisors (white arrow), rostral displacement of the mandibular base of the incisors (turquoise arrow), unilateral molar step mouth with pronounced intraalveolar deformation of the anterior three lower cheek teeth (P3–M1; presumably unilateral).

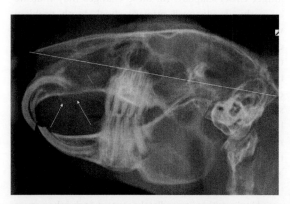

Figure 9.14 Palatal abscess in the maxilla of a three-year-old rabbit (laterolateral view): slight retrograde elongation of the apices of the upper (P3–M2; white line) and lower cheek teeth (P3–M1), significant elongation of the clinical crowns of both maxillary incisors and of the peg teeth, retrograde apex displacement of at least an upper incisor, in the corresponding palatal area formation of a locally restricted bone cavity (abscess; white arrows) and dilation of the nasolacrimal duct (turquoise line).

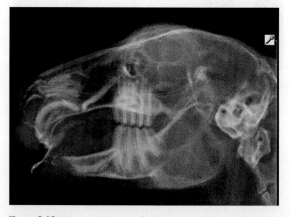

Figure 9.16 Primary incisor malocclusion in a four-year-old rabbit (laterolateral view), contrast study of the nasolacrimal duct; retrograde elongation of at least an upper incisor with secondary compression of the nasolacrimal duct, dentinoid in the tooth socket of a mandibular incisor with periapical osteolysis and normal occlusion in the area of the cheek teeth.

for the progressive narrowing and obstruction of the duct. Occasionally, odontoma-like proliferations may also start to develop which further obstruct the nasal cavity and cause respiratory problems (Figure 9.17).

The pre-stenotic dilated section of the nasolacrimal duct does not drain resulting in persistent, secondary bacterial infections. Any chronic inflammation or obstruction of the nasolacrimal duct (increased watering of the eyes, mostly unilateral, serous or purulent nasal discharge) as well as a (kerato-)conjunctivitis or chronic dacryocystitis that is resistant to treatment is an important indicator of an underlying incisor malocclusion (Figure 9.16) and thus should be indication for a thorough dental examination.

Since the pathological changes are located predominantly intraosseously, radiographs of the head are essential for adequate diagnosis. The nasolacrimal duct should also be flushed on both sides, thereby checking its patency. Saline is the most suitable flushing agent. Apply a local anesthesic eye drop (e.g. Kerakain® eye drops) prior to inserting the fine nasolacrimal cannula and flushing the duct (see Figure 4.8 in Chapter 4). A simple cannula is better suited for rabbits as the punctum lacrimale, which is often poorly visible or not visible at all in an inflamed conjunctiva, can be blindly cannulated more easily. Alternatively, the flexible part of a pediatric peripheral venous catheter is also suitable.

If the irrigating fluid emerging from the nostril is turbid (slightly milky), it indicates a slight purulent infection of the respective duct – whether this is due to the obstruction can only be determined by means of an examination with a contrast agent. If the irrigating fluids contain thicker flecks of pus during treatments, this is a sign of a more severe inflammation or even an intranasal abscess (Figure 9.18). A distension of the cribriform plate may be clinically obvious during palpation (see Figure 5.1 in Chapter 5), as well as a unilateral purulent nasal discharge (see Figure 4.5 in Chapter 4). Eventually, the nasolacrimal duct becomes completely congested by the thick cream-like pus that is typical for rabbits and it cannot be unblocked by flushing. A concomitant feature of chronic infection can be multiple tiny, intracanalicular calculi that contribute to the narrowing of the duct (Figure 9.19). Those calculi tend to

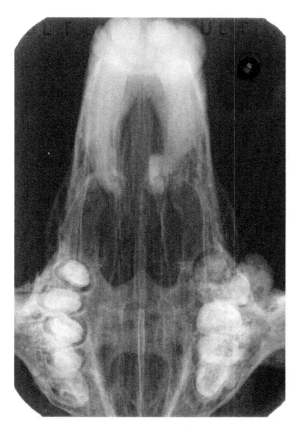

Figure 9.17 Intraoral view of a rabbit with odontoma formation in the area of both maxillary incisors; pronounced apical displacement (on the right), odontoma-like structural change of the first two right cheek teeth (P2/P3), pathological shapes of the rest of the cheek teeth tooth bodies (on the right) and lateral distension of the cribriform plate, indicating a chronic inflammation of the nasolacrimal duct.

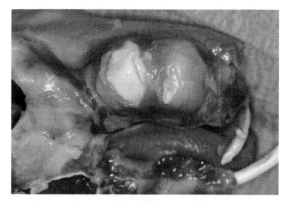

Figure 9.18 Brachygnathia superior in a five-year-old rabbit (specimen) with intranasal abscessation having perforated the outer surface, as a result of a retrograde apex displacement of the right upper incisor with secondary obstruction and purulent inflammation of the nasolacrimal duct.

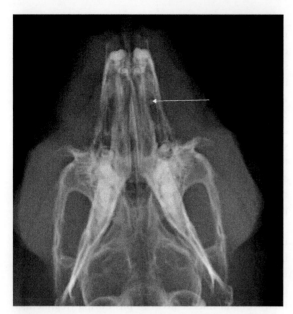

Figure 9.19 Recurring, purulent dacryocystitis in a two-year-old rabbit (dorsoventral view) with small concrement in the right nasolacrimal duct (white arrow) and a two-sided, lateral protrusion of the cribriform plate shortly caudally from the apex of the maxillary incisor, indicating a chronic inflammation of the nasolacrimal duct.

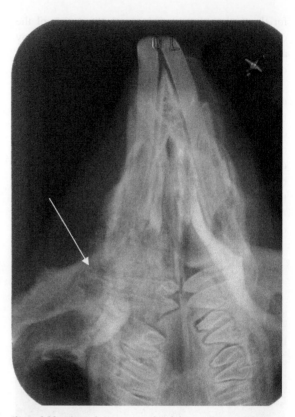

Figure 9.20 Bilateral contrast study of the nasolacrimal duct of a six-year-old guinea pig (intraoral view of the maxilla): no pathological finding on the right side; on the left side there is an interruption of the contrast agent's column where an extensive osteolysis of the maxilla with partial erosion of the outer surface of the first cheek tooth (P4) can be seen. There is also a retrograde displacement of the apex as well as an apical osteolysis (white arrow).

accumulate just before a physiological constriction, i.e. slightly distally from the apical area of the tooth.

When flushing the nasolacrimal duct it is possible to misdiagnose a completed obstructed duct as it may rupture when it is flushed at the site of the obstruction. This will allow the irrigation fluid to flow freely into the nasal cavity despite the peripheral obstruction. In addition, if the pressure is too high during flushing or if the cannula is not handled gently, the flushing fluids may emerge peribulbarly and cause the eye bulb to suddenly protrude from the orbit. If that happens, abort the examination and try again in a few days' time.

When the nasolacrimal duct cannot be flushed or only partially flushed, contrast agents can help to illustrate the intraosseous structure of the duct, its lumen and the exact position of the suspected narrowing or abscessation (see Figure 5.3 in Chapter 5 and Figure 9.20). For dacryocystography, an iodine-containing contrast agent is suitable, e.g. Solutrast® (Iopamidol). A small amount (0.2 ml on each side in rabbits) is injected into the duct without too much pressure immediately prior to the radiographic exposure. Having finished the dacryocystography, the nasolacrimal duct (once) and the eye

(several times) are rinsed with saline solution as the contrast agent can cause severe irritation and a burning pain. In order to protect the conjunctivae, a neutral eye ointment containing vitamin A is applied for one or two days.

If there is only a slight compression of the nasolacrimal duct, the situation may improve after an extraction of the retrogradely displaced incisor, which was responsible for the problem and prevent further compression of the duct. Sometimes the surgery is considered to be too invasive and is not carried out. In the majority of cases, however, there is already a severe obstruction and a chronic-purulent infection of the nasolacrimal duct at the time of first presentation of the patient. The bony part of the duct has often

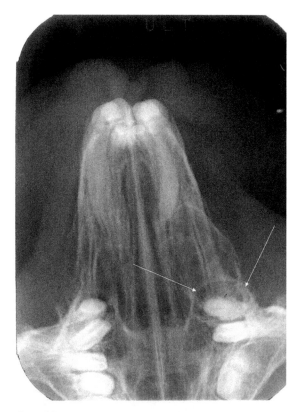

Figure 9.21 Recurring malocclusion of cheek teeth and secondary incisor malocclusion as well as an intranasal abscessation in a four-year-old rabbit (intraoral view of the maxilla); structural change and increased medial displacement of the right incisor, oval bone cavity further caudally in the maxilla and the cribriform plate (abscess originating from the nasolacrimal duct), strong dilation of the periodontium of the first cheek tooth (P2), indicating a purulent periodontitis (white arrow), and structural changes of the caudal cheek teeth (P4/M1). Here further clarification is needed (radiograph of the head in two planes). Moreover, an intraalveolar rotation of the second left upper cheek tooth can be recognized.

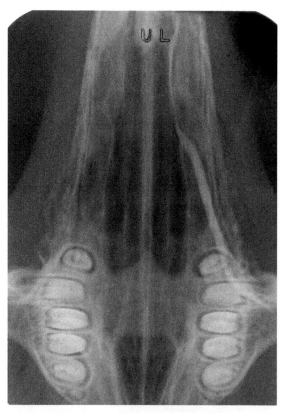

Figure 9.22 Contrast study of the right nasolacrimal duct in a one-year-old rabbit (intraoral view of the maxilla): physiological narrowing of the nasolacrimal duct in the area of the incisor apex and mild dilation of the periodontium of the first cheek tooth (P2).

perforated into the nasal cavity. In those cases, tooth extraction alone will not have much of an effect. This is an indication for a rhino(s)tomy. If larger, tooth-associated intranasal abscesses have formed in the final stage of the disease, then all teeth in the area of the infection need to be extracted in the context of a radical clearance in the area of the abscess (Figure 9.21). This mostly involves the first maxillary cheek tooth (P2), due to the topographic proximity of its apex to the initial section of the bony nasolacrimal duct (Figure 9.22).

Possible differential diagnoses for a persistent infection of the nasolacrimal duct that seems resistant to treatment include: *Pasteurella multocida* causing chronic respiratory infection, a primarily bacterial dacryocystitis that has no dental cause, an intranasal foreign body such as a hay stalk, allergies (rare) or primary pathological changes of the first maxillary cheek tooth, such as a retrograde elongation of the apex with or without periodontal infection.

In herbivorous rodents (guinea pigs, chinchillas and degus), incisor malocclusions mostly have secondary causes (Wiggs & Lobprise, 1995b). The primary cause is also elongation of the cheek teeth. An intraoral elongation of the hypselodont molars causes both jaws to be pushed apart over time. This will inevitably lead to a secondary overgrowth of the incisors. Furthermore, at that stage most incisors are no longer worn down

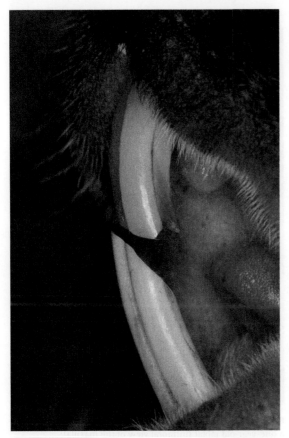

Figure 9.23 Incisor malocclusion in a three-year-old guinea pig (lateral view) with longitudinal splitting of the left maxillary incisor and an indentation of the occlusal surface as well as a slight mandibular prognathism, indicating a malocclusion of the cheek teeth.

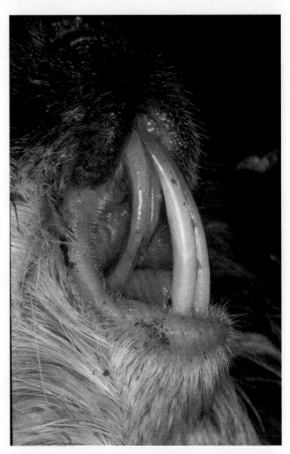

Figure 9.24 Advanced incisor malocclusion in a four-year-old guinea pig with mandibular prognathism and severe overgrowth of all incisors as a result of a primary problem concerning the cheek teeth.

horizontally but instead have an oblique occlusal surface. Sometimes the teeth are also displaced laterally with respect to one another, as a result of a diagonally asymmetrical overgrowth of the molars (see Figure 4.13 in Chapter 4).

At the same time the mandible is displaced more and more rostrally in guinea pigs. The incisors, which at rest are usually at a distance from each other, now immediately occlude with one another. Often the first evidence of a rostral displacement of the mandible is a notch within the occlusal surface of the maxillary incisor(s) (Figure 9.23). As the cheek teeth continue to elongate intraorally, a pronounced mandibular prognathism may develop in an extreme case (Figure 9.24).

Therefore any malocclusion of elongated incisors is a clear indication that there is probably a primary problem of the cheek teeth. This is also true for chinchillas, though here the mandible is displaced caudally in a species-typical fashion (secondary mandibular brachygnathism) (see Section 5.6.3 in Chapter 5, reference lines). Nonetheless, the elongated incisors may still remain in contact. This is because the maxillary incisors, which are more curved, grow toward the elongated mandibular incisors in an arc.

Any change in occlusion of the incisors and the associated abnormal pressures on the apex may damage the germinal tooth tissue (Crossley & Aiken, 2004). This holds true both for herbivorous and for omnivorous rodents. In such cases the newly-formed tooth

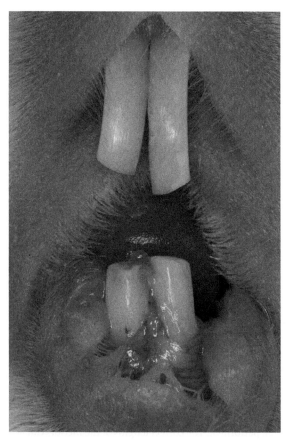

Figure 9.25 Incisor malocclusion in a five-year-old chinchilla with intraoral overgrowth of both upper incisors and slight incisal divergence, shortening of both mandibular incisors with formation of a blunt occlusal surface, pathological tooth color, indicating an apical irritation or infection (lack of pigmentation of the enamel), and hypersalivation.

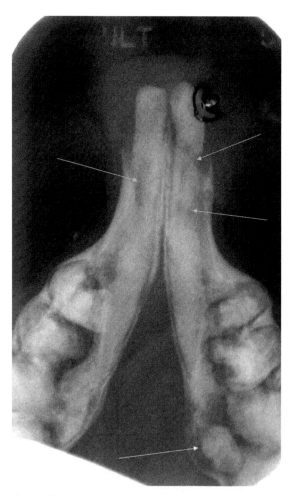

Figure 9.26 Malocclusion of incisors and cheek teeth in a six-year-old chinchilla (intraoral view of the mandible) with severe retrograde displacement and elongation of both incisor tooth bodies which are structurally strongly altered; small isolated tooth fragment on the left apical area with periodontal osteolysis (white arrow), pronounced structural change of all cheek teeth, pathological dilation of the tooth sockets of all incisors and cheek teeth and lytic changes in the area of the tooth bodies of both incisors (turquoise arrows).

substance often has typical transverse grooves and abnormal or patchy discoloration (Figure 9.25). If the eruption of the incisor is also hindered by constant tooth contact, a retrograde displacement of the tooth apex will occur. The tooth apex is displaced further into the bone. In other words, it is displaced toward the palatal bone plate in the maxilla, whilst in the mandible of guinea pigs and chinchillas it is then located ventromedially to the posterior molars or, in smaller rodents, caudodorsally to the last cheek tooth (Figure 9.26). This results in localized pain and abscesses may develop as the changes are progressive over time (see Figure 5.56 in Chapter 5 and Figure 9.35c later). Occasionally, odontoma-like new formations are found in the apical area. In principle those formations may occur in all species, but they are particularly frequent in squirrels and prairie dogs (see Section 9.1.4, pseudo-odontomas).

Treatment

There are two approaches to treating an acquired incisor malocclusion in rabbits: repeated regular shortening of the abnormal incisors or their complete extraction.

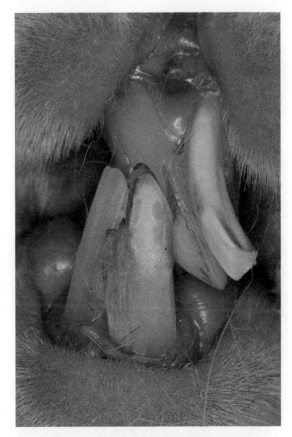

Figure 9.27 Recurring, secondary incisor malocclusion in a seven-year-old rabbit with severe displacement of both upper incisors and an intraalveolar rotation of the left tooth, and marked thickening and partial longitudinal splitting of the left mandibular incisor. There is an indication for intraoral radiographs with subsequent tooth extraction.

There is a higher complication rate (delayed wound healing and postoperative infections) following extraction of some or all of the incisors in older animals with a primarily cheek tooth problem. Frequent regular shortening of the incisors is often recommended instead. This does also depend on the individual case as well as on the particular tooth changes.

If patients suffer from a treatment-resistant, recurring incisor malocclusion where, in addition, the incisors are deformed or structurally altered to such an extent that even after an adequate correction of length of the teeth physiological abrasion is not to be expected in the long term extraction of all incisors is the preferred treatment option (Brown, 1992; Harcourt-Brown, 2002a) (Figure 9.27). There is also an indication for extracting all of the incisors if some or all of the incisors have intraalveolar infection (Figure 9.28a and b). Generally these teeth have marked intraalveolar changes and it does not make sense to try to preserve the remaining incisors in the long term. Intraoral radiographs help to make this decision based on the bony changes seen. It is advisable, however, not to extract all incisors in one session, but to start with the inflamed incisor and then remove the remaining ones as soon as the wound has healed. It is also recommended to use antibiotics to ensure a successful outcome.

If elongated incisors resulting from a primary malocclusion of cheek teeth are to be shortened it is best performed immediately after correction of the cheek teeth. The incisors are shortened to achieve species-specific normal occlusion postoperatively. Following the correction, the mouth is closed, ensuring contact of the cheek teeth, to evaluate whether this has been achieved. The incisor length and position can then be evaluated with respect to one another. If the dentition has been properly corrected, the occlusal edges of the incisors (which are now chisel-shaped again) should be in the correct position and the visible crown heights of both teeth should be identical. If this is not the case, further correction is required.

Postoperative radiographs of the head (laterolateral view) are also useful to evaluate the procedure that has been performed. The correct lengths of the incisors can be accurately evaluated by drawing in the occlusal reference lines. In theory, re-establishing normal incisor occlusion facilitates normal dental abrasion. Unfortunately, this is very rarely effective for longer periods as most patients have dental and jaw pathology that is too far advanced (Figures 9.27 and 9.28a).

Time intervals between tooth-shortening sessions in animals with an acquired incisor malocclusion may vary greatly. They are primarily dependent on the degree of change of the cheek teeth. Incisor shortening may be required more frequently than correction of the cheek teeth and should be managed based on the individual growth rate of the teeth and the pathological changes.

In very advanced dental disease both the incisors and the molars may cease to grow any further and therefore no longer need to be shortened (Figure 9.29). The malformed, elongated incisor crowns are continuously worn down or may fracture in time, but no new tooth substance is formed as the tooth has stopped erupting. This is because the apical germinal cells have undergone severe and irreversible pathological changes. All that

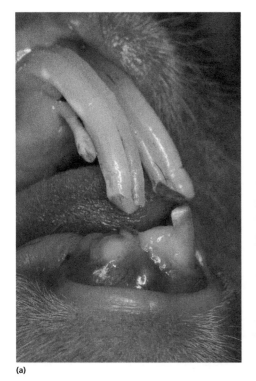

(a)

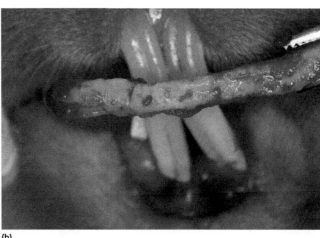

(b)

Figure 9.28 Recurring, secondary incisor malocclusion in a seven-year-old rabbit. (a) Severe overgrowth and enamel hypoplasia of both upper incisors and the visible peg teeth, pathological occlusal plane of all incisors and discharge of pus from the alveoli of the two mandibular incisors, which are clinically strongly shortened. There is an indication for intraoral radiographs as well as an extraction of all incisors. (b) Post extraction of both pathologically changed lower incisors: clearly recognizable apical deformation of the extracted left incisor with typical transverse grooves of the enamel, indicating a chronic apical infection (enamel and dentin hypoplasia). The tooth sac (pulp) is visible in the apical area.

remains are tooth stumps that can be very grotesque-looking and are of no use for chopping up food. Most of these teeth are not painful. Should an infection of the tooth socket occur (with or without loosening of the tooth), it is an indication for tooth extraction.

In the case of an acquired incisor malocclusion, individual incisors may also be mobile. If clinical and radiographic examinations show no indication of an intraalveolar or apical infection, then the affected incisor and its antagonist should be shortened. The aim is to temporarily remove the tooth from occlusion ("immobilization"), which may allow reattachment of the tooth in the tooth socket without any axial pressure. Systemic antibiotics treatment should also be given. This sort of temporary shortening of a tooth may be successful, provided that the mobility is merely due to a trauma. Therapeutic success is rarely achieved as the mobility is usually due to an early infection of the tooth socket. The

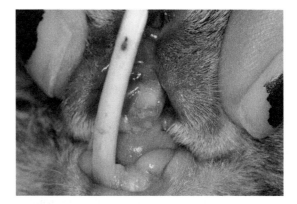

Figure 9.29 Brachygnathia superior in a six-year-old rabbit: growth of the (left) maxillary and mandibular incisor stopped. The right incisors need to be trimmed continuously (every 5 weeks).

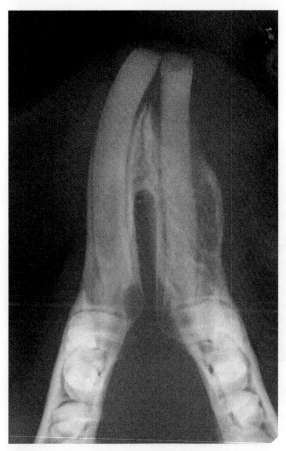

Figure 9.30 Mobile incisor (on the left) in a one-year-old rabbit (intraoral view of the mandible): significant dilation of the tooth socket concomitant with a pathologically altered shape of the intraalveolar tooth body, an indication for tooth extraction.

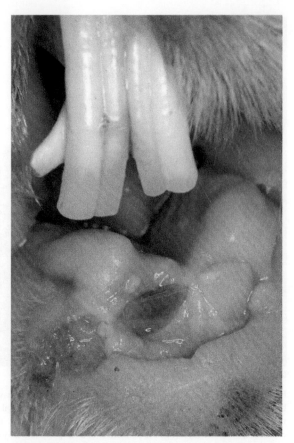

Figure 9.31 Abscess of the (right) mandible in a three-year-old rabbit: pathological discoloration of the right lower incisor as a clear clinical indicator of an apical infection of the tooth root, abnormal elongation and enamel hypoplasia of both upper incisors as well as the right peg tooth and mucosal lesion laterally from the right mandibular incisor (intrusion of the overlong upper incisor).

infection is very difficult to detect radiographically at this stage and it usually only becomes evident when postoperative monitoring radiographs are taken after two to three weeks. If there is clear evidence of infection, tooth extraction is inevitable (Figure 9.30).

Any incisor that shows definitive signs of an intraalveolar or apical infection should be extracted as early as possible in order to prevent further spreading of the infection (Figures 9.31 and 9.34). In the case of a chronic pulpitis (mechanical, infectious or thermal irritation), the disease may be protracted as it is not normally visible on clinical examination. Usually the teeth are painful and the animal is reluctant to use its incisors, resulting in rapid elongation of the tooth despite corrective shortenings. This results in an increased axial load on

the teeth, and ultimately retrograde displacement of the tooth apices. With advancing infection, structural changes of the teeth such as transverse grooves, tooth deformations or discolorations, start to show. These finding are evidence of a more serious chronic (mostly infectious) irritation of the germinal cells. Intraoral radiographs are very useful for specific diagnostics as even slight apical or periodontal changes can be identified relatively easily in their early stages (Figure 9.30). If early symptoms are missed, the initial problem will get worse and will inevitably result in an extensive rostral abscess of the jaw (Figures 9.32 and 9.33).

It is also important to idenitify and extract markedly deformed, malpositioned or structurally altered incisors

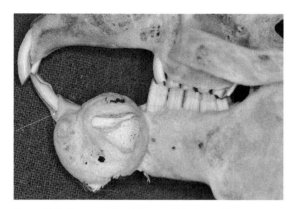

Figure 9.32 Abscess of the (left) mandible in a rabbit (specimen): osseous bone cavity in the rostral area of the lower jaw. The clinical crowns of both mandibular incisors are slightly elongated and incisally offset against each other. The rostroventral tooth socket of the (left) incisor is dilated to a low degree (white arrow). There is an apical tapering of the tooth body of the left mandibular incisor with a structural alteration of the dental hard substance, and a normal occlusion in the area of the cheek teeth.

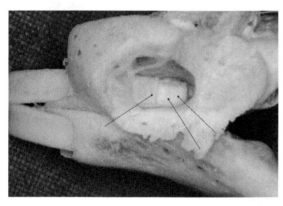

Figure 9.33 Abscess of the (left) mandible in a four-year-old rabbit (mandible specimen, ventral view): extensive bone cavity in the rostral mandibular area, clearly recognizable multiple transverse grooves on the base of the left lower incisor as a result of a chronic irritation of the germinal cells (black arrows).

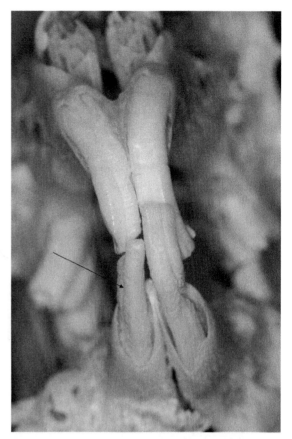

Figure 9.34 Severe malocclusion of the cheek teeth involving formation of an abscess of the lower jaw in a six-year-old rabbit (specimen), pronounced secondary incisor malocclusion, prognathous jaw position, severe structural change (enamel and dentin hypoplasia) and deformation of all incisors, extraalveolar overgrowth of the maxillary incisors, inflammatory dilation of the left mandibular tooth socket, missing longitudinal grooves on the labial surface of the left upper incisor, abnormal occlusal surface of all incisors and a hint of longitudinal splitting of the right mandibular incisor (black arrow).

that can no longer be correctly abraded by their (healthy) antagonists (Figure 9.34) at an early stage, particularly in guinea pigs. An extraction is usually more beneficial for long-term prognosis than repeated shortening and correction. In all cases with incisor changes the intraalveolar area of a tooth should be most thoroughly examined radiographically. This is because infections may easily spread to the anterior two cheek teeth (P4/M1) as well as to the adjacent jawbone, as the apex of the incisor is very close to those two teeth. Frequent complications arising are secondary molar malocclusions whose pathological changes are usually restricted to one side. In order to identify the affected tooth in a guinea pig or a chinchilla, a special exposure for an isolated view of the mandible as described by Böhmer or an intraoral image are required (see Figure 5.56 in Chapter 5). If there are recurrent malocclusions with severe bony changes that are not responding to treatment, euthanasia may be indicated (Figure 9.35a to c).

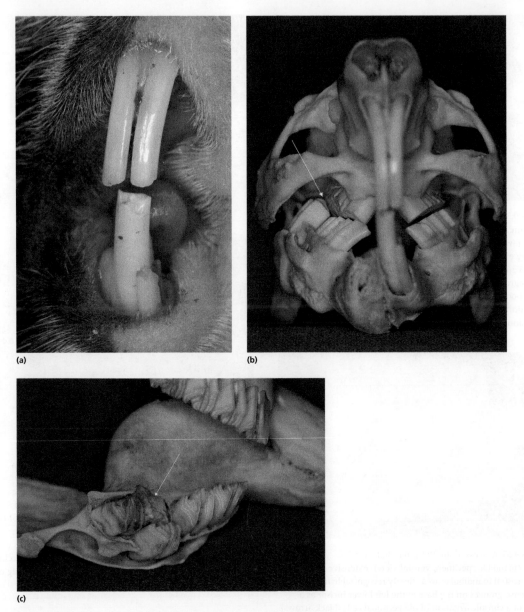

(a)

(b)

(c)

Figure 9.35 Recurring malocclusion of incisors and cheek teeth in a six-year-old guinea pig. (a) The left incisor is thickened and split in the intraalveolar area of the tooth body. The occlusal plane is pathological and the right incisor is missing. There is an indication for intraoral radiographic diagnostics (alternative: isolated radiographic view of the lower jaw according to Böhmer). (b) Looking at the specimen, the malocclusion of the right incisors and cheek teeth can be seen, involving a marked vestibular displacement of the next-to-last molar (M2), a thickening of its extraalveolar tooth body and the formation of a pathological, almost vertical, occlusal surface in the antagonist (white arrow). The clinical crown of the right incisor is missing and there is a thickening and longitudinal splitting of the left lower incisor. (c) The mandible specimen shows an intermandibular thickening of the jaw with a pronounced medial distension of the right mandible as a result of a chronic intraalveolar incisor infection and a lateral displacement of the next-to-last cheek tooth (M2) caused by the apex of the extremely altered incisor (white arrow), which is severely retrogradely displaced.

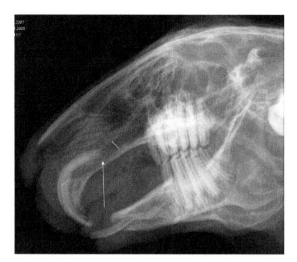

Figure 9.36 Incisor malocclusion in a three-year-old rabbit (laterolateral view) with marked intraalveolar deformation of the lower incisor, intraoral overgrowth and pathological shapes of the two maxillary incisors concomitant with retrograde displacement of the apices toward the palatal plate (white arrow), secondary dilation of the nasolacrimal duct (white line), increased radiopacity of the tympanic bulla and fairly normal occlusion of the cheek teeth.

Due to a secondary enamel and dentin hypoplasia, many incisors that need to be extracted are brittle, which significantly raises the risk of intraoperative, iatrogenic fractures. In addition, those tooth bodies are often very deformed intraalveolarly (abnormal curvature and twists), partially dissolved due to infection or already fractured, and the apices of those teeth are sometimes displaced far retrogradely (Figure 9.36). In the apical area of some incisors (similar to rodents with an elodontoma), an additional proliferation of dental tissue that is rather unstructured and radiodense can be seen or the entire intraalveolar section may be restructured in that way. Those kinds of changes are particularly found in the maxillary incisors of older rabbits (see Figure 9.17). If no trace of a pulp cavity can be identified in the remodeled apex, it is improbable that the incisor will grow any further. In that case, the incisor can be left without a problem after a correction of the dentition has been performed (Harcourt-Brown, 2002a).

In order to identify and record all those dental findings within the alveolus correctly and to be able to evaluate the periapical bone tissue accordingly, a diagnostically conclusive radiograph is always taken immediately prior to a planned tooth extraction (Figure 9.37). Even if there are

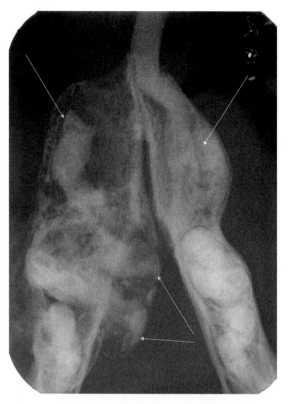

Figure 9.37 Recurring malocclusion of incisors and cheek teeth in a four-year-old rabbit (intraoral view of the mandible), with pronounced intraalveolar deformation and osteoma-like reconstruction of the left lower incisor (white arrow), a structurally altered rest of an incisor in the apical area of the right alveolus (turquoise arrow), high-degree structural change of all visible cheek teeth and retrograde elongation of the first two right lower cheek teeth (P3/P4) with perforation of the medial cortical bone of the jaw (yellow arrows).

no such clinical symptoms, there will often be periodontal or periapical infections that have already spread to adjacent tissues or, in rabbits, to the first mandibular cheek tooth (P3). If these are not detected and included in the treatment, complications with wound healing as well as recurrent abscessation may occur following tooth extraction. If this happens, a second surgery requiring an osteotomy to access the alveolus and associated bone is required to enable systematic local treatment (see Section 9.4.1 below, osteotomy and abscess surgery).

When managing secondary incisor malocclusions with no structural changes to the teeth or infection, of herbivorous rodents, the focus is on treating the primary malocclusion of the cheek teeth. Following correction of the molar dentition, the elongated incisors are shortened with a cutting disc impregnated with diamonds, and the occlusal surface remodeled to a chisel-shaped. After correct trimming of the teeth, the incisors should be at their correct species-specific distance from one another, with their tips located on a horizontal level (see Section 5.6.2 in Chapter 5, reference lines).

9.3 Trimming of incisors

When trimming elongated or incisors with other pathology, e.g. an oblique fracture involving sharp edges or a thickening of the tooth body, complications can be avoided by using a cutting disc impregnated with diamond dust. In order to protect soft tissues (lips and tongue), a suitably-sized wooden spatula can be placed behind the incisors and held by an assistant, whilst holding the head of the animal (Figure 9.38). The cutting disc provides an especially easy way of reconstructing a chisel-shaped occlusal edge that slopes intraorally, after the incisor has been shortened. The rotating disc is positioned at a suitable angle on the occlusal surface before modeling the tip of the tooth accordingly.

Alternatively, suitably shaped and sized diamond burs can be used to trim the incisors, starting from their lateral surfaces, and then remodel a chisel-shaped occlusal surface. There are different recommendations concerning the optimal rotation velocity of the instruments (fast- or slow-rotating micromotor).

> The teeth need to be consistently water-cooled whilst burring as the intense heat can cause a sterile pulpitis or even a pulp necrosis (thermal tooth damage).

When using slow-rotating instruments, a cotton swab soaked in water serves that purpose; it is repeatedly brought into contact with the tooth during trimming. When using fast-rotating turbines, direct water-cooling (integrated water jet) is always employed because of the increased risk of overheating. This is usually no problem if the patient is placed in lateral recumbency and its head is slightly lowered (danger of pulmonary aspiration).

When using the cutting disc, any sharp edges that might be present after trimming can be smoothed relatively easily. When using only a bur, however, this is a bit less comfortable as the device tends to slip off the tooth, leaving the edges more uneven.

Patients with pronounced brachygnathism do not need to have their teeth trimmed to form a chisel shape

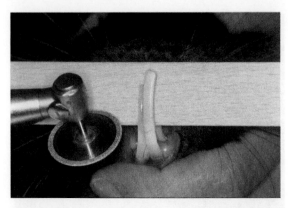

Figure 9.38 Rabbit with elongated mandibular incisors and brachygnathia superior; trimming using a cutting disc impregnated with diamond dust and protection of soft tissue with a wooden spatula.

as the incisors usually do not occlude, even after a correction of length. In such cases, the incisors are more usually trimmed to form a planar shape as this protects the soft tissue better (tongue).

> Elongated incisors should NEVER be clipped.

Clipping regularly causes splits or longitudinal fractures of teeth. If there are also intraalveolar fissures, the pulp cavity can be iatrogenically exposed (see Figure 8.9 in Chapter 8). This isn't visible as the typical central pin-prick hemorrhage at the shortened occlusal surface; instead blood will emerge at the tooth's surface via fine fissures, in a rather linear fashion. If this isn't detected and therefore not treated (vital amputation of the pulp with direct capping), a septic pulpitis can develop which may lead to an apical abscess or an infectious inflammation of the germinal cells (resulting in secondary enamel and dentin hypoplasia). Often a tooth that was iatrogenically injured eventually needs to be extracted. Should the animal's owner be present during such mistreatment, it will be merely a matter of time before he decides to cut costs and trim the incisors himself, using a pair of pliers or even nail clippers.

Trimming the incisors at regular intervals leads to an increased growth rate of the teeth and an coronal extension of the pulp cavity containing the sensitive pulp tissue, beyond the gingival margin (Crossley, 2001b). This will increase the risk of exposing the pulp during shortening of the incisors, particularly when the teeth need to be radically trimmed close to the gum

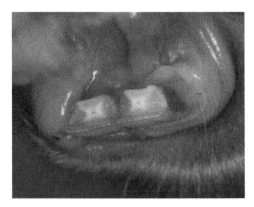

Figure 9.39 Mandibular incisors of a rabbit. The area of the central pulp cavity that is sealed with atubular dentin is clearly visible.

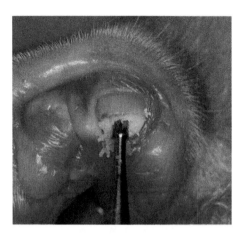

Figure 9.40 After the pulp cavity of a rabbit's right mandibular incisor has been exposed; preparation of a cavity by means of a cylindrical bur and the best possible shaping of overhanging cavity margins so that filling material, which is subsequently inserted, can be rooted better.

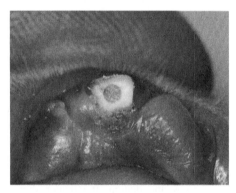

Figure 9.41 Following preparation of the cavity of a rabbit's right mandibular incisor; pulp bleeding has stopped (burring dust).

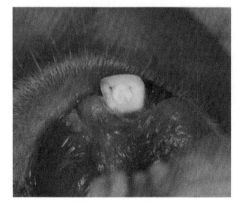

Figure 9.42 After filling the cavity of a rabbit's right mandibular incisor with self-curing calcium hydroxide. There is an indication for sealing of the opened dentin canals with fluoride varnish.

margin. Hence routine shortening of incisors must always be performed very carefully in increments for safety reasons. An imminent opening of the pulp cavity can be noticed as a slight, central discoloration of the dental hard tissue on the surface (Figure 9.39). After initially trimming the incisor down to a point clearly above the level of the gingiva, the tooth is subsequently shortened in increments down to the desired crown height, using the cutting disc impregnated with diamond dust or a suitable bur. In theory, a coronal extension of the pulp cavity can be limited by more frequent, less aggressive shortenings of the incisors. It is questionable whether the owner will agree to this as it significantly raises the costs of treatment.

If the pulp cavity is accidentally exposed (or in case of traumatic fractures), endodontic treatment of the tooth is necessary in order to prevent a pulpitis and a subsequent apical infection. The incisor and its surrounding tissues are thoroughly cleaned and disinfected, e.g. with Betaisodona® (Povidone-iodine) for the oral cavity, before the coronal part of the exposed tooth nerve is resected aseptically, if possible, whilst performing of a cavity preparation (vital amputation; Figures 9.40 and 9.41). When preparing the cavity, a slight incisor wall overhang should be established so that the filling material placed can be anchored more safely. In order to stop the bleeding (which is usually very slight), the ends of tiny paper points or delicate cotton pellets are temporarily placed in the cavity. The paper points are removed and the preparation can then be filled with a thin layer of self-cured or light-cured calcium hydroxide (Figure 9.42). The direct pulp capping procedure stimulates the vital odontoblasts in direct contact with the restoration to form tertiary dentin which, after a while, will cover the coronal margin of the pulp cavity with a dentinal bridge. Below this, the vital pulp will usually retract toward the apex. The calcium hydroxide restoration within the tooth is consistently worn down together with the dentin if the incisors are in occlusion. Healing is supported with systemic antibiotics and nonsteroidal anti-inflammatories.

A final restoration placed over the calcium hydroxide using amalgam or any dental composite as used for brachyodont teeth is not indicated as these substances are too hard when compared with the dentin and enamel of the occluding tooth, which would alter the normal abrasion of the teeth (Wiggs & Lobprise, 1995c). Also, the materials are potentially toxic when swallowed as the tooth erupts and the restoration is displaced.

9.4 Extraction of incisors

Before performing an incisor extraction – whether dealing with a healthy tooth (brachygnathism) or a pathological tooth – the owner must be informed about the risk of iatrogenic intraalveolar fractures, depending on structure, shape and length of the incisor. Complications may occur even when proceeding extremely carefully. Particularly the small peg teeth are at a risk of fracturing. In most cases, however, the short length of the reserve crown allows the apex to be easily luxated with a thin cannula and then removed using delicate, curved mosquito forceps. In addition, the owner should be

aware that one or two incisors may regrow even if the germinal tissue has been removed *lege artis* or devitalized during the incisor extraction. The only way to definitely prevent an extracted tooth from regrowing is to remove the entire pulp with all formative cells (apically adhering "tooth sac") or to destroy any germinal cell that may still be present intraalveolarly (Figure 9.43). On the other hand, if some part of the pulp tissue remains in the tooth socket, then a new, usually deformed, tooth will be formed again after a few weeks or months (Steenkamp & Crossley, 1999) (Figure 9.44). If that happens, a second surgery will be necessary, increasing the costs.

Incisor extraction

Cleaning and disinfection the operating field (teeth, oral mucosa, lips)

Severing of the epithelial connection (18- to 20-gauge needle)

Break down the periodontal fibers (special luxator or 16- to 18-gauge needle)

Continuous luxation of the tooth

"Arc-like" extraction (manually or with a Pean clamp)

Osteotomy of the alveolus in case of complications or primary infections

If possible, no rinsing of the tooth socket (risk of "dry socket syndrome")

Rinsing of the tooth socket and curettage of the alveolus in case of apical infections (additional osteotomy)

Removal of the peg teeth

Analgesia

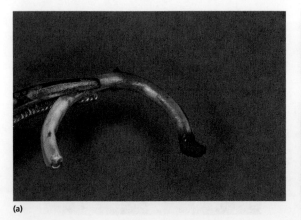
(a)

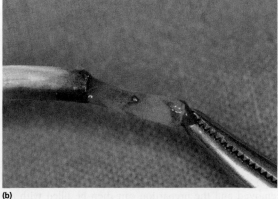
(b)

Figure 9.43 Extracted maxillary incisor in a rabbit: (a) with an apically adhering "tooth sac" (pulp) and (b) with slightly pulled-out pulp.

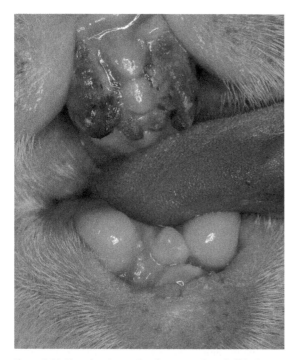

Figure 9.44 Situation 2 months after extraction of all incisors in a six-year-old rabbit: marked structural change of both newly-formed maxillary incisors (insufficient destruction of the germinal cells) and of the peg teeth located medially from there. The mandible is asymptomatic. There is an indication for another tooth extraction after a radiographic check of the intraalveolar tooth body.

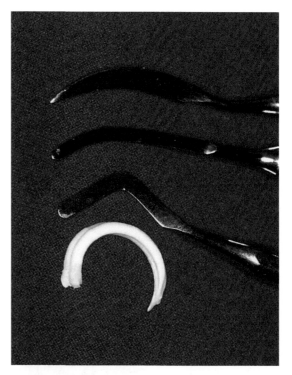

Figure 9.45 Upper incisor of a rabbit with brachygnathia superior and various dental luxators (from top to bottom): according to Crossley and Fahrenkrug, according to Remeeus and Fahrenkrug, and a Heidemann spatula.

If extraction of all incisors is planned, it is best to start with the mandibular incisors before the maxillary ones are removed. The peg teeth are extracted last. As a general rule, an extraction is easier the longer the incisors are at the time of surgery.

Tooth extractions should ideally be performed under aseptic conditions; thus sterile gloves and instruments should be used. In addition, the teeth, the adjacent oral mucosa and the lips are cleaned and disinfected (Betaisodona® or Chlorhexidine® solution for the oral cavity). After performing a local anesthesia (see Section 7.3.2 in Chapter 7, intraligamentary injection or nerve block), a cannula (18- to 20-gauge) or the tip of the scalpel blade is used to cut the gingiva from around the tooth in order to loosen the gingival attachment. To do this, the cut end of the cannula must face the surface of the tooth. Extend the incision into the alveolar socket as this will create space and make it easier to position the tooth luxator into the periodontal ligament. Special

luxators have been developed for use in rabbits that are designed in an arc to breakdown the periodontal ligament fibers (Crossley, 1994). There are different types with blunt or sharp working ends and various degrees of curvature (Figure 9.45). Alternatively, a Heidemann spatula may be used, a conventional spatula for mixing substances in dentistry; its working end can be sharpened with a grindstone in order to facilitate introduction into the alveolus (Böhmer, 2003). This has proven to be successful in tooth extractions, particularly in the the maxilla as it aligns better with the marked curvature of the maxillary incisors (Figure 9.45). By contrast, the specially designed luxators are better adapted to the curvature of the mandibular incisors. Their sharp-edged ends allow easy introduction into the mandibular tooth sockets (Figure 9.46). If the luxator is used to loosen a maxillary incisor, it must be placed carefully into the alveolus in line with the curvature of the tooth structure. Otherwise there will be a risk of perforating the alveolar bone dorsally with the instrument

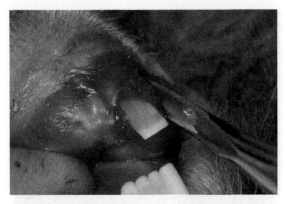

Figure 9.46 Apically infected right mandibular incisor of a two-year-old rabbit: situation after positioning of the luxator in the lateral tooth socket and tearing of the periodontal fibers involving hemorrhaging into the alveolus and secondary loosening of the tooth. The extraction site on the left has healed (removal of tooth 2 months before) and the upper incisors are worn down correctly.

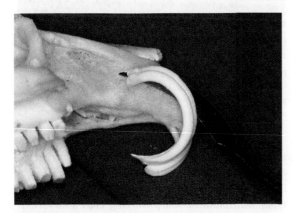

Figure 9.47 Incisor malocclusion in a rabbit (specimen of the maxilla): position of the luxator for a mobilization of the maxillary incisor. There is a risk of perforating the nasal cavity if the tip of the instrument is guided too steeply.

and to perforate the nasal cavity (Figure 9.47). The resulting epistaxis acutely obstructs respiration and secondarily predisposes the rabbit to an iatrogenic, usually purulent rhinitis. Alternative instruments that can be used for tooth extractions are long cannulae (16- to 18-gauge), which are bent into shape to match the curvature of the teeth (bend the cannula to the shape based on the radiographs) (Harcourt-Brown, 2002b).

In order to loosen the tooth, the luxator is introduced into the periodontal space on all four aspects of the tooth, applying a slight, consistent pressure. Work

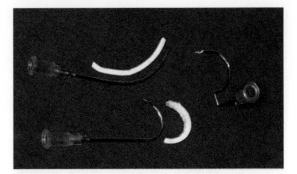

Figure 9.48 Cannulae for a curettage of the empty alveoli of the mandibular and maxillary incisors. The curvature corresponds to the curvature of the extracted incisor tooth body.

from the mesial aspect around the tooth, finishing with the palatal/lingual surface (Figure 9.46). Pressure is maintained for approximately 20 seconds at each point, causing the fibers to tear (Crossley, 1994). The intraalveolar bleeding resulting from this helps to destroy more fibers and helps to continuously loosen the incisor as it pushes the tooth structure in the opposite direction.

If the tooth is sufficiently loose, grip it with two fingers before gently rocking the tooth in a see-saw movement with a slight simultaneous rotation. Alternatively, Pean forceps may be used to carefully grip the incisor. Provided the tooth is sufficiently loosened, it will then be possible – either manually or by means of those forceps – to pull it out of the alveolus, applying gentle continuous traction whilst moving the tooth in a curved direction, the same as the curvature of the tooth. It is advisable to remain patient and not to tilt the tooth as this can easily lead to intraalveolar fracturing. Following extraction check whether the tooth is complete and whether the germinal tissue (and pulp), which usually adheres to the tooth apex as a small lump of tissue has also been removed – if not, the tooth may regrow (Figure 9.43).

If there are remains of the pulp or germinal sac in the tooth socket, they need to be destroyed. This can be achieved by curetting the apical alveolar area with a cannula that has been bent into shape based on the shape of the extracted tooth (Böhmer, 2003) (Figure 9.48). Occasionally, at least for the mandibular teeth, the germinal tissue can be grasped and removed using fine, curved mosquito forceps, which are introduced deeply

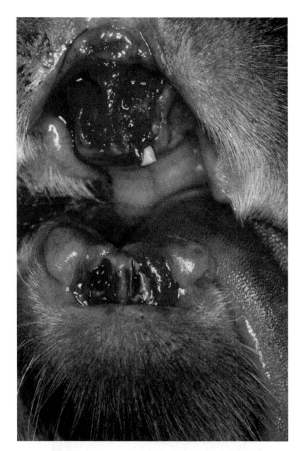

Figure 9.49 Situation in a rabbit after incisor extraction. The left peg tooth is still left to be removed.

into the empty tooth socket (Steenkamp & Crossley, 1999). Alternatively, the alveolus can be curetted out with a small, sharp curette. This is usually not possible for the maxillary incisors as the alveolar sockets are more markedly curved. The extracted tooth itself may also be used. Its apical section is moistened with iodine solution and then reintroduced into the tooth socket and pushed against the base of the alveolus for about 20 to 30 seconds, making rotating and seesawing movements (tooth intrusion) (Steenkamp & Crossley, 1999). The sharp apical edges will destroy the germinal tissue, preventing regrowth of the tooth (see Figure 2.3 in Chapter 2).

Having extracted the four large incisors, the peg teeth are then extracted (Figure 9.49). Their individual shapes vary greatly; they are either short and relatively straight or longer and slightly curved, just like the large incisors.

They can be luxated using fine cannulae. These are introduced deeply into the alveolus on all four sides of the peg teeth, with the cutting face pointing toward the tooth at an acute angle. Since the peg teeth are rather thin, they tend to fracture easily while being loosened. If any of their tooth fragments have remained in the alveolus during this, they can be identified relatively easily, loosened by a slight dilatation of the alveolus and then extracted.

Following any tooth extraction, the alveolus usually fills with blood that slowly coagulates, thus largely occupying the hollow space within the bone. Postoperative flushing of the tooth socket should not take place unless it is absolutely necessary to avoid disrupting this clot. This can significantly delay healing (alveolitis sicca or "dry socket syndrome"). If however, there are intraalveolar infections that require consequent postoperative wound irrigation, this is not the case. Suturing the socket by placing gingival sutures is not necessary and it may also prevent early detection of postoperative complications such as intraalveolar infection.

Intraalveolar fractures of a tooth can occur if the extraction is rushed, or the instruments are not used correctly (incorrect levering movements, tilting the tooth). This usually happens in the area of the apex as the walls of the tooth are particularly thin at the apical foramen. In some cases the remaining fragment, which has already been loosened but is still present in the alveolus, can be skewered or impaled by turning a pointed instrument (for example a Hedström file or nerve broach) that has been introduced into the wide-open pulp cavity. It can then be extracted by constantly tugging and making small tilting movements. If this fails because the tooth base has not yet been sufficiently loosened during the extraction attempt, it must be assumed that the tooth is going to regrow.

In that case, the removal of the tooth is suspended and postponed to a later stage. After four to six weeks, the newly-formed incisor will usually have reached a length that allows its removal in a second session. Depending on the extent of trauma to the tooth apex that occurred during the primary mobilization of the tooth, the regrown incisor can be structurally altered (enamel and dentin hypoplasia). Often there will be additional intraalveolar deformations and dental narrowings predisposing the tooth again to iatrogenic fractures. Hence special caution must be taken during a second attempt to extract an incisor. If necessary, an osteotomy of the tooth socket can be performed (see Section, osteotomy and abscess surgery).

However, not all incisors that have fractured intraalveolarly during an extraction attempt will regrow correctly. A possible reason for this is the fact that eruption of the regrowing tooth is hampered by intraalveolar scar tissue such that the tooth cannot erupt or can only erupt incompletely from the alveolus (Steenkamp & Crossley, 1999). In that case, the most prominent radiographic feature is an intraalveolar, mostly unstructured, dentinoid. If the jawbone that surrounds the tooth is not inflamed, it can be left and monitored for longer time.

Another possible reason that teeth are not reformed after an intraalveolar incisor fracture during an extraction attempt is due to an iatrogenic devitalization of the pulp. This will happen if, during an extraction attempt an incisor has already been markedly mobilized prior to fracturing, the pulp would have become irreversibly damaged. Non-vital tooth fragments that remain in the tooth socket like this become "foreign bodies." As a result they almost always lead to an intraalveolar infection and thus need to be removed. In order to completely extract tooth fragments and prevent a bony infection, an osteotomy of the tooth socket is performed (see Section 9.4.1, osteotomy and abscess surgery).

Occasionally a tooth fragment positioned relatively deep in the tooth socket will regrow after an incisor extraction, despite the germinal cells having been correctly destroyed. If such an intraalveolar tooth structure, which usually is severely abnormal in shape, is detected during a radiographic follow-up examination, check whether there is inflammation or localized infection present. If the dentinoid does not cause any long term problems and remains in the tooth socket with the rest of the socket filled with cancellous-like bone it is unlikely that complications will arise as the growth of the tooth-like material has usually been arrested and will not be expected to grow any further (Figure 9.50). Nonetheless, the patient will need regular monitoring. However, if radiographs show any changes indicating localized infection (usually seen as a periodontal radiolucency), the tooth fragment needs to be removed (Figures 9.51 and 9.52).

If a single maxillary or mandibular incisor is extracted, extraction of the opposite incisor is usually not indicated at that point. Experience has shown that the single remaining tooth will sufficiently abrade the two

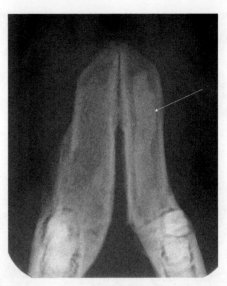

Figure 9.50 Situation in a two-year-old rabbit after extraction of the lower incisors 4 months before (intraoral view of the mandible); regrown left incisor (white arrow) and unproblematic position in the jaw, thus no indication for extraction.

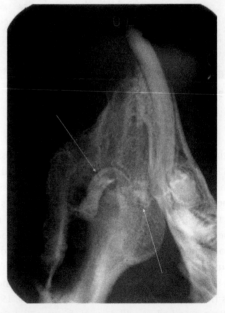

Figure 9.51 Situation in a three-year-old rabbit (intraoral view of the mandible) 2.5 months after extraction of all teeth of the right lower jaw. There are two newly-formed dentinoids: a roundish, nonirritating structure in the jawbone in the area where the apex of the incisor used to be and more elongate dental tissue on a level with the first cheek tooth (P3; white arrows). Due to the slight periodontal osteolysis, there is indication for extraction.

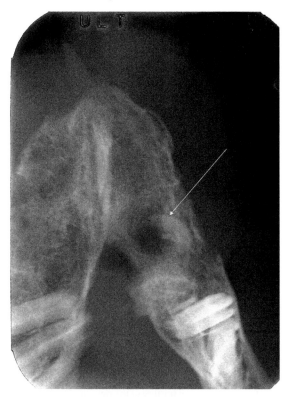

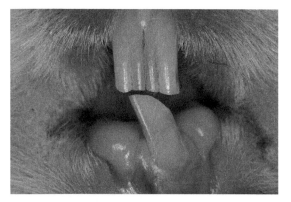

Figure 9.53 Situation in a three-year-old rabbit 3 months after extraction of the right lower incisor. The left mandibular incisor is tilted slightly mesially. The occlusal plane is oblique, but apart from this there is normal occlusion.

Figure 9.52 Situation in a six-year-old rabbit (intraoral view of the mandible) 2.5 months after bilateral extraction of the lower incisors and cheek teeth (right P3/P4). As there is regrown dentinoid on the left side with apical osteolysis (white arrow), there is an indication for extraction of the dentinoid. The rostral part of the right half of the jaw is without pathological findings.

antagonists – both in rabbits and in rodents. The occlusal plane, however, changes in most cases. The occlusal edge of individual or all teeth is no longer horizontal but slightly oblique instead (Figure 9.53) and the remaining incisor tilts slightly toward the extraction site as it lacks support from the neighboring tooth. As a result of the pressure changes on all incisors due to the asymmetry secondary pathological changes can occur in the apical area. Patients are regularly monitored ideally requiring intraoral radiographs as well as a clinical examination. Intraoral radiographs detail the intraalveolar area of teeth and facilitate a more thorough evaluation.

Since incisors are usually only extracted if they become non-functional or even hamper an animal's feeding (brachygnathism), most patients do not have problems adapting to the new postoperative situation. They usually

take little time in getting used prehending chopped-up food with their lips. Many of them will have adopted that way of feeding whilst they were suffering from the more severe types of incisor malocclusion before their current therapy. The incisors of rabbits, however, do not just serve to chop up suitable pieces of food. They provide support in grooming as they are used to pluck dead hairs. Hence there can be fur problems such as tangled hair after an extraction. In such cases, the owner is required to provide care by regularly brushing the fur.

9.4.1 Osteotomy and abscess surgery

Often extensive infections or jaw abscesses in the apical areas of pathological mandibular incisors cannot be sufficiently resolved by merely extracting the affected incisor – despite ongoing local treatment including regular flushing of the tooth socket and the administration of antibiotics (Figure 9.54). There is a risk of the infection spreading further within the bone, without any accompanying clinical symptoms until an abscess of the mandible forms and spreads to the adjacent premolar (P3). A ventral osteotomy of the infected tooth socket will allow immediate access to the center of infection, which can then be allowed to heal by secondary intention and regular monitoring.

An osteotomy is also indicated in the case of an extraction of mandibular incisors that are fractured or completely abnormal in shape and structure (Figure 9.55). The procedure is also necessary when removing mandibular incisors showing signs of resorption due to

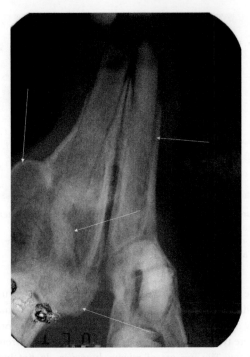

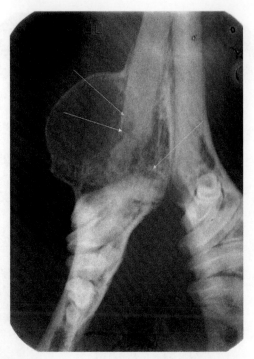

Figure 9.54 Rostral abscess (on the right) in a two-year-old rabbit (intraoral view of the mandible): right incisor with severe apical deformation and a periapical distension of the jawbone (white arrows), slight dilation of the left incisor tooth socket (rostrolateral part) (turquoise arrow), the first right mandibular cheek tooth (P3) is missing and there is an indication for extraction of the right incisor to go along with ventral osteotomy of the jaw as well as radical abscess surgery. Regular checks of the left incisor, or an extraction of that tooth in the case of clinical loosening, should be performed.

Figure 9.55 Rostral abscess of the jaw in a two-year-old rabbit (intraoral view of the mandible): presumably inflamation-related, apical transverse fracture of the right lower incisor (white arrow), bone cavity protruding laterally in that area, small lytic changes of the right incisor rostrolaterally from the fracture site (turquoise arrow), slightly blurred translucency in the mesial apical area of the decently retrogradely elongated first right cheek tooth (P3; yellow arrow) and an indication for tooth extraction with ventral jaw osteotomy as well as radical abscess surgery.

infection and inflammation (Figure 9.56a and b) or when there is remaining dental tissue in the alveolus after an incomplete tooth extraction (Figure 9.57). Preoperative radiographs are required to identify abnormalities prior to surgery (intraoral images or isolated views of the mandible in guinea pigs and chinchillas, as described by Böhmer). The osteotomy will allow access for both removal of teeth or their remains with minimal risk of complications and an optimal postoperative healing period.

Unless the jaw has already become partially osteolytic due to infection (which often provides some access to the tooth socket; Figure 9.58), the alveolus is opened in the deepest possible area, using a small suitably-sized bur (Figure 9.56c). The area of the osteotomy can then be enlarged as needed by means of

fine Luer bone rongeur forceps and the dental tissue can be removed without complications (Figure 9.56d and e). The intraalveolar center of infection can be flushed and cleaned via the osteotomy site over the course of several days or weeks if necessary; afterwards it can be plugged with iodoform gauze previously soaked in a mixture of sugar and an appropriate local ointment (Figure 9.56f). This allows the tooth socket to heal from within the oral cavity while the infected alveolar area can be kept open ventrally for as long as needed and treated according to individual requirements.

While an osteotomy is always recommended in the case of an extraction of purulent mandibular incisors, tooth extraction can sometimes be done without an

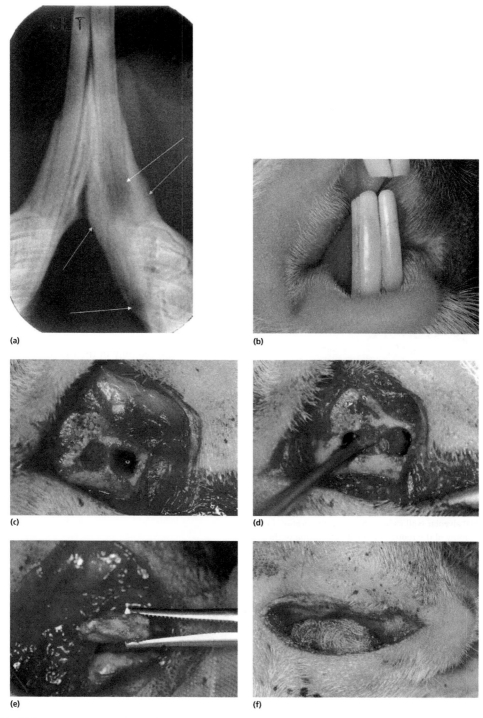

Figure 9.56 Thickening and splitting of the left lower incisor in a two-year-old guinea pig. (a) The intraoral view of the mandible shows an intraalveolar and apical lysis of the left incisor (white arrows) and inflammatory bone proliferations in the area of the rostral mandible (turquoise arrows). There is an indication for a tooth extraction with ventral osteotomy of the mandible. (b) The clinical picture shows the thickening and splitting of the right lower incisor. (c) Situation during the operation: ventral osteotomy of the incisal alveolus with two drillings. The lower jaw is slightly distended in the apical area and structurally changed superficially (blurred bone structure on the left of the picture). (d) Situation during the operation: ventral osteotomy of the incisal alveolus; both drilling holes have been connected by removing the bridge in between with narrow Luer bone rongeur forceps, which allows a relatively broad access to the tooth socket; infected alveolar tissue is removed with a fine curette. (e) Situation during the operation after tooth extraction: removal of the apical tooth section above the osteotomy area. (f) Situation during the operation: alveolus packed with iodoform gauze; the wound area is temporarily sutured for 2–3 days.

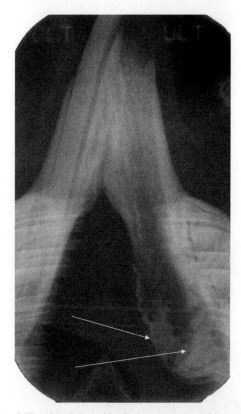

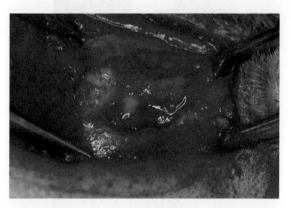

Figure 9.58 Rostral abscess of the lower jaw in a two-year-old guinea pig. Situation during the operation: ventral view on to the area of abscess; inflammatory ventral osteolysis of the left incisor socket. Further below dental tissue belonging to the incisor can be seen, while pus discharges from the alveolus.

Figure 9.57 Delayed wound healing in a two-year-old guinea pig following excision of an abscess of the lower jaw with extraction of the (left) incisor (intraoral view of the mandible): apical residue of dental tissue after incisor extraction approximately 3 weeks before and undulated tooth structure near the medial alveolar wall (white arrows), an indication for a ventral osteotomy of the tooth socket with extraction of the tooth residue.

accompanying osteotomy in the case of removal of the maxillary incisors. Since the alveoli open downwards, any exudate is able to drain rather well via the empty tooth socket (contrary to the lower jaw). An intraoral lateroventral or an extraoral dorsolateral osteotomy of the alveolus will be necessary, however, if the infection is involving more of the upper jawbone (see Section 11.1.6 in Chapter 11, abscess).

CHAPTER 10

Changes of the Cheek Teeth

10.1 Hypselodont cheek teeth

In rabbits, the syndrome of an acquired malocclusion affecting the cheek teeth does not usually occur before the age of approximately three years, and almost four years in guinea pigs. Chinchillas can be even older at the time when their owners first notice possible dental problems. The clinical picture is characterized by changes in shape, structure and position of the cheek teeth with resulting changes to the occlusal plane and thus the functionality of the dentition (Table 10.1).

10.1.1 Lagomorphs
Etiology

The exact etiology of the acquired malocclusion has not yet been clarified. Two of the most important factors proposed in the pathology of hypselodont cheek teeth are metabolic bone disorders involving a disturbance of the sensitive calcium phosphate metabolism, and insufficient wear of the cheek teeth (Harcourt-Brown, 2002a; Crossley & Aiken, 2004). In addition, there have been reports about a genetic predisposition in rabbits stating that male lop-eared dwarf rabbits in particular are more frequently affected by an acquired malocclusion (Turner, 1997).

Calcium phosphate homoeostasis is mainly regulated by parathyroid hormone, calcitonin, vitamin D and the amount of calcium and phosphate, respectively, that is nutritionally available and actually absorbed. Apart from this, thyroid hormones, oestrogens, corticosteroids and somatotropin play a major part in maintaining that delicate balance. For example, an experimental study has shown that in animals with a corticosteroid-induced osteoporosis, the teeth had a tendency to be displaced and suffer deformations due to the poor bone structure, even when the strain on them was normal (Ashcraft, Southard & Tolley, 1992).

If the calcium content of the blood decreases, parathyroid hormone release is increased, which stimulates calcium mobilization from the bone, and thus bone resorption. Blood tests confirm higher levels of circulating parathyroid hormone in response to low serum calcium levels. This was demonstrated in a study where rabbits that were kept outdoors in a more natural environment had significantly lower parathyroid hormone levels compared to indoor rabbits presenting with an acquired malocclusion (Harcourt-Brown & Baker, 2001).

A calcium deficiency can also be caused by selective eating behavior, particularly when rabbits are offered commercial food mixtures ad libitum. Rabbits often prefer ingredients such as corn (maize) or peas, which are low in calcium, while refusing pellets that contain minerals and vitamins but are not as palatable (Harcourt-Brown, 2002a).

Physiological aging processes or pregnancy and lactation may also influence the structure and strength of bone and teeth, as may chronic disorders of the gastrointestinal tract, the liver and the pancreas (Julius, 1997; Harcourt-Brown 2002a).

A deficiency of vitamin A, protein or magnesium can also negatively affect the tooth quality. All three are absolutely necessary for normal bone growth and for undisturbed formation of dental tissue (Harcourt-Brown, 2002a).

It has been proven in rabbits, that if the delicate balance is disturbed, it will lead to poor mineralization of the entire cranial skeleton and a loss of alveolar bone, which is crucial for tooth stability (Spuzjak, 1989; Wu et al.,

Dentistry in Rabbits and Rodents, First Edition. Estella Böhmer.
© 2015 John Wiley & Sons, Ltd. Published 2015 by John Wiley & Sons, Ltd.

Table 10.1 Frequent symptoms and findings in malocclusions of rabbits and herbivorous rodents.

Frequent symptoms	Intraoral findings
• Reduced general condition • Poorly groomed skin and fur, particularly in chinchillas • Selective feeding: preference for soft food • Dysphagia • Anorexia, purely due to pain or as a result of extensive intraoral findings • *Foetor ex ore* (bad breath) caused by gingivitis/stomatitis • Digestive problems such as high-degree gastrointestinal bloating and recurring colic • Bruxism, pain-related • Diarrhoea • Faecal changes: smaller and harder scybala (chinchillas) • Hypersalivation due to intraoral lesions of soft tissue caused by tooth spurs or tooth "Bridge formation" • Abnormal opening of the jaw due to intraoral tooth overgrowth • Mandible prognathism in guinea pigs • Passive loss of food already chewed, possible tongue entrapment • Primary or secondary incisor changes • Multiple ventral distensions of the mandible due to retrograde tooth displacements • Lumps/swellings in the area of the head, caused by abscesses • Epiphora, possibly with purulent discharge from the eyes in the case of a secondary bacterial infection • White, crusty material in the medial canthus=crystals from dried lacrimal fluid • Nasal discharge, serous to purulent • Exophthalmos, mostly unilateral	• Dental overgrowth of individual or various teeth • Tilting of individual or various teeth • "Bridge formation" (tongue entrapment typical of guinea pigs) • Typical lingual or buccal injuries to the soft tissue and hypersalivation • Lingual and buccal tooth spurs in individual or various teeth • Changed orientation of the enamel folds, tooth rotation in chinchillas • Altered occlusal surface of individual teeth, crippled or giant teeth in guinea pigs • Carious or other (caries-like) resorptive change of the occlusal surface • Increased interdental areas, periodontal disease and gingivitis • Food impacted intraalveolarly and intradentally • Inactivity-related discoloration of occlusal surface and enamel (darker color in a row of teeth) (guinea pigs, chinchillas) • Local enamel and dentin defects (mostly sharp-edged) • Generalized enamel and dentin hypoplasia (soft, white dental substance) • Longitudinal splitting of cheek teeth • Toothless alveoli filled with food debris and hairs: partial or complete loss of teeth • Irregular occlusal plane, wave mouth • Shorter individual teeth

1990; Gilsanz, Roe & Antunes, 1991; Harcourt-Brown, 1996, 2002a). Poor ossification can be seen radiographically as a clearly visible, granular appearance of the cranial vault (parietal calvarium), as well as loosening and deformation of teeth, retrograde displacement of individual cheek teeth and teeth penetrating the adjacent jawbone (Figure 10.1). Hence a radiographic examination is of crucial importance for the diagnosis of a metabolic bone disorder and a nutrition-related, secondary hyperparathyroidism in rabbits (Harcourt-Brown, 2002a).

Apart from metabolic disturbances, insufficient wear of the hypselodont cheek teeth plays a major part in the etiology of acquired malocclusion. As a result of insufficient dental wear, intraoral elongation of teeth will occur, followed by retrograde displacement of the tooth apices as well as curving and deformation of the tooth structure as the disease progresses (Harcourt-Brown,

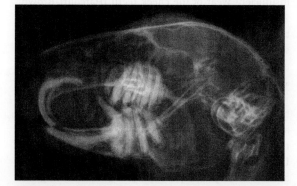

Figure 10.1 Radiograph of an advanced malocclusion of incisors and cheek teeth in a four-year-old rabbit (laterolateral view) with pronounced demineralization of the entire cranial skeleton, intraalveolar deformation of the tooth structure of all incisors, structural change as well as intraoral elongation of all cheek teeth (missing lamina dura and loss of the intradental enamel line) and an intraoral rostral spur of the first lower cheek tooth (P3).

2002a; Crossley & Aiken, 2004) (see below). This results in an established acquired malocclusion. This theoretical scenario is supported by an experimental study in which a precisely determined amount of pressure was applied to the maxillary incisors of a rabbit over several hours (Steedle, Proffitt & Fields, 1983; Proffitt & Sellers, 1986). It was found that a weight of less than 0.5 g was enough pressure to inhibit physiological tooth eruption and a weight of 2.5 g could lead to a retrograde displacement of the tooth apex.

Rabbits that are mostly kept indoors and fed cereal-based, high-energy mixed food as well as some additional hay and vegetables are most likely to be affected by tooth elongation. Those animals hardly need to chew their food, which quickly leads to an elongation of cheek teeth and thus a malocclusion. By contrast, wild rabbits that browse or graze all day rarely suffer from dental problems. This suggests that sufficient dental wear is an extremely crucial, if not the most important, factor for the maintenance of healthy dentition. It was shown that pet rabbits, regardless of species, that live outdoors all year round and are thus left to graze freely are very rarely affected by malocclusions. Likewise, the risk of developing a malocclusion decreases if animals that are kept indoors are predominantly fed a lot of fresh grass, hay and vegetables (Harcourt-Brown, 2002a).

However, a deficiency of fibrous, abrasive food and insufficient mastication are not the only reasons for the development of an acquired malocclusion. For example, the disorder never affects laboratory animals or commercially kept rabbits, although these are usually fed solely on pellets or, if any hay is available, only in small amounts of hay. In an experiment, large laboratory rabbits (New Zealand rabbits) were fed exclusively on liquid food without subsequently developing malocclusions (Latour et al., 1998). Bruxism may play a crucial part here in ensuring sufficient dental wear or the molars might have stopped growing due to the lack of mechanical stimuli – which (based on the author's own experience) is what happens to the antagonists of cheek teeth after extraction. All this proves that continuous growth of hypsodont teeth is influenced by a multitude of different factors, many of which are still unknown.

Pathogenesis

Rabbits' molars are formed and precisely interlocked (see Section 3.1.3 in Chapter 3) in such a way that they continuously wear down and shape each other whilst grinding down, or actually cutting up, the food. If the teeth are insufficiently worn down due to the insufficient rough fiber in the food, the delicate balance between tooth growth and wear is broken and an elongation of the clinical tooth crown results from this. As a consequence of the intraoral elongation of the teeth, the cheek teeth, which normally are slightly spaced apart from the opposite arcade while at rest, now occlude with their respective antagonists. By contrast, occlusion of the incisors remains unchanged at this point.

This produces an increase in occlusal pressure, not only at rest. At the same time, the maxilla and the mandible are pushed further apart in an unphysiological fashion. This can be seen radiographically when the lines of the floor of the mouth and palatal bone are no longer convergent. In the medium to long term an overgrowth of the incisors inevitably occurs. This secondary malocclusion of the incisors is very common in rabbits and can be regarded as a primary indicator of a malocclusion of the cheek teeth (see Section 9.2 in Chapter 9).

The intraoral growth of the cheek teeth will progress until the tone of the masticatory muscles (at rest) significantly hampers or largely stops the intraoral overgrowth (Crossley & Aiken, 2004). The teeth will then elongate more slowly. The increase in occlusal pressure, which is caused by the elongation of the clinical crown and the simultaneous increase in basic tension of the jaw muscles, will not stop the physiological tooth eruption completely. The increase in interdental occlusal pressure, however, leads to a partial change of the direction in which the affected cheek teeth protrude. Retrograde displacement of the apices occurs due to the constantly increasing pressure on the tooth apices, which is transferred via the longitudinal axis of the teeth (Harcourt-Brown, 2002a; Crossley & Aiken, 2004). At the same time, curvature of the teeth also occurs (see Figure 10.52 later). The germinal zone of each cheek tooth will be displaced deeper and deeper into the adjacent jawbone as the apical alveolar bone is destroyed due to compression. The tooth seems to be growing in the wrong direction (Wiggs & Lobprise, 1995b).

There is resorption and replacement of bone at the tooth apex, which occurs at the same time as the retrograde displacement of the tooth apices. If this is an equal process, all teeth will keep a relatively normal shape while the retrogradely displaced germinal zones will remain enclosed by a thin bone lamella – the alveolar bullae are still "covered" (Figure 10.2). Clinically, these bony changes result in the ventral (ventromedial) border of the mandible, becoming uneven. Each of the displaced tooth apices forms a small, readily palpable bony prominence, which usually is not painful, provided that the lamina dura and the mandibular cortex remain intact despite the retrograde displacement.

If, however, the bone is perforated completely as a result of the increasing elongation of the entire tooth, the sensitive periosteum is disrupted, and the alveolar bullae are now exposed ("uncovered") resulting in localized pain (Figure 10.3). A certain degree of remodeling of the periapical bone is partly physiological in rabbits and can also be found in older, healthy wild rabbits. The process is considered to be pathological whenever the apices of the cheek teeth are exposed and the teeth exhibit additional changes.

Interestingly, the alveolar bullae are exposed in all young rabbits ("babies"). Over time, they are covered by a thin bony lamella (Figure 10.4). This process may be negatively influenced by a mineral deficiency during the period of growth, predisposing to the development of a malocclusion.

Retrograde displacement of the tooth apices, as well as the abnormal occlusal pressure conditions, are

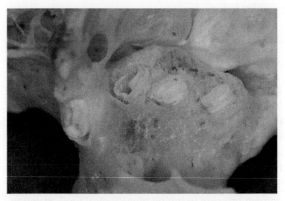

Figure 10.3 Left orbit of a three-year-old rabbit with advanced malocclusion and exposed alveolar bullae (P4–M2).

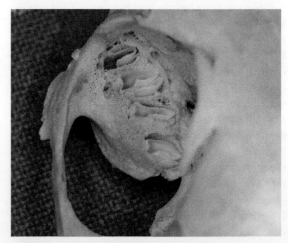

Figure 10.4 Left orbit of a three-week-old rabbit with normal occlusion and extensively exposed alveolar bullae (P4–M3).

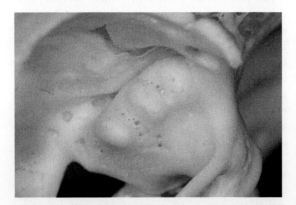

Figure 10.2 Right orbit of a wild rabbit with normal occlusion: covered alveolar bullae of the last four maxillary cheek teeth (P4–M3).

concomitant with a chronic irritation of and damage to the germinal cells, and thus an aseptic pulpitis (Crossley & Aiken, 2004). This greatly impairs the tooth-building function of the apical germinal tissue, leading to the formation of predominantly dysplastically changed dental hard tissue (enamel and dentin hypoplasia). The teeth have a glassy, brittle appearance with typical fissures on the tooth surfaces. They also have a tendency to curve and they are prone to deformations as well as to intra- or extraalveolar fractures (Figure 10.5). The dental hard substance takes on a yellow hue.

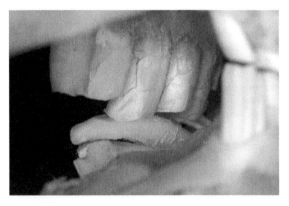

Figure 10.5 Advanced malocclusion in a six-year-old rabbit (right maxillary row of cheek teeth, medial view) with severe enamel and dentin hypoplasia of all molars, severe malformation and elongation as well as rostral tilting of the last two mandibular molars (M2/M3).

Due to the pressure-related damage done to the germinal cells, the physiological folding of the enamel and dentin may also be lost, or the crown enamel, which is altered as well, will no longer be able to connect the individual dentin columns tightly enough. Affected cheek teeth are therefore often split/fracture longitudinally. In rabbits, the split parts of the tooth are almost of the same size (predisposition due to bilophodonty); in guinea pigs, splitting is mostly less symmetric (different size of both dentin columns) (Figure 10.6a and 10.34 later). This splitting of teeth is the result of an apical, pressure-related or infectious irritation and has nothing to do – as could be presumed – with a traumatic origin (e.g. increased chewing pressure) (Figure 10.6b). Chewing with split teeth is very painful so the affected animals preferentially grind their food using teeth on the contralateral side. This results in elongation of the split cheek teeth to the point where the crown ultimately fractures completely. There is a progressively deteriorating quality of teeth and bones and an additional risk of infection spreading periodontally, ultimately resulting in the formation of an abscess (Figure 10.7).

At intraoral examination, in the early stages of a malocclusion, elongation of the cheek teeth is often considered to be less severe compared to the secondary intraosseous changes (Figures 10.6 and 10.7). In less experienced hands, the elongation of the clinical crown may not even be recognized. Hence most rabbits with elongated cheek teeth do not present for treatment until

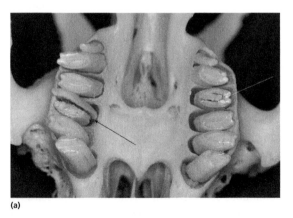

(a)

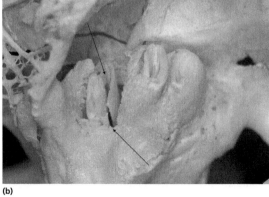

(b)

Figure 10.6 Malocclusion in a one-year-old rabbit. (a) Maxilla specimen: longitudinal splitting of the third left cheek tooth (P4; black arrow), elongation of the clinical crown with slight enamel and dentin hypoplasia of all cheek teeth, generalized pathological dilation of the desmodontium of all teeth and hint of a splitting of the fourth right cheek tooth (M1; white arrow). (b) Left orbit specimen (dorsal view): marked retrograde elongation of the apices of the cheek teeth (P4-M2) with perforation of the alveolar bullae, extensive defect of the cortical bone of the split premolar (P4; black arrow).

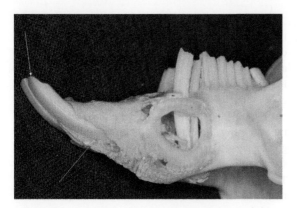

Figure 10.7 Example of a (left) mandibular abscess in a three-year-old rabbit (mandible specimen): proliferation of the rostral bone with lateral destruction of the jaw, longitudinal splitting and retrograde apex displacement of the first cheek tooth (P3), slight shortening of the clinical crown of the left incisor (white arrow) and mesial loss of the alveolar bone (turquoise arrow).

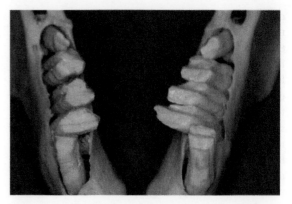

Figure 10.8 Malocclusion in a six-year-old rabbit (mandible specimen) with pronounced lingual twisting and tilting of the middle left lower cheek teeth (P4–M2), resulting secondary extension of the occlusal surface, slight changes of the same kind on the right (P4/M1), severe enamel and dentin hypoplasia of all cheek teeth (more pronounced on the right than on the left) and generalized dilation of the desmodontium with loss of the lamina dura (more pronounced on the right than on the left).

an advanced stage of disease has been reached; this is when animals exhibit anorexia, or an abscess of the jaw, or more dramatic secondary changes of the incisors (Figure 10.7).

In order to recognize the early stage of a cheek tooth malocclusion, which is seen as intraoral tooth elongation, and to ascertain the intraosseous changes that have already occurred (and to treat them early) laterolateral skull radiographs of the head are helpful. With the help of the dorsal reference lines according to Böhmer and Crossley that have been described in Section 5.6 of Chapter 5, the often surprising extent of the intraosseous findings can be objectively depicted. This will allow early treatment involving correction of the dentition, improvement of husbandary and diet etc., whereby the continuously advancing processes will probably not be stopped but at least will be significantly delayed.

As tooth elongation advances, the slight physiological curvature of the cheek teeth becomes more pronounced. The teeth become altered structurally (concave bucally in the maxillary arcades and concave lingually in the mandibular arcades; see Figure 10.52 later). As a consequence of that increasing curvature, there is insufficient wear of the whole occlusal surface of the teeth despite the extensive laterolateral jaw movements. This is due to the contact area of the teeth increasing and being displaced as a result of the tooth curvature

(Figure 10.8). At this point, tooth spurs start to form – buccally in the maxilla and lingually in the mandible – which are typical of rabbits and can be very pronounced (Harcourt-Brown, 2002a; Crossley & Aiken, 2004). Secondarily, there are extremely painful injuries to the buccal mucosa and the tongue, which may lead to anorexia and hypersalivation.

Many of these patients, on reflexion, will have episodes where they may have eaten poorly and salivated more for a short time before improving again, only for the primary symptoms to return. The reason for this episodic nature of the disease is due to scarring of the tongue following the chronic irritation (Figure 10.9). Primarily, a relatively small tooth spur leads to a painful lingual lesion that is associated with acute salivation and anorexia. Many animals will also refuse to drink from a bottle at that point in time due to the pain. If the patient does not present for tooth trimming, the symptoms will go away for a while as the tongue forms a local scar that is superficial at first. Pain-related anorexia and salivation will return as soon as the tooth spur – owing to the continuous dental growth – again reaches the sensitive lingual tissue under the scar tissue. That scenario can be repeated several times and explains why many rabbits do not present for examination until they have severe lesions or even splitting of the tongue. The same types of changes may also occur on the buccal mucosa.

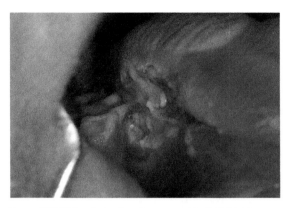

Figure 10.9 Malocclusion in a four-year-old rabbit (right row of cheek teeth) with lingual spur formation in the second and third cheek teeth (P4/M1) due to a primary intraalveolar twisting of the tooth, recent and older scarred lesions of the tongue visible, an indication for maximal shortening of the teeth.

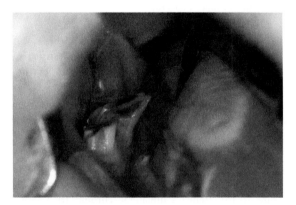

Figure 10.10 Malocclusion in a six-year-old rabbit (right row of cheek teeth) with lingual spur formation in the second and third cheek teeth (P4/M1) due to an intraalveolar tilting of teeth, secondary lesion of the tongue, reddish, fasciated foliate papilla visible distally, an indication for maximal shortening of teeth.

In the early stage of a malocclusion, the curvature of the cheek teeth and the corresponding formation of tooth spurs are still slight. Both findings, however, progressively become more pronounced. The increased intraalveolar curvature of the entire tooth that is associated with tooth elongation leads to increasing pressure, both on the lingual edge of the mandibular molar and on the buccal edge of the maxillary molar during occlusion and grinding of food, respectively. This further increases the curvature of the cheek teeth and the extent of tooth spur formation

(Figure 10.10). If only the protruding dental spurs or spikes are removed in the context of corrective dentistry, such as trimming of teeth and correction of the occlusal plane, those edges will rebuild within a few weeks. Even a maximal shortening of all cheek teeth down to the gum-line will only delay the progression of the tooth-curvature to a small degree, but will not halt it.

Tilting and intraalveolar curvature of individual cheek teeth are increased if the patients are fed grains instead of fibrous food, as those grains will have to be crushed. This will increase the axial load, especially on the middle cheek teeth on both sides of the jaw, further raising the extent of pathological changes. The second (P4) and the third mandibular cheek teeth (M1) are particularly affected by this.

An increasing retrograde displacement of the sharp-edged apices ("uncovered" alveolar bullae) is concomitant with an irritation of the sensitive periosteum (Harcourt-Brown, 2002a; Crossley & Aiken, 2004; see Figure 10.3). When the mandibular tooth apices, which are now exposed transosseously, are palpated (ventral cortical bone of the mandible), the patients exhibit a pronounced localized pain or at least a sensitivity to pressure. If an even more pronounced curvature of the teeth, due to the lack of tooth support owing to the loss of the lamina dura, adds to the elongation of the entire tooth, then the mandibular molars can perforate the mandible laterally (Figure 10.11).

Corresponding to their normal curvature, the mandibular cheek teeth will usually perforate the cortical bone of the jaw ventromedially. Thus the retrogradely displaced, often exposed, apex of the first premolar (P3) is usually located in the rostral, intermandibular area near the symphysis (see Figure 4.9 in Chapter 4). That finding is often bilateral and can be seen especially well on intraoral images (see Figures 9.37 and 9.55 in Chapter 9). Likewise, the small last molar (M3) often perforates the rabbit's mandible, primarily medially (see Figure 4.10 in Chapter 4 and Figure 10.12). The retrograde displacement of the apices, however, which predisposes to abscess formation, is often overlooked clinically as many examinations (palpations) are often restricted to the ventrolateral border of the mandible. Furthermore, such changes are often difficult to verify due to superimposition on the classic four radiographic views of the head. The changes are often diagnosed at a later stage once the mandible has been resorbed due to

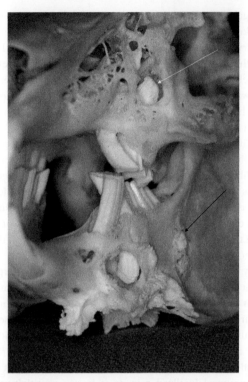

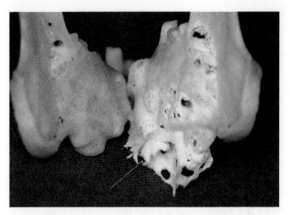

Figure 10.12 Mandible specimen of a two-year-old rabbit (caudorostral view) with severe retrograde elongation of the last right lower cheek tooth (M3), a ventromedial perforation of the cortical bone of the jaw, an exposed apex (white arrow), a marked expansion of the jaw as a result of a secondary abscess formation and a diffuse bony distension of the left medial cortical bone of the jaw.

Figure 10.11 Unilateral malocclusion with abscess formation in the (left) lower jaw in a two-year-old rabbit (specimen): significant elongation of the clinical crowns of all cheek teeth, marked displacement and tilting (buccally in the upper jaw, lingually in the lower jaw) of all cheek teeth except for the first lower cheek tooth (P3), perforation of the lateral and ventral cortical bone of the mandible at the apex of the second lower cheek tooth (P4) together with the formation of multiple bone proliferations (abscess area), extensively exposed apex of the retrogradely elongated second upper cheek tooth, as a result of an osteolysis of the facial tuberosity (P3; white arrow), retrograde displacement of the last lower cheek tooth (M3) with perforation of the lateral mandibular cortical bone (black arrow).

infection and a larger mandibular abscess has perforated the outer cortex of the jaw (Figure 10.13a to c).

The same types of pathological changes involving retrogradely displaced and exposed apices are also found in the maxilla, the facial tuberosity and the ventrorostral part of the orbit (Figure 10.11). Due to the buccally concave curvature of the molars, the tooth apices in the maxilla mainly undergo a dorsolateral displacement. In a retrograde displacement of the first upper cheek tooth (P2), the tooth penetrates deeper into the maxilla, encroaching on the upper part of the nasolacrimal duct,

which runs intraosseously here (Figure 10.14). In advanced malocclusions, proliferative and destructive bone reactions take place in the apical area of the premolar (P2) occasionally causing narrowing of the nasolacrimal canal. Occasionally a therapy-resistant, chronic-purulent dacryocystitis or even an intranasal abscess will develop as a result of a compression-related drainage disturbance or the spread of a primarily apical tooth infection to the adjacent nasolacrimal duct (see Figure 4.3 in Chapter 4, Figure 9.21 in Chapter 9 and Figure 10.15). Hence a unilateral, chronic, treatment-resistant conjunctivitis or a rhinitis may be indicative of not only an apical incisor problem but also an advanced cheek tooth malocclusion, and it should always be an indication for a thorough dental examination, including radiographs. In these cases, the cribriform plate typically bulges forward and outwards (dorsoventral radiographs), giving the rostral part of the skull an asymmetric appearance, both clinically and radiographically.

Only pathological alterations of the first upper molar (P2) may result in pathology associated with the nasolacrimal duct. The apex of the second upper premolar (P3) is usually not in the proximity of the nasolacrimal duct in the case of retrograde displacement of the apex. With retrograde elongation, the tooth typically curves concavely outwards, thereby perforating the lateral wall of the lacrimal bone (facial tuberosity) species-specifically (Figure 10.16a and b). This results in various prolifera-

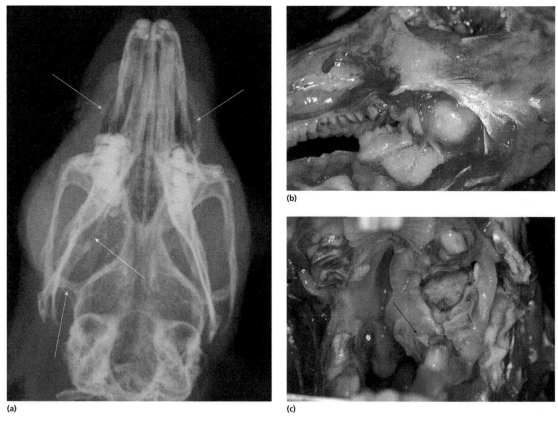

Figure 10.13 Abscess of the (left) mandible originating from the last cheek tooth (M3) in a three-year-old rabbit. (a) Dorsoventral view: medial bone proliferation with extensive osteolysis of the caudal mandibular cortical bone (white arrow), significant swelling of soft tissue visible laterally, pathological dilation of the temporomandibular joint (yellow arrow) and a bilateral distension of the cribriform plate (turquoise arrows). (b) Specimen: As well as a primarily medial abscess, there is also a lateral abscess and a pustule the size of a cherry located below the masseter muscle (resection of the rostral part). (c) Specimen (rostrocaudal view into the oral cavity): severe swelling of soft tissue of the left temporomandibular joint, which is also involved secondarily in the inflammation, and extensive necrosis in the jaw angle. The tooth causing this abscessation is tilted lingually (M3; black arrow).

tive or osteolytic changes of the zygomatic process and the formation of dental abscesses.

The apices of the last four maxillary cheek teeth (P4–M3) are located intraorbitally in the ventrorostral area of the orbit, in other words in immediate proximity to the tear glands and the eye (Figure 10.3). Their germinal zones, which are small, round, partially connected bone protrusions bulging forward into the orbit, are normally covered by a thin bony lamella. With retrograde overgrowth of the caudal maxillary cheek teeth, the apices are displaced further and further into the orbit until ultimately the alveolar bullae are exposed and often become secondarily infected. This results in the formation of retrobulbar abscesses (see Section 11.2 in Chapter 11).

Since the last maxillary cheek tooth (M3) is normally rather small and short, it plays only a minor role in these kinds of changes. Only very rarely will it be the only tooth to perforate the intraorbital bone lamella – mostly infections will spread to that small tooth secondarily from the adjacent molars.

Since pathologically altered cheek teeth differ from healthy molars in terms of hardness and, usually, shape as well (often those teeth are softer but thicker), the teeth are subject to different degrees of dental wear. This results in a "step mouth" (exsuperantia dentium), in rabbits (Figure 10.17). This condition is rarely found in herbivorous rodents as their jaw excursions during grinding of the food are mostly rostrocaudal. The lateral grinding movements of lagomorphs, however, lead to

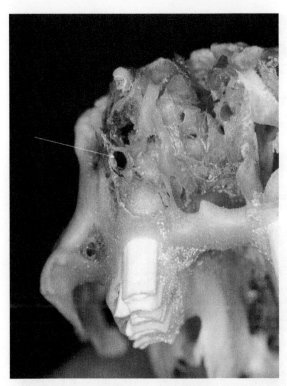

Figure 10.14 Specimen of the right maxillary row of cheek teeth in a rabbit (rostrocaudal view; transverse section slightly rostrally from the first upper cheek tooth, P2): oval opening of the bony part of the nasolacrimal duct located dorsolaterally from the premolar (transverse cut; white arrow).

the cheek teeth being ground continuously over time so that they are exactly compatible with each other, i.e. the cheek teeth that are pathologically shortened and elongated interlock exactly. The precise, tenth-of-a-centimeter-perfect alignment can often be astounding indeed.

The amount of wear of an individual tooth or several teeth in one of the jaw halves can also be reduced due to unilaterally decreased masticatory pressure or even a lack of grinding activity (unilateral dental overgrowth). Possible causes of this are painful disorders or infections of individual teeth, the periodontal tissues or the entire jaw (e.g. abscess, tumor).

Acquired malocclusions of rabbits are always progressive and, in principle, cannot be stopped; at best they can be slowed down a bit. In the long term, however, the germinal cells are likely to be increasingly destroyed causing dental growth to cease. Hence regular trimming of teeth is no longer required in the terminal stage of the disorder (Harcourt-Brown, 2002a). The markedly altered clinical crowns tend to fracture and the gingiva grows

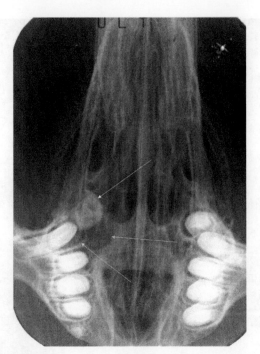

Figure 10.15 Intranasal abscessation (on the left) in a three-year-old rabbit with chronic rhinitis and anorexia (intraoral view of the maxilla): extensive, inflammatory resorption of the palatally displaced first left cheek tooth (P2; white arrow), osteolysis of the maxilla recognizable caudomedially from the tooth (rostrolateral part of the palatal process; turquoise arrow), significant dilation of the desmodontium of the second left cheek tooth, which is slightly rotated intraalveolarly (P3; yellow arrow), bilateral distension in the area of the cribriform plate and slight lateral displacement of the second right cheek tooth.

over the embedded tooth which remains quiescent in the jaw (Figure 10.18). A few teeth are preserved intraorally as mostly discolored yellowish, severely malformed stumps. However, it is enough to allow the animals to sufficiently chop up soft food that they prefer, and eat it.

10.1.2 Herbivorous rodents
Etiology and pathogenesis

While principal factors of the etiopathogenesis of malocclusions are basically the same in lagomorphs and herbivorous rodents – and the symptoms are also similar – there are still species-dependent differences, for example, hypovitaminosis C in guinea pigs.

There have been many reports of a certain correlation between an intraoral overgrowth of the cheek teeth and dietary deficiency of vitamin C in guinea pigs (Brown & Rosenthal, 1997; Klaus & Bennett, 1999; Gorrel &

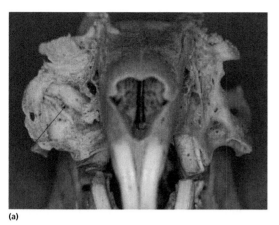 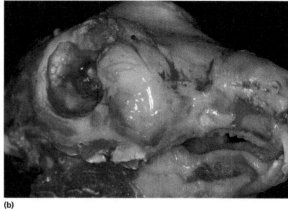

(a) (b)

Figure 10.16 Abscess of the (right) upper jaw in a rabbit. (a) Specimen, rostrocaudal view: second upper cheek tooth (P3; black arrow) elongated retrogradely, displaced and concavely curved buccally and extensive destruction of the right facial tuberosity with pronounced secondary bone proliferations; bilateral malocclusion of the cheek teeth. (b) Postmortem specimen, view from the right: extensive distension in the area of the facial tuberosity.

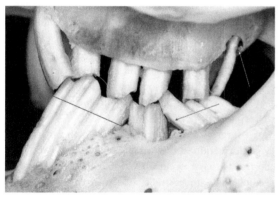

Figure 10.17 Advanced malocclusion and significant step mouth in a two-year-old rabbit. Specimen, left row of cheek teeth, lateral view: the first lower cheek tooth is pathologically thickened and has an abnormal occlusal surface with loss of the lateral alveolar wall of the last upper molar (M3; white arrow). The third mandibular cheek tooth (M1) is missing, causing the pathological mesial tilting of the two posterior lower cheek teeth (M2/M3; red arrow); enamel hypoplasia of all teeth and dilation of all approximal areas in the upper jaw.

Verhaert, 2006; Kotaniji, 1927). Likewise, it is presumed that an existing malocclusion can be worsened by vitamin C deficiency (Schaeffer & Donnelly, 1997; Brown & Rosenthal, 1997). The cause of this is presumed to be a collagen defect that results from the vitamin deficiency. Since collagen is needed for the intraalveolar anchoring of the teeth, which is solid but flexible at the same time, that kind of defect leads to a weakening of the periodontium and presumably a secondary tilting of the molars. Since the cheek teeth

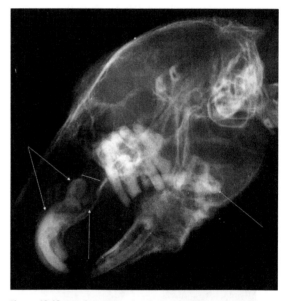

Figure 10.18 "End-stage" malocclusion in a seven-year-old rabbit (laterolateral view): severe demineralization of the entire cranial skeleton, odontoma-like restructuring of the maxillary incisors (white arrows), lower cheek teeth partially reabsorbed and no longer able to be verified, severe structural alteration of all upper cheek teeth as well as the remaining mandibular molar (M3; turquoise arrow), step mouth, ventral bulging of the palatal plate (yellow arrow) and severe dilation of the bony nasolacrimal canal (white line).

are no longer correctly abraded as a result of this, a secondary malocclusion develops. In addition to the displacement of the teeth, problems with the continuous eruption of teeth are also said to occur. In order for a healthy guinea pig's cheek teeth to be completely replaced with new tooth substance within the space of only 40 days, a continuous tooth protrusion involving repeated reconstruction processes in the area of the plexus intermedius is needed. Vitamin C plays an extraordinarily important part in this (Fish & Harris, 1935).

However, vitamin C deficiency can have a negative effect not only on the periodontium but also on the dental hard tissues (Mickoleit, 2004), for example, damage to the odontoblasts of the incisors with a concomitant secondary inhibition of the dentin production has been shown, as has a dilatation of blood vessels and hemorrhage of the pulp (Figure 10.19). Enamel production, however, was not primarily influenced or inhibited by hypovitaminosis C (Boyle, 1938). Hypoplastic enamel formation occurred as the physiological forces acting on the tooth were transferred directly – a consequence of the collagen defect – on to the enamel-forming ameloblasts via the abnormal fibrous tissue of

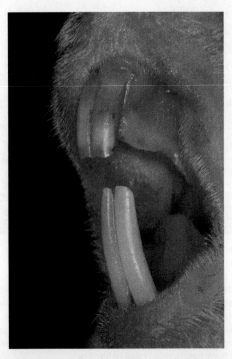

Figure 10.19 Hemorrhage of the pulp cavity of the left maxillary incisor in a six-month-old guinea pig with normal occlusion (seen as pink discoloration of the maxillary incisor). Bleeding is the result of a chronic undersupply of vitamin C (hypovitaminosis C).

the periodontal ligament. This resulted in locally restricted or more extensive enamel defects. A determination of the enamel–dentin ratio provided evidence for the fact that only the production of dentin and not enamel was compromised by vitamin C deficiency. That ratio was 3:4 in animals with healthy incisors, whereas guinea pigs with a vitamin C deficiency resulting from a reduced dentin production had a ratio of 3:1 or 4:1 (Boyle, 1938).

It has been discussed that excessive selenium uptake could also be a possible cause of an excessive growth of cheek teeth in guinea pigs (Williams, 1976). Both an excess and a deficiency of selenium is said to result in a disturbance of collagen formation. This again compromises the complex reconstruction processes of the periodontal tissue, thus causing – just like vitamin C deficiency – a general weakening of the periodontal fibers. Guinea pigs have no selenium reservoirs and are therefore particularly dependent on a continuous supply of selenium. Provided that sufficient vitamin E is supplied, 0.08 mg of selenium is required per kg of food (Jensen, 2008). A deficiency of both vitamin E and selenium can lead to myopathies that may also affect the jaw muscles (Hill et al., 2009). Those kinds of deficiencies, however, are very rare in pets.

An overgrowth of cheek teeth involving a typical bridge formation of the mandibular premolars was reported to have occurred at nine large guinea pig breeding mills in Australia, due to excessive fluoride content of the food (chronic fluoride poisoning) (Hard & Atkinson, 1967a, b). Not only the molars but also the incisors were affected. The fluoride was incorporated into the dental substance, causing the teeth to become harder and thus to be insufficiently abraded. All cheek teeth had rough plaques of dental calculus on their lateral surfaces.

Furthermore, vitamin A is important for the formation of healthy tooth substance. For example, vitamin A deficiency was reported to lead to an atrophy of odontoblasts in the area of the cheek teeth of guinea pigs, causing insufficient dentin production (Pohto, 1939). Vitamin A also influences tooth eruption. This was proven in rat incisors (Fredericia & Gudjonsson, 1936). In the case of a vitamin A deficiency in young animals, the average tooth growth rate of 3.3 mm per week was down to 2.5 mm per week after three weeks, and merely 1.5 mm after that.

The main etiological factor, however, that leads to a primary elongation of cheek teeth in herbivorous rodents is insufficient dental wear resulting from feeding a high-calorie food that is also not abrasive enough. This means that too little time is spent eating the amount of food that is needed; in addition, the teeth are strained in an abnormal way during the consumption of pellets (Crossley et al., 1998). Contrary to rabbits, the cheek teeth of guinea pigs, chinchillas and degus occlude immediately at rest. In the case of an intraoral tooth elongation – if only a slight one – the axial occlusal load acting on the cheek teeth increases at rest (Crossley et al., 1998). Due to an increased resistance, the teeth cannot grow normally because their continuous eruption is disturbed. Tooth growth happens mostly at night when the teeth are not used. As a result of the increased axial load, the typical retrograde displacement of the tooth apices occurs. In chinchillas, that displacement occurs even before intraoral tooth elongation has manifested itself clinically (see Figure 5.35 in Chapter 5). Those early stages of a malocclusion are usually not recognized. Thus early radiographic examinations using the reference lines for a correct evaluation of the bony changes are very important.

Wild animals eat a lot of sparse, rough plant material with a high silicate content (dry grasses), which is also covered in dust and sand due to the dryness of their habitat. The food has a low energy content, which means that the animals consume a lot and spend a long time eating in order to ensure enough energy uptake. Constant grinding of that kind of highly abrasive, low-energy food means that dental abrasion is sufficient, which is what the teeth of guinea pigs, chinchillas and degus have been inherently designed for. This also explains why chinchillas that are kept in a zoo and fed a natural diet less frequently suffer from malocclusions (Crossley, 2001a).

Stress that is caused, for example, by being held in captivity also plays a part in the etiology of malocclusions. High concentrations of corticosteroids have a negative influence on the quality of the odontogenic tissue and the periodontal ligament fibers, indirectly influencing continuous tooth eruption. Immune suppression plays a major part, particularly in chinchillas. For example, approximately one-third of animals examined in a study had hyperplasia of the adrenal glands (Crossley & Miguelez, 2001). Chinchillas, who are very

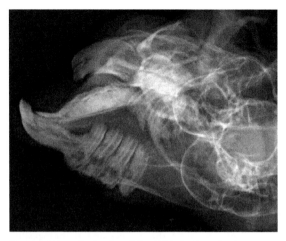

Figure 10.20 Malocclusion of the (left) cheek teeth of a six-year-old chinchilla (isolated view of the left lower jaw as described by Böhmer) with multiple resorptive lesions of all cheek teeth. In the apical area of the tooth, dental tissue is well preserved, which is why a protrusion of normal tooth substance is possible. There is an indication for maximal shortening of the teeth as well as an antibacterial therapy.

susceptible to stress, very often also suffer from periodontal disorders that can become very severe. During the terminal stage of a species-specific periodontitis, extensive secondary intraalveolar tooth resorptions occur in most cases (see Figure 9.26 in Chapter 9 and Figure 10.20).

Another consideration is that the supply of minerals for pets is usually optimal, meaning that the teeth are well-mineralized and thus are worn down less – an effect that is enhanced by food that is hardly abrasive (pellets). Wild animals, by contrast, are more likely to suffer from mineral deficiency, causing the teeth to be worn down more quickly (Crossley, 2001a). This theory is based on the observation mentioned above that in guinea pigs who received too much fluoride, the resultant tooth substance became harder, resulting in insufficient dental abrasion and an elongation of the cheek teeth over time (Hard & Atkinson, 1967a, b). In addition, it has been found that many macerated skull specimens of guinea pigs with malocclusions have extremely well-mineralized bones. Many skulls even exhibited additional hypertrophic calcifications (see Figure 5.32a and c in Chapter 5 and Figure 10.56 later). This is in stark contrast to the hypocalcifications that are very prominent in the corresponding rabbit specimens (Figure 10.1).

For example, in a comparison of the skulls of 10 healthy chinchillas and 10 chinchillas with malocclusions from farms that had a history of that disorder, radiographs and postmortem examination showed that all chinchillas with a dental problem had excessively mineralized teeth and bones (Sulik et al., 2007). Typical radiographic evidence of osteosclerosis were skull bones that were thickened overall and radiopaque, particularly in the area of the sutures. As a result of the excessive mineralization of the teeth, no pulp cavity could be verified within the dental substance, which was also significantly more radiopaque (pulp fibrosis), both in the incisors and in the cheek teeth. All of the altered teeth were also elongated (intraoral overgrowth and retrograde displacement of the apices) and pathologically worn down. The blunt occlusal edges of the incisors were excessively mineralized and did not show any abrasion. Moreover, there were one or two alveolar abscesses or a periostitis in the area of the molars – all of these findings were also frequently seen in pet chinchillas suffering from malocclusions (see Figure 8.14 in Chapter 8 and Figure 9.26 in Chapter 9). Contrary to this, healthy teeth were usually less mineralized and had a clearly visible pulp canal as well as a physiological occlusal plane (Figure 10.21).

An osteosclerosis, which involves a condensation of cancellous bones and diminished medullary spaces, can be caused by an increase in osteoblast activity or a reduced bone resorption due to a chronic infection or extreme strain on the bones. Those changes can be isolated or systemic and thus generalized. Possible causes are fluoride, lead or phosphate poisoning (Sulik et al., 2007).

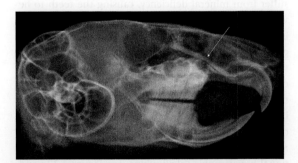

Figure 10.21 Contrast study of the nasolacrimal duct in a six-year-old chinchilla with normal occlusion (laterolateral view, skull specimen). The anatomical proximity of the duct to the apex of the first maxillary cheek tooth (P4; white arrow) becomes clearly visible.

The more one is concerned with the etiology of malocclusions, the more difficult it is to answer whether guinea pigs and chinchillas primarily suffer from eburneation (ostitis ossificans) and a concomitant tooth hardening. The technical term denotes an excessive bone formation originating in the medullary space and the periosteum (increase of the compact bone at the expense of the spongiosa). Many macerated specimens exhibit such changes and indications of those changes can also be found in many radiographs (see Figure 5.32a in Chapter 5). A localized or generalized bone hypertrophy leads to an increase in bone hardness, but at the same time the dynamic resilience decreases. This could explain why retrograde perforations of the cortical bone by the apices occur. Further research will clarify that situation.

Pathology

In rodents with hypselodont cheek teeth (guinea pigs, chinchillas and degus), the pathological changes of teeth and jawbone are in principle the same as in lagomorphs. There are, however, certain species-specific differences (see below). Tooth elongation in guinea pigs and chinchillas, for example, more rarely results in tooth spur formation (which is typical for rabbits) or a curving of individual teeth. Degus, however, exhibit these kinds of change, most often in the form of a lingual tooth spur in the first lower premolar (P4) (Figure 10.22). The most frequent pathological findings in all three species are those concerning several or even all cheek teeth in a jaw quadrant or several quadrants. The changes concern both the shape and length of the molars and the structure of the tooth substance. In addition, there are corresponding secondary processes in the jawbone.

The affected teeth of guinea pigs and chinchillas curve buccally in the maxilla and lingually in the mandible (intraoral finding; see Figure 5.40d in Chapter 5 and Figure 10.23). This leads to a widening of the occlusal surfaces of the affected molars and results in sharp-edged tooth elongations that point in the direction of the cheek and the tongue and mostly extend over the entire occlusal surface. Painful injuries to the soft tissue result but are sometimes a bit difficult to identify; understandably, they lead to hypersalivation and anorexia. Curvature of teeth is rarer, however, in degus (intraoral finding; Figure 10.22). These animals mostly exhibit a step mouth, which can be extremely pronounced in comparison with other species. Mastication in degus

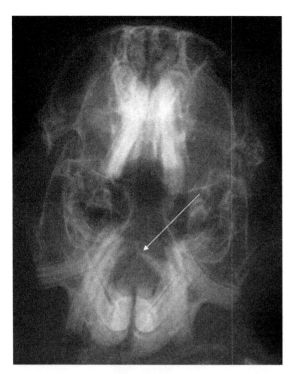

Figure 10.22 The same patient as in Figure 9.12 (in Chapter 9), a degu (rostrocaudal view) with severe malocclusion of cheek teeth: the lingual tooth spur of the first left lower cheek tooth (P4; white arrow), severe retrograde elongation of all lower cheek teeth with perforation of the cortical bone of the jaw and exposed apices, and elongation of the left upper cheek teeth.

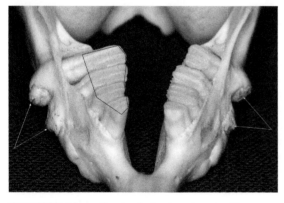

Figure 10.23 Advanced malocclusion in a six-year-old chinchilla (mandible specimen) with severe lingual tilting and retrograde elongation of all right cheek teeth and secondary, lateral perforation of the cortical bone of the jaw (M2/M3; white arrows), secondary widening of the occlusal surface (black lines) and retrograde displacement of the last two left molars (M2/M3) with perforation of the lateral cortical bone of the jaw (turquoise arrows).

must be associated with laterolateral jaw excursions, otherwise those kinds of findings would be impossible. More precise studies on this have not been undertaken.

Intraoral elongation of cheek teeth, which occurs when dental abrasion is insufficient, will – independent of species – push the lower and the upper jaw further and further apart (wider angle of mouth opening) and will inevitably lead to an overgrowth of the incisors. Hence secondary malocclusion of the incisors is always an indication of a primary problem concerning the cheek teeth. In guinea pigs, the rather steeply inclined occlusal plane of the molars (approximately 40°) and the caudorostral convergence of the rows of cheek teeth cause the mandible to be displaced rostrally, parallel to the intraoral elongation of the teeth. The elongated incisors no longer occlude correctly due to the displacement of the jaw. The incisors contact one another instead of having the normal space between them as seen normally. Their occlusal surfaces also change. In the case of more severe malocclusions, a mandibular prognathism may even develop where the elongated mandibular incisors occlude rostral to the maxillary incisors, which are also elongated (see Figure 4.13 in Chapter 4 and Figure 9.24 in Chapter 9).

The situation in chinchillas is an entirely different story. Although in these animals the mandibles converge rostrally, the mandible is displaced more and more distally with an increasing intraoral elongation of the cheek teeth (see Figure 5.37 in Chapter 5). The clinical result of this is a relative mandibular brachygnathism. Here, too, the angle between the jaws becomes wider so that the incisors get longer and longer, resulting in secondary incisor malocclusions. Since the maxillary incisors are more markedly curved, their elongation results in the teeth growing distally into the oral cavity; there they will make indirect (blunt) contact with the correspondingly elongated mandibular incisors (see Figure 10.24 and Figure 10.29 later).

Jaw displacement is rather rare in degus. The kind of displacement needed for it to occur is hardly possible theoretically due to the stepped formation of the pathologically altered occlusal plane. Some animals, however, exhibit a slight caudal displacement of the mandible that is similar to the findings in chinchillas; here the individual steps of the dentition still interlock exactly. The lack of dental wear leads to the first upper cheek tooth forming a very pronounced rostral spur (see Figure 9.11 in Chapter 9). If teeth are tilted or curved

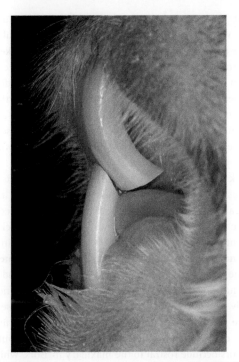

Figure 10.24 Incisor malocclusion in a six-year-old chinchilla with intraoral overgrowth of the maxillary and mandibular incisors and abnormal occlusal contact. The abnormal occlusal surface and the curvature of the maxillary incisors indicate a primary malocclusion of cheek teeth.

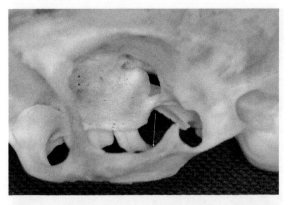

Figure 10.25 The same patient as in Figure 9.11 (in Chapter 9), a degu with malocclusion of cheek teeth (left orbit specimen): distal spur in the occlusal area of the last upper cheek tooth (M3; white arrow) and distal concave curvature of the tooth with slight retrograde elongation into the orbit.

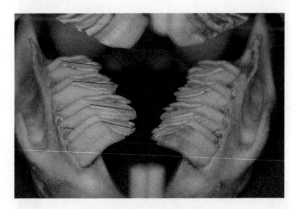

Figure 10.26 Severe lingual tilting of all lower cheek teeth of a four-year-old guinea pig (specimen, rostral view) with rostral bridge formation as well as buccal spurs of the maxillary teeth; secondary pathological enlargement (widening) of the chewing surface (black lines).

additionally, a lingual spur causing a secondary lesion of the tongue, which resembles the findings in rabbits, can develop here (Figure 10.22). The slight jaw displacement implies that the occlusal surface of the last upper molar is no longer worn down in its entirety either. This leads to typical, distally orientated spurs that are also very sharp (Figure 10.25). This tooth may also penetrate the orbit with retrograde displacement.

A rostral jaw displacement in guinea pigs implies that the third maxillary molar will no longer have an antagonist and that it cannot be sufficiently abraded. The consequences are buccal tooth spurs that cannot be seen very well (intraoral examination) and are therefore easily missed (see Figure 10.55 later). Moreover, both first cheek teeth in the mandible now lack a suitable antagonist. Due to the normal curvature, which is enhanced by the pathological overgrowth of the teeth, the two mandibular premolars which now hardly occlude, start to grow toward each other – uni- or bilaterally. As soon as they are in contact, they form a tooth

bridge, which is typical of guinea pigs. When this happens, the premolars may either just touch each other with their tips or may grow past each other by some distance. The tooth bridge will trap the tongue underneath (tongue entrapment) and prevent normal swallowing of food (see Figure 3.15 in Chapter 3 and Figure 10.26). The animals are not able to manage to push the food bolus up against the palate with the base of their tongue and then send it into the pharynx. This is made even more difficult by the marked spreading of the jaws (Figure 9.24 in Chapter 9). The animals will still take up food by themselves and chew it, although

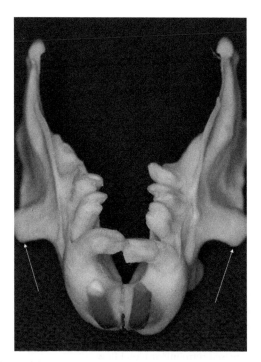

Figure 10.27 Malocclusion of cheek teeth in a three-year-old degu (mandible specimen) with slight lingual tilting of all cheek teeth and a rostral tooth bridge formation (P4); retrograde displacement of the apices of the last two cheek teeth with significant lateral protrusion of the respective cortical bone of the jaw (M3; white arrows).

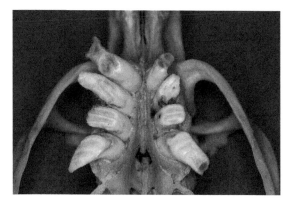

Figure 10.28 Advanced malocclusion of cheek teeth in a ten-year-old chinchilla (maxilla specimen) with large buccal spur formation of almost all cheek teeth; intraalveolar rotation of the first two cheek teeth (P4/M1; altered occlusal pattern) and carious lesions on the distal surface of the first two left cheek teeth (P4/M1).

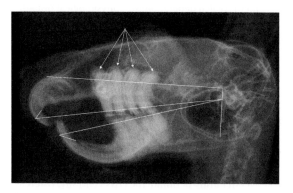

Figure 10.29 Advanced malocclusion of cheek teeth in a six-year-old chinchilla (laterolateral view) with intraoral overgrowth and retrograde elongation of all upper cheek teeth, particularly the last two molars (M2/M3; acting as fulcrum); pathological caudal occlusal plane and secondary incisor malocclusion.

this becomes very difficult for them. They will not, however, be able to swallow the food mush because of the restricted mobility of their tongue. Hence the food, which has been half-chewed, will fall back out of their mouths after a few rather listless grinding movements. At the same time, the animals frequently wipe their mouths with their front paws while opening the mouth widely.

Mandibular tooth bridges rarely occur in degus and not at all in chinchillas (Figure 10.27). The pathology of a cheek teeth malocclusion in chinchillas is predominantly in the maxilla (apices), whereas in degus changes mainly affect the apical portion of the mandibular molars (high-degree retrograde tooth elongation; Figure 10.22). Many chinchillas with malocclusions, however, exhibit similar clinical symptoms as guinea pigs with a tooth bridge formation: food falling out of the mouth, typical wiping movements with the paw and increased salivation. The cause of this are very painful, buccal tooth spurs of the upper molars or an occlusal

correction that has not been performed correctly (Figure 10.28). Especially in chinchillas with their extremely long, narrow, poorly accessible oral cavity, the last upper cheek tooth is often not trimmed sufficiently. Thus it will act as a fulcrum and the animals will not be able to close their mouths correctly. The oral cavity remains partially open and the incisors, which were trimmed down to the correct heights, are spaced far from one another (Figure 10.29). If the patients try to close their mouths more by contracting their jaw muscles more strongly (chewing attempt), the result is a luxation of the temporomandibular condyle (temporomandibular hyperextension). The animals try to reposition it by opening their mouths wide. Guinea pigs will show identical symptoms after nonprofessional occlusal correction (still overlong caudal molars).

In laterolateral radiographs of the skulls of guinea pigs, chinchillas and degus intraoral tooth elongation can be recognized from an increasing divergence of the palatal and mandibular bone plates (see Section 5.6 in Chapter 5, reference lines), as well as from an increasing clinical approach or even contact of the incisors, which are normally apart at rest.

As well as the intraoral tooth elongation, there is always a concomitant retrograde displacement of the tooth apices into the adjacent jawbone, due to the increased axial load of the cheek teeth. This can be seen clearly on laterolateral skull radiographs, using the appropriate reference lines (Figure 10.29). There are species-specific predilection sites for that retrograde displacement, which depend on the (physiological or pathological) curvature of the teeth. Secondary abscesses are frequently formed in those areas in particular. In guinea pigs and chinchillas, such predilection sites are the lateral maxillary area (the nasal bone in the proximity of the nasolacrimal duct), the orbit and the ventrolateral cortical bone of the mandible (see Figures 5.32d and 5.40d in Chapter 5). By contrast, degus mainly exhibit – apart from a displacement of the apices of the maxillary and mandibular incisors – a retrograde displacement of the lower cheek teeth (Figure 10.22). The first two cheek teeth mostly perforate the jaws ventrally, whereas the last two molars perforate the lateral wall of the jaw (see Figure 9.11 in Chapter 9). In degus, the pathology affecting the maxillary molars is never as pronounced as in the mandible. There is usually a significant discrepancy here (Figure 10.25).

The constant bone resorption and simultaneous apposition of new bone substance below the tooth apex causes the apical part of the tooth to be continuously displaced further and further into the adjacent jawbone. In the early stage of a malocclusion, the germinal tissue is still covered by an albeit thin layer of cortical bone even as retrograde displacement increases. Since the animals often exhibit hardly any clinical symptoms whilst local bone changes can be quite marked, it is thought to be relatively painless and thus rather unproblematic. However, if the tooth apices perforate the apical layer of bone and reach the sensitive periosteum, pain and therefore clinical symptoms will increase (exposed

alveolar bulla) (see Figure 4.7 in Chapter 4 and Figure 10.54 later). In these cases, not even an optimally performed correction of the dentition brings the desired success or at least even short-term clinical success. The cause of the sustained anorexia will often not be recognized without further radiographic diagnostics.

In the caudal area of the upper jaw, a retrobulbar abscess – rising periodontally or spreading from one tooth to the other – can develop as a result of a simultaneous apical infection of the last two molars (M2/M3). These changes are rare in degus, compared to guinea pigs or chinchillas. The exophthalmos resulting from this is usually not as pronounced in guinea pigs and chinchillas as it is in rabbits, at least in the early stage. Both eyes need to be compared very carefully in order to detect a mild eye protrusion. In chinchillas with changes on both sides, a slight bulb protrusion may be difficult to detect as the animals normally have slightly protruding eyes (Crossley et al., 1998). Sometimes that protrusion is exaggerated when the animal becomes excited, due to an increase in blood pressure involving an increased retrobulbar blood flow.

If there is a suspected clinical asymmetry of the two eyes, the cheek teeth – apart from the eyes – should be examined particularly thoroughly. In all three animal species, there is an absolute indication for radiographs, which can help identify apical infections of the cheek teeth. The last two upper molars in particular are usually involved as their apices will be located deeply within the orbit when retrograde displacement occurs (Figure 10.30a). Such changes are extremely rare in degus. If there is some pathology, in most cases only the last upper molar which is curved caudally will be affected (Figure 10.25). The protrusion mostly becomes more pronounced over a period of a few months, during which the animals present for tooth trimming time and again, until ultimately an exposure keratitis with a subsequent panophthalmia develops – just as in rabbits. After appropriate radiographic examination, involving isolated views of the maxilla as described by Böhmer, not only is enucleation required but also extraction of the affected cheek tooth. In most cases it is the only way to ensure that the wound area will heal completely without complications or persisting deep infections. Otherwise often a persistent intraoral fistula will be formed. Unfortunately it is unclear why both chinchillas and degus much more rarely suffer from extensive apical abscessations, in spite of generally identical pathological

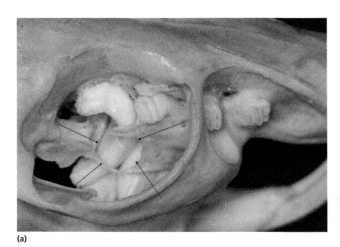

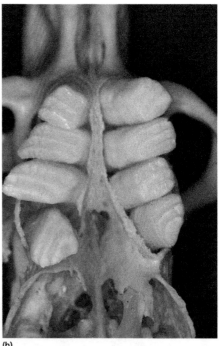

(a)

(b)

Figure 10.30 Severe malocclusion in a five-year-old chinchilla. (a) Specimen, right orbital area: marked retrograde elongation of all cheek teeth and exposed alveolar bullae; marked, distally concave curvature of the last molar (M3) with extensive resorption of the laterodistal alveolar wall (black arrows). The opening of the bony nasolacrimal duct is visible dorsorostrally from the second cheek tooth (turquoise arrow). (b) Maxilla with advanced malocclusion; significant elongation of the clinical crowns of all upper cheek teeth, buccal spurs of the middle right molars (M1/M2), marked intraalveolar rotation of the last right cheek tooth (M3) with altered orientation of the occlusal pattern (enamel folds orientated almost longitudinally) and slight rotation of the first left cheek tooth (P4).

changes of the apices of the maxillary (and also the mandibular) cheek teeth as in rabbits.

In parallel to the inflammatory apical processes in guinea pigs and chinchillas, the entire shape and structure of the affected cheek tooth, which has retrogradely penetrated the orbit, also change. This can be recognized from a pathological pattern of the occlusal surface of the respective tooth during a thorough intraoral examination (see Figure 2.8 in Chapter 2).

In chinchillas, an intraalveolar rotation of the tooth occurs together with retrograde elongation (mostly with a typical perforation of the lamina dura), due to the reduced resistance of the alveolar wall, which is now partially resorbed. The intraalveolar rotation of the tooth is associated with an intraoral change of the pattern of the occlusal surface (pathological orientation of the enamel folds; Figures 10.28 and 10.30b). As can be seen in intraoral findings, the enamel crests now

have an oblique or even rostrocaudal orientation in contrasts to their usual transverse (i.e. buccopalatal) orientation.

The types of rotations of guinea pig cheek teeth, which are more securely anchored in the jaw and generally larger in structure, are rather unusual, due to the more complex structure and the normal curvature of the teeth. There are, however, frequent changes to the overall structure of the occlusal surface of a pathologically altered cheek tooth – in very different ways and to various degrees. Most commonly the affected tooth becomes unnaturally wide (Figure 10.31). At the same time, it is often unnaturally smooth and has an altered coronal surface in that additional, abnormal enamel folds are formed or the physiological "lophs" have an different orientation from the normal. There are also thickenings of individual dentin bodies (dentin columns). Apart from the altered pattern of the occlusal

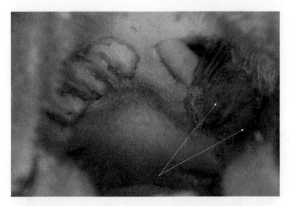

Figure 10.31 Intraoral view of the maxilla of a four-year-old guinea pig with advanced malocclusion; pathologically altered and markedly widened occlusal surface of the last two left cheek teeth (M2/M3; white arrows) are clinical indicators of a severe, presumably inflammatory, changes of their apices.

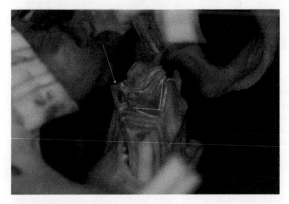

Figure 10.32 Malocclusion of cheek teeth in a six-year-old guinea pig (specimen, left mandibular occlusal plane): severely altered occlusal surface of the last two cheek teeth (M2/M3) with 90° angulation of the occlusal surface (white lines), indicating a pathological finding in the area of their apices, and expansion of the lingual alveolar area of the last molar (M3; turquoise arrow).

surface, a steep buccal tooth ridge, which is mostly orientated at a 90° angle toward the occlusal plane, can be recognized in some guinea pigs (Figure 10.32).

Those specific changes are important indicators of the precise localization of the more severe, painful processes occurring in the jaw, which are often responsible for a sustained anorexia despite treatment. The extent of the changes can be further identified using radiographic examination with specific positionings (e.g. an isolated view of the maxilla or mandible as described by

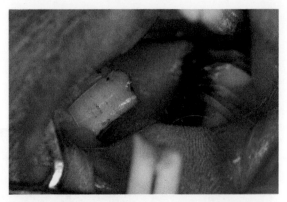

Figure 10.33 Malocclusion of cheek teeth in a three-year-old guinea pig (intraoral view, left mandibular row of cheek teeth): dark discoloration of the occlusal surfaces of all left cheek teeth, indicating insufficient wear, moderate degree of bridge formation of the anterior cheek teeth (P4), unsymmetrical dental wear, lingual tilting of the entire left row of cheek teeth and oblique occlusal plane of the mandibular incisors.

Böhmer). The information obtained can then be used to discuss further treatment and prognosis.

In chinchillas and guinea pigs, painful tooth rows that are not being used during mastication and therefore are not being abraded can be recognized from the discoloration of their occlusal surfaces, which are significantly darker or even black (Figure 10.33). A discoloration may also appear in individual teeth that are not in occlusion. The insufficient abrasion of molars that are altered in this way also results in a tendency for occlusal caries development (see Figure 12.12 in Chapter 12). All these clinical findings may indicate the localization of the primary painful, intraosseous cause of the malocclusion.

The apices of the last two upper molars of guinea pigs, chinchillas and degus are located intraorbitally. By contrast, the apical areas of the anterior two upper cheek teeth are located in the maxilla (nasal surface). In the case of a retrograde displacement of the latter, the likely consequences are compressions of the nasolacrimal duct, whose bony portion runs in the immediate proximity of the tooth apices (see Figure 9.20 in Chapter 9 and Figure 10.21).

If there is a suspected narrowing of the nasolacrimal duct, it can be flushed in principle as in rabbits, although this is very difficult because the structures are very tiny. Conventional cannulae designed for the nasolacrimal duct are too large to be used here. The plastic parts of pediatric peripheral venous catheters are better suited. Both guinea pigs and chinchillas have two lacrimal puncta that are located close to the medial canthus on the upper and lower margins of the eyelid (see Figure 4.7 in Chapter 4). In chinchillas, the narrow-lumened, tiny ducts that run from there to the rostrum come together to form a larger canal, which disappears in the lateral area of the maxilla close to the fossa infraorbitalis (entrance to the bony nasolacrimal duct; Figure 10.30a). In guinea pigs, by contrast, the nasolacrimal duct runs in a short, bony canal in the immediate proximity of the eye before running rostrally along the lacrimal bone. After that, the nasolacrimal duct re-emerges in the area of the apices of the anterior two upper cheek teeth before disappearing in the rostrum dorsorostrally from the premolar, which is similar to the situation in chinchillas (Figure 10.34b). A degu anatomy is similar to that of a chinchilla.

As for guinea pigs, a chronic infection of the tooth apex may not only lead to the formation of a structurally altered, mostly thickened or otherwise misshapen tooth. It may also result in a scenario where the individual dental substances (dentin, enamel and cementum) no longer form a normal compound. As described above for rabbits, this results in a secondary longitudinal splitting of the affected bilophodont cheek tooth. This bifurcation of the tooth body is not traumarelated (e.g. caused by biting on a hard piece of food or foreign material), but is the consequence of a chronic irritation or a subclinical infection of the tooth-forming germinal cells. The latter continue to produce dental substances, but the individual dentin lamellae are not adequately connected with one another via a relatively thick layer of crown cementum as well as a thinner peripheral enamel bridge. In addition, the dentin column(s) is (are) mostly altered structurally (Figure 10.34a and b). Such findings may easily be overlooked without specific radiographs including isolated views of the lower and upper jaws, as described by Böhmer.

While longitudinal splitting of the cheek teeth is relatively frequent in guinea pigs, it is very rare in chinchillas and basically unknown in degus. The reason for this is the structure of the chinchilla's trilophodont cheek teeth, which is more compact overall, with the individual dentin bodies tightly connected to each other in an almost square shape, and without any lateral indentations filled with larger amounts of cementum (as can be found in rabbits) (see Figure 3.21 in Chapter 3). The structure of the teeth is even simpler in degus, whose cheek teeth only have a bilateral, slight indentation. The dentin body, which is always shaped in a figure-of-eight in the mandibular teeth and L-shaped in the maxillary teeth, is covered by a relatively large, cuff-like enamel layer (see Figure 3.24 in Chapter 3). That layer is considerably resistant to longitudinal

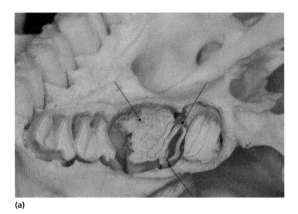

(a)

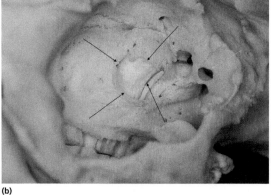

(b)

Figure 10.34 Malocclusion and retrobulbar abscessation in a four-year-old guinea pig. (a) Specimen, right maxillary row of cheek teeth: pathologically altered occlusal surface of the next-to-last cheek tooth (M2; black arrows), thickening of the rostral dentin column and longitudinal splitting of the distal tooth body, pronounced dilation of the desmodontium, indicating a chronic periodontitis, and pathologically altered tooth body of the last molar (M3). (b) Specimen, right orbit: severe intraorbital displacement of the apex of the last three cheek teeth (M1–M3) and perforation of the lateral cortical cover of the alveolar bulla of the next-to-last intraalveolarly split molar (M2; black arrows). The first part of the short first section of the bony nasolacrimal duct is visible in the area of the lacrimal bone (turquoise arrow).

splitting. Tooth indentations that are primarily filled with crown cementum (as in rabbits) predispose to longitudinal splitting.

In guinea pigs, longitudinal splitting of teeth mostly involves the entire length of the cheek tooth structure. There are, however, occasional cases of tooth chipping that are restricted to the clinical crown or partial crown fractures. The primary cause of those is insufficient mineralization of the dental substance or enamel and dentin hypoplasia, which also leads to the formation of structurally altered, less-resistant crown cement. Those defects of the dental hard substance, which are mostly generalized, cause the teeth to become more brittle overall. An additional, crucial element involved with tooth splitting is the particular structure of the W-shaped molars of guinea pigs. Especially in the case of an additional elongation of the clinical crown (in other words an intraoral tooth overgrowth), pathologically altered crown cement is washed out too quickly from between the double-walled enamel folds, which are located buccally in the mandible and palatally in the maxilla (Figure 10.35). The intradental enamel folds are now insufficiently filled, predisposing the tooth to pathological separations or fractures of the intraoral tooth structure. By contrast, those kinds of changes are very seldom in the molars of chinchillas, whose molars have a more compact structure (less cementum).

Concomitant with the intra- and extraoral tooth elongation, the longitudinal axis and thus the intraoral

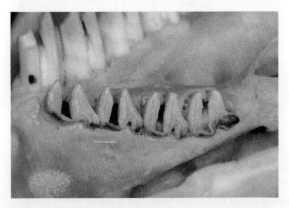

Figure 10.35 Early malocclusion in a two-year-old guinea pig (specimen, right maxillary row of cheek teeth): severely washed-out crown cementum between the dentin lamellae of the anterior three cheek teeth (P4–M2). The resulting gaps are partially filled with foreign material. There is a predisposition to pathological tooth splittings as well as a periodontitis.

shape of the affected cheek teeth changes. The teeth become more curved and hereby form a much wider (broader) occlusal plane (see Figure 5.40d in Chapter 5 and Figure 10.26). This is due to the abnormal occlusal pressure (increase of pressure on certain parts of the affected tooth). Such an abnormal curvature or tilting of single teeth can be caused as well by local periodontal disease (food impaction), with a local loss of the alveolar bone supporting the tooth or a generalized bone weakness, which may have metabolic causes if more teeth are involved. As a result of the abnormal pressure on the entire tooth, the tooth apex is often secondarily displaced retrogradely. In the lower jaw of guinea pigs and chinchillas, it mostly perforates the outer cortical jawbone – partially or completely – so that the displaced apex will often be exposed (uncovered alveolar bulla). When this occurs the animals start to exhibit more severe clinical symptoms as the pain-sensitive periosteum is irritated and perforated. In the case of an additional infection, mandibular abscesses of the teeth will develop, which will mostly affect the caudal area of the jaw in these animals, meaning they are mostly located underneath the masseter muscle. In principle, however, any cheek tooth can be affected (see Figure 8.1b in Chapter 8).

Both the tilting of the tooth body and the lateral apex displacement, with a subsequent perforation of the mandible, will cause a sustained and irreversible change in the direction of tooth growth (in all species), as well as alter the width of the abnormal occlusal surface (Figure 10.23). Hence in such cases, correcting the occlusal surface and the length of teeth will only bring temporary therapeutic success. A long-term re-establishment of normal occlusion is no longer possible, so the treatment is purely palliative. If individual teeth are affected, tooth extraction might be considered.

The tooth displacement leads to an increase in the periodontal ligament space, which is opposite to the direction of tilt, and an increase of the interproximal areas between the teeth. Food particles impact the tissue, resulting in a secondary periodontitis (see Figure 8.13a in Chapter 8). As an example of this, see also Section 12.1 in Chapter 12. In addition, there is no physiological "self-cleaning" of the dentition due to the abnormal surface structure and angulation of the entire occlusal surface and the elongation of all or individual cheek teeth. Soft plaques are formed near the gingiva, leading to an additional, inflammatory response of the peridontium, particularly in guinea pigs and chinchillas. The resulting deep gingival pockets can become impacted with food particles as well as hair, further worsening the periodontitis. Since a progressive loss of the alveolar bone supporting the tooth occurs concurrently, the tilting or loosening of the tooth increases, and a vicious cycle starts that is very difficult to control or treat.

Typical pathology of the cheek teeth in guinea pigs

Malocclusions in guinea pigs are presumed to be primarily related to inappropriate feeding and improper husbandry. Hence food that is not abrasive enough plays the biggest role, along with a lack of or not enough sunlight. It is still unclear to what extent genetic causes and other environmental influences that have already been discussed are involved. What is clear is that many guinea pigs – just like chinchillas – that are kept indoors suffer from an acquired malocclusion. It is striking that some of these animals are even related to each other (siblings, direct offspring). There is a lack, however, of exact scientific studies on that subject.

As mentioned above, the most frequent findings in guinea pigs with a malocclusion are bridge formations of the mandibular premolars and a rostral displacement of the mandible, which may even lead to mandibular prognathism in extreme cases. Very sharp or pointed buccal spurs frequently develop on the upper molars, and they tend to be missed during correction of the dentition.

Also relatively typical of guinea pigs, and rather frequent, are structurally deformed and/or split cheek teeth (crippled or giant teeth), which have already been discussed above. Either an individual tooth or several molars may be affected (Figure 10.31). Those changes always worsen the general symptoms of a malocclusion further (intraoral tooth elongation and retrograde growth of the cheek teeth). An altered occlusal surface that can be identified on oral inspection is an important clinical indicator of a malocclusion. Since the apices of the affected cheek teeth – mostly the last two molars – are always retrogradely displaced to a high degree and exposed apically (uncovered alveolar bulla), this leads to intense pain. Often there are concomitant, localized, apical microabscessations. If those kinds of findings are not recognized due to insufficient or poor diagnostic radiographs, patients will still exhibit sustained clinical symptoms of a malocclusion even though dental

correction was optimally performed. The expected success of treatment fails to materialize "for no reason." Hence any postoperative, inexplicable anorexia or dysphagia should be a reason to critically re-evaluate the dental treatment that was performed. For this, not only is a thorough intraoral examination needed but also radiographs including the use of the correct reference lines. The structure and the apical area of each individual tooth can be exactly evaluated once again. If there is any doubt, specific positionings such as isolated views of the lower and upper molars of guinea pigs as described by Böhmer (Figure 10.36a and b) can be used to clarify inconclusive findings. If the suspicion of an apically altered crippled or giant tooth is confirmed, an extraction of the tooth is the only option for long-term therapeutic success. This is not only because of the painfulness of the apical processes but also because of the fact that a molar that has been altered in that way can never be correctly abraded by its antagonist. The risks of a tooth extraction are assessed in every single case (prolonged healing period, secondary tooth displacement, possible need for repeated dental treatments).

If early apical infections are not recognized, the initial, localized infection will inevitably become a more extensive periodontal abscess with time. These tooth-associated jaw abscesses in guinea pigs frequently affect the posterior (retrobulbar) area of the maxilla (Figure 10.34b). In the mandible, abscesses mostly occur in the area below the masseter muscle as the two last molars are primarily affected. As the infection continues to spread, the masticatory muscle undergoes liquefactive necrosis, resulting in a continuously extending abscess (see Figure 8.1b in Chapter 8). If, however, an apical infection of the anterior two cheek teeth is present, a readily palpable fluctuant mass is usually present in the rostroventral area of the mandible. In most of those cases the incisors are also affected secondarily, or even primarily. More extensive bony involvement of the mandible (bony lysis with widespread bony apposition), which are typical of rabbits, are rather rare in guinea pigs.

An apical infection or severe retrograde elongation of the first two maxillary cheek teeth can lead to a compression of the nasolacrimal duct, and thus epiphora. This may result in the crystallization of the lacrimal fluid (seen as whitish salt crusts) at the medial canthus. A local irritation of the masseter muscle (infra-orbital part) can also be caused by a retrograde tooth displacement

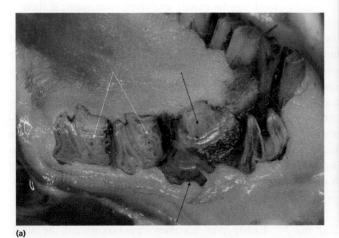
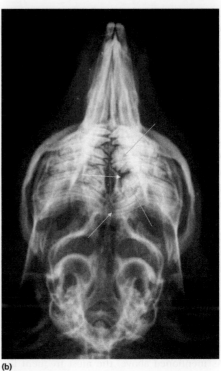

(a)   (b)

Figure 10.36 Advanced malocclusion of cheek teeth in a five-year-old guinea pig. (a) Specimen, left maxillary row of cheek teeth: structurally altered second cheek tooth (M1; black arrows), widening of the occlusal surface and buccal tooth spur; slight morphological change of the occlusal surface of the last two molars (M2/M3; white arrows) and thickening of the respective rostral dentin columns, indicating an apical irritation of the germinal cells of all three affected molars (M1–M3). (b) Isolated view of the maxilla as described by Böhmer: structural change of the apices and the tooth bodies of the two middle left cheek teeth (M1/M2; turquoise arrows), periapical lysis in the area of the next-to-last left upper molar (M2; white arrow) and retrograde elongation of the last maxillary cheek tooth (M3; yellow arrow).

(see Figure 5.32c in Chapter 5). This can lead to a pain-related dysphagia or general symptoms of a malocclusion that become progressively worse. Occasionally there is localized pain.

Typical pathology of the cheek teeth in chinchillas

Chinchillas – just like guinea pigs and degus – originate from the western part of South America and were bred mainly for fur in the early years of the last century (Crossley et al., 1998). Some animals were captured and bred, and a certain amount of inbreeding occurred. After that, chinchillas were also used as laboratory animals before they were increasingly turned into pets. The fact that a majority of today's chinchilla population are the offspring of very few different individuals may have an influence on the relative frequency of malocclusions in that species.

The first publications on tooth disorders in chinchillas appeared in the 1980s of the last century (Harkness & Wagner, 1983; Webb, 1985; Wiggs & Lobprise, 1990; Emily & Penman, 1994; Crossley et al., 1998). Compared with wild chinchillas, today's pets have altered skull measurements (16% longer and 6% wider) and their cheek teeth are approximately one-third longer. Measurements yielded length averages of 5.9 mm for the molars of wild animals, 6.6 mm for zoo animals and 7.4 mm for "healthy" pets. That value increased to an average of 10 mm in chinchillas with a malocclusion. This proves that, in general, all captive chinchillas are already suffering from at least an early stage of malocclusion (Crossley & Miguelez, 2001). Healthy wild animals have a smooth mandible and their good cortical cover prevents penetration of the cheek teeth apices into the orbit, whereas those kinds of changes can be found in almost all pets that appear to be "healthy."

A genetic predisposition for disorders of the dentition has not been confirmed. Hence it is supposed that malocclusions in chinchillas are mainly related to nutrition and husbandry (Crossley et al., 1998; Brenner et al., 2005). Consequently, malocclusions can be prevented with proper nutrition (Brenner et al., 2005). Since almost all pet chinchillas receive the wrong food, a large proportion of these animals suffer from pronounced acquired malocclusions. A study found that 35% of all animals presumed healthy had significantly elongated cheek teeth and thus early dental disease (Crossley & Miguelez, 2001). In contrast to guinea pigs, chinchillas rarely suffer from primary incisor malocclusions; secondary changes involving the cheek teeth are predominant.

Particularly during the early stages of malocclusion, many chinchillas exhibit a pain-related, serous eye discharge – with or without concomitant anorexia – that is resistant to treatment (Figure 10.37). It is caused by a retrograde displacement of the apices of the maxillary cheek teeth. Physiological (micro-)movements of the molars are transferred directly on to the periapical periosteum during normal chewing, leading to a painful local irritation (Crossley et al., 1998). During these early stages, pain can often be successfully relieved with analgesics (Crossley, 1995a). Moreover, maximal trimming of cheek teeth can reduce the pressure acting on the apices, for a little while.

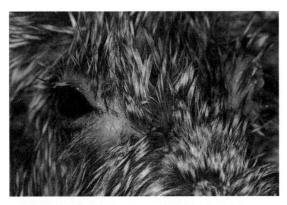

Figure 10.37 Epiphora, periocular dermatitis and bilateral rostral swelling in a six-year-old chinchilla. There is a suspected cheek tooth malocclusion with a retrograde displacement of the maxillary tooth apices.

Unfortunately the symptoms, which are fairly typical of dental disease, are often misinterpreted, and only a presumed eye disorder is treated. Epiphora, however, should always be recognized as a possible indicator of an early malocclusion and thus be an indication for a clinical examination, and most importantly a radiographic examination of the dentition. Laterolateral skull views usually yield clear evidence of a maxillary retrograde tooth displacement when reference lines are used. Intraoral examination, by contrast, can be difficult as most pathological findings are very slight and tend to be missed, particularly if the practitioner is inexperienced in dealing with this species (see Figure 3.22 in Chapter 3).

The species-specific dominance of the retrograde tooth displacement can be explained by the fact that due to the relatively steep position of the cheek teeth (inclination of approximately 10°), a very slight intraalveolar tooth overgrowth will already be enough to stop tooth eruption (Crossley & Miguelez, 2001; see Figure 3.23 in Chapter 3). A progressive intraoral tooth elongation further increases the vertical pressure acting on the molars and the tooth apices are ultimately retrogradely displaced. There is also intra- and extraalveolar curvature of teeth, which are always more pronounced in the upper jaw than in the lower jaw (see Figure 5.40d in Chapter 5). As a result of this, a secondary widening of the occlusal surface occurs. In addition, there is a pathological angulation of the occlusal plane. Intraalveolar tooth rotations that alter the occlusal pattern of enamel folds is often visible intraorally. The elongated clinical crowns of the molars will then protrude far into the oral cavity instead of being flush with the gingiva. The accompanying mandibular brachygnathism is species-specific (see Figure 5.37 in Chapter 5).

Just like guinea pigs, chinchillas also experience a painful, local irritation of the infraorbital part of the masseter muscle. In the case of a severe retrograde displacement of the apices of the two anterior upper cheek teeth, the normal ample lumen of the infra-orbital canal is markedly narrowed and the masticatory muscle function is hampered. A secondary compression of the nearby nasolacrimal duct is just as frequent. The animals exhibit clinically persistent epiphora, sometimes involving purulent-opaque lacrimal fluid. In contrast to rabbits, pathological changes associated with the apices of both maxillary incisors more rarely affect the nasolacrimal

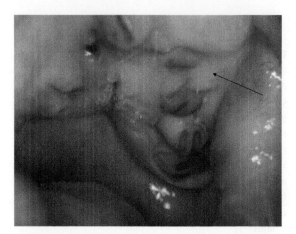

Figure 10.38 Advanced malocclusion in a twelve-year-old chinchilla (left maxillary row of cheek teeth): elongation of the clinical crowns of all cheek teeth, discharge of pus from the tooth socket of the first molar (M1; black arrow), altered occlusal enamel pattern of all cheek teeth's chewing surfaces as a result of an intraalveolar tooth rotation, pronounced gingival hyperplasia and pathological tooth discoloration.

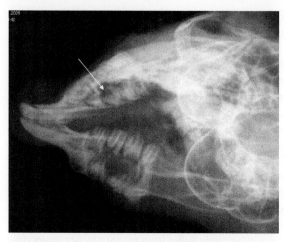

Figure 10.39 Advanced malocclusion in a five-year-old chinchilla (isolated view of the left mandible as described by Böhmer): pronounced, resorptive, intraalveolar lesions of all cheek teeth. Some of the clinical crowns are completely isolated (M1/M2) and the contralateral side is also affected (white arrow). There is an indication for an isolated view of the right mandible.

canal of chinchillas, even though the canal runs just as close to the apices.

Retrobulbar abscesses are very rare in chinchillas in comparison to guinea pigs and rabbits, even in the case of the most severe intraorbital tooth pathology. The same is true for 'classic' abscesses of the mandible originating from the cheek teeth. Most commonly, mandibular abscesses are a result of a primary apical incisor inflammation that can spread to the premolars because of the close anatomical proximity of the tooth apices (see Figure 9.26 in Chapter 9).

A predominant finding in many chinchillas with advanced malocclusions is a generalized osteolysis of the jaw, which usually will not only destroy the entire bone but also result in resorption of the cheek teeth (see Figures 8.13 and 8.14 in Chapter 8). Pus may ooze out of one or several sockets with slight occlusal pressure on the cheek teeth (Figure 10.38). To evaluate the full extent of pathology, the lower or upper jaw is radiographed separately (views described by Böhmer). Often the findings will be so severe that euthanasia may be the only option (Figure 10.39).

When chinchillas with advanced intraoral and intraosseous findings first present for treatment, treatment is purely palliative. Maximal trimming of cheek teeth is supposed to re-establish intraoral normal occlusion with a planar, horizontal occlusal surface (see

Section 8.2 and Figure 8.12b in Chapter 8). The required trimming is determined by using the reference lines. Trimming of the cheek teeth may slightly reduce both the axial load of the molars and the associated apical pain (Crossley, 2001a). The apical, intraosseous changes, however, remain irreversible and will progress, albeit at a slower pace after radical shortening of the cheek teeth, a finding based on the author's experience. It is advantageous if the first-time trimming of the cheek teeth is performed when the apices are still covered with a thin bone lamella. Hence it is crucial that intraosseous changes are diagnosed as early as possible.

Even after trimming teeth *lege artis*, recurrences are always possible in chinchillas with severe malocclusions; these may require further corrective treatment, usually every three to four months. The further advanced the pathological changes are, the shorter the time intervals between dental treatments should be. Even if a patient were free of symptoms for longer periods, intervals between individual trimmings must not be too long as axial loads of the cheek teeth will quickly increase excessively, causing the apical findings to worsen unnecessarily. More frequent treatments at regular intervals provide a more favorable long-term prognosis (Crossley, 2001a).

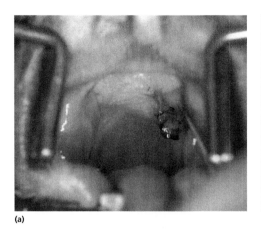
(a)

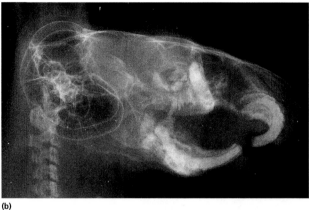
(b)

Figure 10.40 End stage of a malocclusion in a fifteen-year-old chinchilla. (a) Intraoral findings: there is only one tooth left in the left upper jaw and that tooth is markedly altered structurally. (b) Laterolateral view: most extreme structural change of all cheek teeth. The tooth bodies are largely resorbed; severe enamel and dentin hypoplasia of the dental tissue still present and a pronounced retrograde displacement of all incisor apices with a bilateral protrusion of the palatal bone plate.

Since all malocclusions are progressive, the germinal cells are likely to be destroyed in the long term, leading to cessation of growth of the affected teeth, which would otherwise grow throughout life. This is sometimes found to occur in older chinchillas. In such cases, all that is left in the jaw are a few "tooth stubs" that hardly resemble normal teeth structurally. The rest of the cheek teeth will often have disintegrated due to infections or they are roundish, nonirritating dentinoids present in the jawbone (Figure 10.40a and b).

In almost any stage of malocclusion in chinchillas, a diffuse hypertrophy of the maxillary gingiva can lead one to falsely believe that the upper cheek teeth are not altered, or even elongated, intraorally as they remain flush with the gingival margin (see Figure 3.22 in Chapter 3). Lateral radiographs of the head using the reference lines, will help in evaluating the individual situation. While the cause of that species-specific gingival hyperplasia remains unclear, chronic gingivitis and periodontitis play a major part.

Many chinchillas suffer from carious-like changes of the cheek teeth and odontoclastic resorptions close to the gingiva (Crossley, 2001a; Crossley, Dubielzig & Benson, 1997). While carious defects typically lead to localized, brownish discolorations of the occlusal surface and the interproximal area, odontoclastic resorption of teeth is characterized more by an appearance of the lateral surfaces of the teeth resembling moth damage (Figure 10.41). Caries in chinchillas is caused by

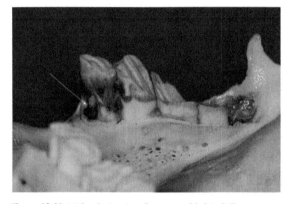

Figure 10.41 Malocclusion in a five-year-old chinchilla (specimen, right mandibular row of cheek teeth, medial view) with caries lesions of the lingual surface of the first cheek tooth, which is significantly elongated intraorally (P4; white arrow), and pathological occlusal surface of all molars (P1–M3).

pleomorphic, either gram-positive or gram-negative bacteria and affects all three of the tooth-forming substances – enamel, dentin and cementum. In principle, hypselodont teeth are relatively resistant to carious defects as they grow continuously. Chinchillas, however, that are chronically ill often receive food that contains a lot of sugar, such as raisins or infant cereal, which seems to predispose them to caries lesions. By contrast, odontoclastic tooth resorptions can be linked to chronically recurring periodontitis that is always concomitant with a malocclusion (Figure 12.1 in Chapter 12).

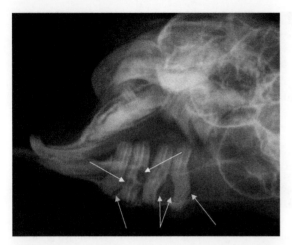

Figure 10.42 Malocclusion in a six-year-old chinchilla (isolated view of the left mandible as described by Böhmer) with a resorptive dental lesion in the area of the mesial and distal intraalveolar surface of the second cheek tooth (M1; white arrows), slight apical displacement and distal lysis in the basal area of the first cheek tooth (P4; turquoise arrow), curvature of the tooth and periodontal bone dissolution (osteolysis) in the intraalveolar section of the two posterior cheek teeth (M2/M3; yellow arrows).

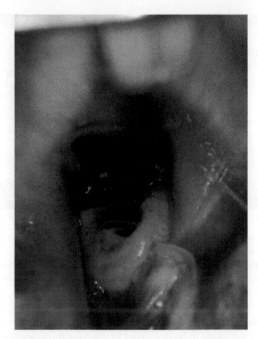

Figure 10.43 Malocclusion in a ten-year-old chinchilla (intraoral finding, left mandibular row of cheek teeth): slight stepped and darkly discolored occlusal surface, indicating insufficient dental wear, often a result of painful intraalveolar resorptions of dental substances.

Primary intraalveolar tooth resorptions are a frequent finding in chinchillas with chronic-recurrent advanced stage malocclusions (Figures 10.20 and 10.42). These mostly multiple, caries-like dissolutions of the tooth structure can affect both the upper and the lower cheek teeth. Usually this is more frequent and more pronounced in the mandible, and the typical inflammatory dissolutions of the dental hard substance mainly affect several adjacent molars. Mild changes, however, can often be detected in individual cheek teeth (early stage). In such cases, further examinations need to show whether they are typical odontoclastic resorptions – it is an evident suspicion anyway. Affected teeth may appear to be completely unchanged intraorally except for a minor elongation of the clinical crown or they may exhibit a darkly discolored occlusal surface resulting from the reduced tooth abrasion due to pain (Figure 10.43). In most cases several teeth in different jaw quadrants are affected.

These fairly typical lesions (that may also occur in guinea pigs and degus) can be seen very clearly on radiographs especially with the isolated views of the lower and upper jaws. Often there is hardly any dental tissue remaining in the middle intraalveolar section of a tooth, in other words between the tooth apex and the extremely short clinical crown. These areas have been completely dissolved, presumably as a result of the chronic desmodontal inflammation (Figure 10.39). Most tooth sockets of the affected cheek teeth are also expanded and filled with pus that may discharge into the oral cavity from around the tooth (severe purulent periodontitis; Figure 10.38). Since several neighboring molars are usually affected, the teeth are often devoid of any attachment or support and are loose within an expanded mandible or (more rarely) maxilla (see Figure 8.13a in Chapter 8). During the terminal stages of the disease, there will often be hardly any normal tooth substance left that can be identified on the radiographs. The predominant findings are scattered tooth fragments irregularly positioned within the jaw and are sometimes ankylosed with the jawbone (Figure 10.40b). Interestingly, some of the patients also suffer from chronic infections of other organ systems such as the kidney or liver. Even intraabdominal abscesses have been identified when postmortem examinations were performed. Hence there is reason to believe that the infection is able to spread to other organs via the bloodstream. The exact causes of the tooth resorption are still largely unknown, but chronic periodontitis certainly plays a major part here.

Treatment of these changes that are extremely painful and progressively destroy the entire tooth structure is basically not feasible. However, experience has shown that a cheek tooth can regrow under certain conditions: if the tooth apex has remained vital and the germinal cells are still functioning. Those conditions involve really radical tooth trimming including resection of the entire clinical crown that is in most cases already isolated from the apical rest of the tooth (Figure 10.39), as well as antibiotic and analgesic therapy. This will reduce the local inflammation, although destruction of the tooth socket and the mandible, respectively, cannot be corrected. Hence it must be decided in each individual case whether treatment is possible at all (in the case of a preserved apex), and whether it is in the best interest of the patient. Euthanizing the animal may often be the best alternative.

Remarkably, many affected chinchillas "quietly suffer" for a relatively long time. More severe clinical symptoms typically do not occur until sharp buccal spurs causing secondary lesions of soft tissue form on the occlusal surface or when there is involvement of the periodontium (Figure 10.44). It is only then that the animals show their pain by eating less. Most findings

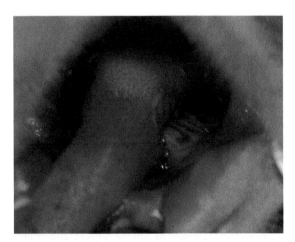

Figure 10.44 Malocclusion in a chinchilla (intraoral finding, left mandibular row of cheek teeth): slight elongation of the clinical crown of all cheek teeth including a formation of lingual spurs, secondary tongue lesion and abnormal angulation of the occlusal plane (10° outwards).

remain undetected before this point as there are usually no visible abscesses and intraoral findings alone often appear to be less dramatic. However, when radiographs are taken, sometimes one cannot help but wonder how the animals would have been able to eat at all during the previous few months. It is these cases that provide ample evidence of how important it is to perform a thorough radiographic examination of the dentition as early as possible. It is the only way to accurately trim the altered cheek teeth during the early stages of malocclusion and that has been proven to have a long-term positive influence on the disease or may at least delay its course.

Typical pathology of the cheek teeth in degus

Degus – just like guinea pigs and chinchillas – are purely herbivorous rodents and exhibit a typically extreme need for gnawing. They also inhabit the Andean mountains of northern and middle Chile. While the pathology of malocclusions of the cheek teeth of guinea pigs and chinchillas has been described and discussed in good detail in numerous publications over the last few years, there is little information on dental disorders in degus. That information comes from rather short, hardly informative notes in a few textbooks and a small number of other papers. A more recent study on malocclusions, however, showed that many pet degus suffer from undiagnosed dental disorders. In the study, 36% of all animals that had presented for other problems had an additional dental problem (Jekl, Hauptman & Knotek, 2006, 2008).

The etiology of malocclusions in degus is still completely unclear. It is presumed that – just like in guinea pigs and chinchillas – both diet-related insufficient dental wear and metabolic bone diseases as well as possibly poor husbandry play a certain part (Jekl, Hautman & Knotek, 2008). However, it has not yet been explained why it is mainly the apices of the mandibular cheek teeth exhibit a pronounced retrograde displacement in degus (with or without a perforation of the alveolar bone and the jawbone). This results in the formation of multiple swellings of the ventrolateral mandibular border (main dental finding), which, amazingly, are usually painless and thus the degu does not show any symptoms (see Figure 9.12 in Chapter 9 and Figure 10.22). By contrast, a retrograde displacement of the upper cheek teeth is rather rare and relatively subtle if present.

Just like chinchillas, degus often do not present for treatment until severe intraoral tooth elongation has caused a more severe step mouth, or when lingual or – more rarely – buccal tooth spurs have formed as a result of a tilting of the teeth (Figure 10.27) (Jekl, Hauptman & Knotek, 2008). The spurs cause soft tissue injuries which are painful resulting in the animals salivating more and refusing to eat by themselves.

A species-specific peculiarity of degus is the fact that many of them suffer from odontoma-like changes of the incisor apices (see Section 9.1.4 and Figures 9.11 and 9.12 in Chapter 9). These benign, mostly apical proliferations of dental substance are associated with a pronounced retrograde displacement and an elongation of the maxillary or mandibular incisors. Secondary cheek teeth problems may arise from that.

Due to the relatively upright position of the cheek teeth (<10° angulation) as well as the simpler structure of the molariform teeth (no central enamel folds), self-cleaning of this species' dentition is very good. That, together with the lack of marked tilting of the teeth, which can cause secondary pathological periodontal pockets, leads to the fact that periodontopathies and secondary loosening of teeth are rather rare in degus. According to the author's experience, however, inflammatory odontoclastic resorptions of the intra- and extraalveolar dental substance are frequently found – just like in chinchillas (Figure 10.45). They are very painful and there is an extremely cautious long-term prognosis as several teeth are usually affected. If only one individual tooth is affected an extraction of that tooth may be considered. True carious tooth defects of the occlusal surface are very rare indeed as the tooth surface is relatively smooth, aggravating caries development.

Although a severe retrograde displacement of the apices of the mandibular cheek teeth, which leads to a complete destruction of the lower jawbone (multiple perforations), must be extremely painful, many degus lack clinical symptoms despite the marked changes. Just as with chinchillas, most patients do not present for treatment until they refuse to eat due to painful intraoral lesions of the soft tissue. Often one is astonished (as is the owner) about the extent of "secondary changes." The anterior two cheek teeth (P4/M1) mostly perforate the mandible ventrally whereas the last two molars (M2/M3) mostly perforate the jaw laterally. The animal's lethargy is either astonishing or – which is more

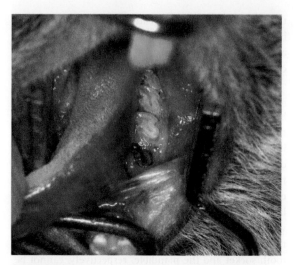

Figure 10.45 Malocclusion in a four-year-old degu (intraoral finding, left mandibular row of cheek teeth): dark discoloration of the first cheek tooth (P4) as a clinical indication of painful, apical infection or intraalveolar lysis of the tooth bodies and slight pathological alteration of the mesiolingual occlusal surface of the second cheek tooth (M1).

probable – the affliction is not recognized. This is further proof of the fact that seemingly undisturbed feed intake of flight in prey animals does not mean that everything is "okay" with them.

10.2 Brachyodont cheek teeth

Due to their brachyodont cheek teeth, which do not grow throughout life, rats, mice and hamsters suffer from dental disorders much more rarely than rabbits and herbivorous rodents. However, massive overgrowths of incisors often occur as a result of wrong feeding and housing conditions (insufficient possibilities for gnawing). The owners notice the animals' secondary problem in feed intake and thus the patient is presented for treatment. Carious and periodontal disorders of the cheek teeth, however, tend to be overlooked. They seem to be much more frequent than previously thought. For example, in a more thorough examination of older rat head specimens, 5 of 15 skulls had carious and periodontal changes to varying degrees. That study may not be representative, but it suggests that such kinds of disorders are not uncommon.

Diagnosis is often difficult as rodents with periodontal or apical infections as well as carious tooth defects often

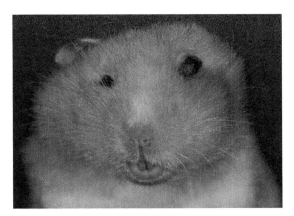

Figure 10.46 Dental abscess in the upper jaw of a one-year-old hamster with a diffuse swelling of the left half of the face.

do not exhibit any recognizable symptoms during the early stages. The problem will start to be obvious only after a secondary abscess of the jaw or the cheek has developed (Figure 10.46; see Section 12.2.3 in Chapter 12). The animals continue eating (other than in case of an incisor problem) and appear to be rather alert – depending on the extent of the bone changes. Just as in rabbits, small rodents are prey and flight animals and thus hide any pain rather efficiently.

Hence the brachyodont cheek teeth of small rodents should be subject to examination more frequently, if only for prophylactic reasons. If periodontopathies are found they need to be treated. Periodontal disorders that have primarily been induced by plaque are supposed to be the most frequent indication for an abscess-associated tooth infection necessitating extraction in small rodents with brachyodont teeth (Gorrel & Verhaert, 2006) (Figures 10.47 to 10.49). In some cases such an invasive procedure can certainly be avoided with early periodontal diagnosis and treatment.

Another complication is the fact that a proper examination of the dentition is only possible under anesthesia as the patient is difficult to restrain due to its highly defensive behavior and susceptibility to stress, as well as the fact that the teeth are so small. An exception to this are hamsters whose mouths can be opened wide (by approximately 120–180°) without even a sedation while holding the animal by the scruff of the neck, offering a good view of the oral cavity.

There have been very few clinical reports on age-related changes of teeth and tooth sockets in rodents with brachyodont teeth. One recent study described an

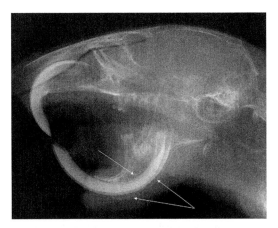

Figure 10.47 Loss of the clinical crowns of several teeth in the upper and lower jaw of a one-and-a-half-year-old hamster (laterolateral view): intraalveolar residue of tooth roots (white arrow), diffuse osteolysis in the area of the alveolus of a lower incisor (white double arrow), almost complete dissolution of the associated periodontal mandibular bone and intraoral overgrowth of the maxillary and mandibular incisors.

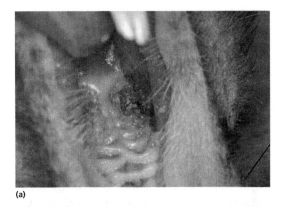

(a)

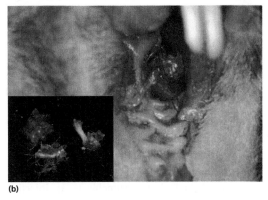

(b)

Figure 10.48 Abscess of the maxilla in a two-year-old hamster. (a) Intraoral finding: loosening of several cheek teeth of the right maxilla. (b) Situation after extraction of the infected molars.

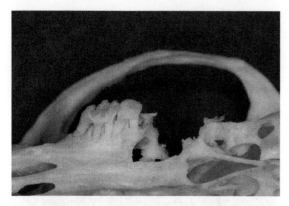

Figure 10.49 Abscess of the maxilla in a two-and-a-half-year-old rat (specimen, left maxillary row of cheek teeth): extensive osteolysis of the maxilla in the area of the missing M3, with a secondary penetration of the orbit.

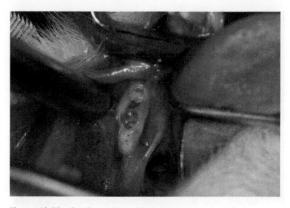

Figure 10.50 Cheek tooth problem in a two-year-old chipmunk (intraoral finding, left mandibular row of cheek teeth): loss of the entire crown of the second (M2) and part of the first cheek tooth (M1); accordingly, roots that have remained in the jawbone are visible.

inflammatory loss of alveolar bone that is "not uncommon" in older laboratory animals (Nishijima et al., 2009). The alveolar bone of hamsters is also reported to continuously decline as a result of the physiological aging process, with the length of cheek teeth being reduced concomitantly (Miles & Crigson, 2003). This leads to a more frequent secondary loss of individual or various cheek teeth in older animals. This can be seen more often in specimens of hamsters that were also kept as pets (Figure 10.47). Not much is known about the etiopathogenesis of these processes, which presumably result from a periodontitis. It is not only pet rodents but also wild animals that may suffer from periodontitis. A three-year-old wood mouse, for example, was found to have undergone an age-related loss of alveolar bone with a secondary partial loss of the molars (Keil, 1966).

Squirrels with malocclusions primarily suffer from disorders of the incisors, but there are also (much rarer) pathological changes of the cheek teeth (Figure 10.50). For example, in a study on dental disorders of red squirrels (*Sciurus vulgaris*) found dead in the United Kingdom, 7 of 91 animals had pathological dental findings (Sainsbury et al., 2004). Excessive wear of several cheek teeth was verified in one particularly old animal, while two other squirrels had an incisor overgrowth. Another animal exhibited partial anodontia (all cheek teeth were missing), due presumably to an infection with a parapoxvirus. Three other squirrels had suffered from dental abscesses of the jaw originating from diseased incisors.

10.3 Trimming of cheek teeth and occlusal correction

10.3.1 General remarks
Basics and possible complications
During trimming of the cheek teeth, adequate protection of soft tissue needs to be ensured, which can be accomplished by using spatulae (see Figure 8.5 in Chapter 8). Should iatrogenic defects of soft tissue occur nonetheless or should there be primary mucosal lesions caused by tooth spurs, they are best covered with a chlorhexidine adhesive gel (Gingisan®) after cleaning and disinfection of the affected area. Suitable analgesics should also be administered. Although intraoral injuries are very painful, they do have a good healing ability.

When performing intraoral treatment, there is always a risk of injuring the relatively large venous vessels at the angle of the jaw; injuries are mostly caused by extensive movements while using the instruments (see Figure 8.3 in Chapter 8 and Figure 10.51). The oral cavity will fill up with blood in a very short time and, depending on the positioning of the patient, there is a danger of aspiration or obstruction of the respiratory pathways. In order to keep the trachea open and ensure free breathing, the head of the patient is lowered as soon as possible or the animal's thorax can be lifted accordingly. At the same time, the tongue is pulled far out of the oral cavity before placing a suitably-sized cotton swab in the angle of the jaw and applying slight pressure on the area. This will help to compress the

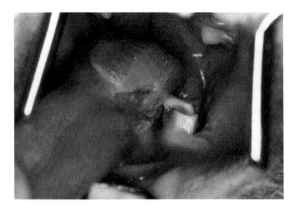

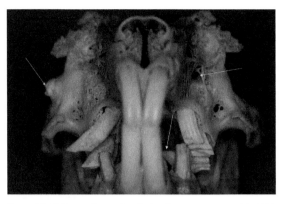

Figure 10.51 Recurring malocclusion in a six-year-old rabbit (left mandibular row of cheek teeth) with a lingual tilt and a secondary spur formation of the second cheek tooth (P4) with a severe injury to the tongue, chronic scarring and extensive loss of tissue in the lateral body of the tongue. The branch of the maxillary vein is visible in the jaw angle.

Figure 10.52 Recurring malocclusion in a seven-year-old rabbit (specimen): severe intraoral tooth elongation of all upper and lower cheek teeth, pronounced enamel and dentin hypoplasia of all molariform teeth (except for the ones in the left upper jaw quadrant), pronounced buccal curvature of the right upper cheek teeth and strong lingual tilt of the third left lower cheek tooth (M1; white arrow), generalized expansion of the maxillary tooth sockets and perforation of the facial tuberosity by the retrogradely displaced apex of the second right upper cheek tooth (P3; turquoise arrow). On the left side, the infraorbital foramen can be clearly seen (yellow arrow) dorsally from the premolar (P2).

blood vessel and stop the hemorrhage within the shortest amount of time. Mouth gags and cheek dilators can be removed before slightly closing the upper and lower jaws while the cotton swab remains in position. Bleeding normally stops after an average of two to three minutes. If the oral cavity starts to fill up with blood again, the saturated cotton swab is replaced with a new one while slightly increasing the amount of pressure on the jaw angle. As soon as bleeding has been successfully stopped, the mouth can be carefully reopened and cleaned with smaller cotton swabs. The area of the bleeding is checked again, and further treatment is best postponed as experience has shown that intraoral manipulations and a maximal opening of the oral cavity lead to renewed bleeding.

Subtle versus radical trimming of cheek teeth

There is great controversy as to what extent the cheek teeth ought to be trimmed in the context of occlusal treatment. In other words, should it be a radical approach burring the tooth crown down to the gum margin (Bennett, 1999; Crossley & Aiken, 2004) or should only the tooth spurs as well as individual elongated teeth be trimmed before slightly smoothing the entire occlusal surface (Harcourt-Brown, 2002a)?

In cases of an acquired form of malocclusion, it could be considered better in principle to radically trim the cheek teeth down to the gum line in order to extend the time intervals between dental treatments. This has

been confirmed, but not in rabbits (Harcourt-Brown, 2002a). An argument in favor of a subtle cheek tooth trimming is the fact that rabbits will be more able to consume fibrous food postoperatively and thus abrade their cheek teeth better if the teeth are not shortened too much. This method, however, seems not to be recommended for elongated cheek teeth, which are more markedly curved (concavely buccally in the upper jaw and concavely lingually in the lower jaw) (Figure 10.52). Depending on the extent of tooth curvature, only a part of the occlusal surface is abraded following subtle tooth trimming, and a new tooth spur soon forms. In order to delay that for as long as possible, it does seem to be advisable to radically trim the clinical crown of more markedly curved teeth as this will allow the entire occlusal surface to be abraded again, at least temporarily.

Another consideration is that maximal trimming of cheek teeth will decrease the axial strain on the retrogradely displaced tooth apices and significantly reduce the pain during grinding of food – at least temporarily. Following moderate tooth trimming, by contrast, the axial load will remain relatively constant. This can cause the retrograde displacement of the apices to progress

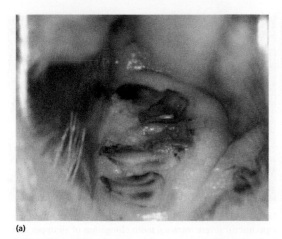

(a)

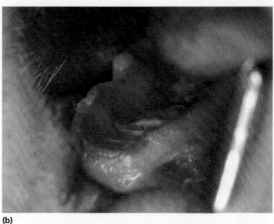

(b)

Figure 10.53 Recurring malocclusion in a twelve-year-old chinchilla (left maxillary row of cheek teeth). (a) Judging merely from the clinical examination, the cheek teeth appear hardly elongated intraorally as a pronounced gingival hyperplasia is present; pathological enlargement (widening) of the occlusal surface of all cheek teeth with typical, buccal spurs. Radiographs help to correctly assess the severe intraoral tooth overgrowth (reference lines), which is why tooth trimming is necessary. (b) Following adequate tooth shortening down to below the level of the hyperplastic gingiva to obtain a physiological length of the cheek teeth. The redundant gingiva needs to be resected; this is done using a small scalpel blade.

faster, particularly if the cortical cover of the alveolar bullae has already been perforated. When deciding about the most sensible extent of correction of the dentition, take into account that maximal trimming of teeth can stimulate their growth. However, this has only been confirmed in experimental examinations of incisors and should not be extrapolated for the cheek teeth without further investigation (as we see that growth of the antagonists stops after extractions of cheek teeth). There is also a constant risk in maximal trimming, i.e. almost complete resection of the atubular dentin, of inadvertently opening the tubular, innervated dentin as well as the pulp cavity. This is particularly true for pathologically altered cheek teeth in which the coronal dimensions of the pulp cavity vary greatly (as it does in incisors).

If the molars are trimmed very radically, hypertrophic gingival tissue or an inflammatory, swollen buccal mucosa may overlay the tooth stubs while the animals are trying to grind food between their cheek teeth. This can lead to postoperative, pain-related anorexia, which often seems inexplicable. Such kinds of proliferations of the gingival mucosa are particularly frequent in chinchillas. In order to prevent complications in the case of gingival hypertrophy, the gingiva should be resected its normal level using a scalpel following tooth trimming (Figure 10.53a and b).

Also, keep in mind when carrying out radical shortening of the teeth of rabbits in the terminal stages of an acquired malocclusion that at some point the tooth growth ceases and any substance that has been removed will not regrow. These animals may not be able to grind down raw fiber sufficiently with their teeth for the rest of their lives as the teeth are simply too short to occlude with one another physiologically (Harcourt-Brown, 2002a).

In order to regain intraoral normal occlusion in guinea pigs with severe elongation of cheek teeth, the upper molars are trimmed down to the level of the gingiva while the normal physiological angulation of the occlusal plane is recreated, if possible. If this succeeds, the maxillary cheek teeth will mostly protrude somewhat further beyond the level of the mucosa palatally than they will buccally. The lower molars are also trimmed accordingly (higher on the lingual side than on the buccal side). Likewise for chinchillas, the most radical possible shortening of cheek teeth is usually recommended (Crossley & Aiken, 2004). An argument in favor of such an extreme approach is that experience has shown that maximal shortening of cheek teeth reduces the abnormally increased pressure on the tooth apices (which are mostly severely displaced retrogradely) and thereby reducing the local, intraosseous pain significantly (see Figure 8.12a in Chapter 8 and

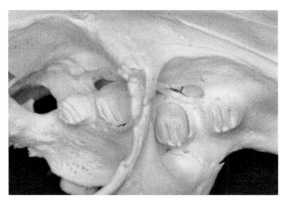

Figure 10.54 Recurring malocclusion in a fourteen-year-old chinchilla (specimen, right orbital area): severe retrograde elongation of all upper cheek teeth with a perforation of the cortical cover of the alveolar bullae (P4–M3).

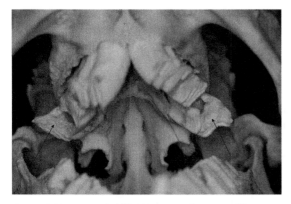

Figure 10.55 Recurring malocclusion in a five-year-old guinea pig (maxilla specimen, rostrocaudal view): asymmetrical tooth wear (clinical crowns of the cheek teeth longer on the right than on the left) and pronounced structural changes of the occlusal surfaces of the last two molars (M3; black arrows), leading to a suspected primary retrograde tooth elongation with perforation of the alveolar bullae. Pronounced vestibular deviation of all cheek teeth with formation of sharp buccal spurs in the area of the last two molars (M3) and a generalized dilation of the outer tooth sockets with inflammatory bone proliferations (on the right).

Figure 10.54). This is generally true for all patients with markedly curved, tilted or displaced cheek teeth that often show a dental growth disturbance (Figure 10.55). Radical shortening of the teeth may at least delay any further displacement of the entire tooth structure and thus may often extend the time interval between dental treatments. The author's experience has shown that this is true for guinea pigs and chinchillas.

Since the length of the incisors always depends on the length of the cheek teeth, the former need to be trimmed down to a relatively low level after more radical shortening of the molars. In order to avoid the tubular, innervated and thus sensitive dentin becoming exposed during shortening of the incisors and cheek teeth, the dental material should be removed very carefully in increments. An imminent opening of the pulp cavity is usually seen as a slight, central discoloration of the tooth body (see Section 9.3 in Chapter 9).

Proper trimming of cheek teeth

Regardless of whether one decides to trim the teeth moderately or radically, it can be difficult to exactly evaluate – depending on individual as well as species differences – how much tooth substance needs to be removed to re-establish normal occlusion and thus physiological grinding ability. The reference lines by Böhmer and Crossley that are described in Section 5.6 in Chapter 5 have proven extremely helpful here. When drawn on to preoperative radiographs, they mark the exact course of the individual, physiological occlusal plane. All cheek teeth, and then all incisors, should be trimmed down to at least that level if one decides to perform a subtle correction of the dentition (see Figure 5.37 in Chapter 5). By contrast, if the radical approach is chosen then even more dental substance needs to be removed. This can be up to one-third of the entire tooth structure, particularly in guinea pigs and chinchillas (see Figure 8.12a in Chapter 8).

The corrected dentition can be evaluated rather well, even clinically, immediately postoperatively. The position and length of the incisors that have been trimmed down to a suitable, physiological length subsequent to a correction of the cheek teeth are used for orientation. Proper trimming – at least as far as the length of teeth is concerned – can be confirmed if the following is found following completion of the procedure for incisors and cheek teeth. There is a species-specific normal occlusion of the incisors (physiological length and position of the incisors), while at the same time when the mouth is completely closed, the cheek teeth also occlude against one another with normal contact. If the molars have not been shortened sufficiently, the incisors will be too long and their positions will not be quite correct either (prognathism). Further trimming of the cheek teeth will be necessary in that case.

If – particularly in guinea pigs and chinchillas – the jaws remain slightly open after tooth trimming whilst

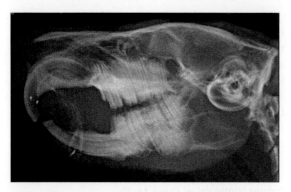

Figure 10.56 Malocclusion in a six-year-old guinea pig (laterolateral view). Postoperative radiograph following trimming of the cheek teeth: the jaws cannot be closed properly as – unilaterally – the last mandibular cheek tooth (M3) has not been trimmed enough. That tooth exhibits additional structural changes of the tooth substance, as does the next-to-last mandibular molar (M2). The incisors have also not been trimmed enough. There is an indication for an isolated radiographic image of the lower jaw as described by Böhmer as well as retrimming of the posterior cheek teeth and all incisors, for reconstruction of a typical chisel-shaped biting edge. Additional hypercalcification in the area of the orbit can be seen.

the incisors that were trimmed down to their normal physiological lengths do not occlude normally, the cause will often be insufficient shortening of the last upper and/or lower molar (Figure 10.56). If the rostral part of the jaw is pushed together with force during the postoperative check of the occlusion, then both temporomandibular joints will subluxate (overextension) as the last, elongated cheek tooth will act as a fulcrum. This will give the impression that everything is correct, resulting in a serious misjudgment of the tooth trimming. Many patients will then exhibit sustained postoperative problems during food intake unless the last (mostly mandibular) molar is again corrected accordingly. The animals will keep wiping their lips with their paws, open their jaws wide sometimes (as if they were luxated) and salivate excessively. Normal uptake of food is impossible although the patients mostly seem to have a good appetite. Due to insufficient or even complete lack of tooth contact and thus dental wear of the incisors and the premolars, those teeth will regrow extremely quickly so that another treatment will be necessary after a relatively short time interval. At this stage, the overall intraosseous findings may be much more problematic than at the time when the animal was first presented for

treatment (Figure 10.54). In order to prevent such complications, tooth trimming can be critically re-evaluated in the case of any unclear clinical finding (or on a routine basis). This is achieved by determining the exact course of the occlusal plane on a postoperative radiograph of the head in a laterolateral view by using the correct reference lines.

The clinical symptoms that have just been described ("opened" mouth) are basically identical in guinea pigs with a significant incisor overgrowth as a predominant feature (severe prognathism) and a pronounced bridge formation of the premolars if only those teeth that are visibly affected are trimmed – these are the incisors and the anterior lower cheek teeth that grow toward each other, entrapping the tongue underneath them (see Figure 3.15 in Chapter 3). Often this sort of incorrect tooth trimming is performed without sedation using any kind of forceps disregarding the unique hardness of the teeth. Due to a lack of basic knowledge and an omission of radiographic diagnosis, which would be desperately needed in those cases, the overall problem of a severe malocclusion is not detected during the examination of those patients. Hence no attention is paid to the last, also elongated, mandibular and maxillary molars (M2/M3). Those teeth act as a fulcrum, and the last upper cheek tooth often has buccal spurs as well, which are difficult to identify even under anesthesia and hard to access anyway (Figure 10.55). Particularly in guinea pigs, the painful buccal lesions of the soft tissue caused by the tooth spurs are often the reason that patients still suffer from prolonged anorexia having undergone dental correction.

If only the incisors of those patients are trimmed and the tooth bridge is "simply" removed, the animals will mostly be more able to swallow their food again postoperatively as tongue mobility is back to normal. However, as has been described, they will usually not be able to close their jaws properly. Their mouths remain partly open and the shortened incisors and cheek teeth, all of which are at a distance from their respective antagonists, will quickly regrow owing to a lack of dental abrasion. Those "inexplicable recurrences," which keep occurring after increasingly shorter time intervals, can be demonstrably prevented if trimming of cheek teeth is principally performed under anesthesia, and subsequent to good diagnostic radiographs. All other treatment options are obsolete and must be strictly refused.

10.3.2 Lagomorphs

In principle, treatment of choice for lagomorphs with an acquired malocclusion is an attempt to re-establish intraoral normal occlusion by remodeling the species-specific, physiological length, shape and angulation of the occlusal plane (Harcourt-Brown, 2002a; Crossley & Aiken, 2004; Gorrel & Verhaert, 2006). This is achieved by shortening the cheek teeth and subsequently correcting the length of the incisors. The primary goal of those measures is to ensure normal function of the teeth and the entire dentition so that the animal will be able to eat by itself again. However, this does not equate to reestablishing completely normal occlusion as in most cases there will be additional intraosseous changes that cannot be influenced directly or reversed, such as perforations of the apical alveolar bone, curvature and tilting of teeth or structural changes of the tooth substance as well as the jawbone.

Therefore it is basically impossible to cure a malocclusion. Repeated, maximal trimming of the hypselodont cheek teeth can only slow down the changes that are hidden intraalveolarly which are always progressive, but it will not be able to halt them. The earlier therapy is commenced the better the long-term prognosis (importance of the reference lines). Likewise, any local or generalized pain is only reduced temporarily or removed for a short time at best. Thus dental treatment will always be only palliative. In many cases with advanced changes, euthanasia will be the kindest option for the patient.

Repeated occlusal corrections, however, will only help long-term therapeutical management if other factors that may worsen a situation are recognized and eliminated permanently. A good example is a cheek tooth with an apical infection. If that localized, painful process is not diagnosed and thus incorporated in treatment (tooth extraction), the patient will exhibit prolonged anorexia despite having undergone optimal intraoral correction of the dentition, or will present again for tooth trimming after a very short time (see Figure 1.2a in Chapter 1). Since rabbits avoid the painful area during mastication, there is much more strain on one side of the mouth and the teeth of any jaw quadrant that is not actively involved will become elongated again due to insufficient wear after a very short time. All that leads to a pronounced asymmetry of the entire dentition, which in turn has repercussions on the intraosseous structures. A vicious cycle begins.

Often the overall situation of a patient appears to be confusing if only the intraoral findings are considered (see Figure 11.30a in Chapter 11). A plausible explanation for such cases will always be the presence of more advanced intraosseous findings (which is purely hypothetical without concomitant radiographic examination). Since those findings cannot be influenced primarily, it is often wrongly assumed that treatment would not differ from repeated tooth shortening. These problem cases usually solve themselves when the patient eventually presents again with an acute abscess formation. The abscess may now be too extensive for the owner to allow surgery or even inoperable in the most severe cases. This may be an extreme example, but it is certainly no extraordinary case.

In summary, it must be stated that elongated cheek teeth of rabbits can no longer "simply be shortened." In many cases this procedure is obsolete and should be a thing of the past. In order to really be able to decide whether an intraoral correction of the dentition is sufficient in any given case (for classic cases of acquired malocclusion) or whether further therapeutic measures need to be taken due to an additional, mostly localized, painful process, well-founded preoperative diagnostics are needed. An indispensable part of that is a radiographic examination of the skull as this is a relatively easy and convenient way of recording findings that are not visible clinically (which is true for more than 80% of all changes) in a very accurate way.

Radiographs may not only help to find the precise causes of a tooth elongation – particularly in patients with an unclear or unknown medical history – but also offer a possibility of managing pathological findings that may already be present. Intraosseous changes may get much worse within just a few weeks. If only the cheek teeth are repeatedly trimmed without recognizing the further changes, one may question the increasingly shorter time intervals between individual dental treatments. This also shows that shortening the cheek teeth without preoperative radiographs is really unacceptable. The risks of not identifying important pathology are simply too high.

Thus the first – and most important – step in a planned dental workup is a careful interpretation of diagnostically conclusive, current radiographs. If it has not been possible to image the head without sedation in at least four planes, those images with incorrect positionings are repeated under anesthesia, and additional radiographs are taken if necessary (special positionings for a better view of individual teeth or areas of the jaw, as well as intraoral images). When interpreting the radiographs, the appropriate reference lines are used to record the extent of malocclusion and the progression of various changes objectively so that they can be compared with earlier findings.

In addition, the lines provide important reference points for how much tooth substance currently needs to be removed from the cheek teeth as well as the incisors, in order to achieve a largely normal intraoral occlusion. As an alternative to the reference lines, individually correct lengths of cheek teeth can also be determined by means of an exact measurement of individual molars using a periodontometer (Schumacher, 2007). That technique, however, appears to be somewhat more difficult for everyday use as there are currently only comparative values for the lengths of the cheek teeth of medium-sized rabbits, and the teeth of guinea pigs, chinchillas and degus have not been measured at all (in addition, weight values vary considerably here).

Since each dental patient is different, it is difficult to set up guidelines for an optimal treatment that are strict and reasonable, except for the most important general rule: "Any treatment is to be preceded by a diagnosis!" Practitioners must formulate a treatment plan that is sensible for each individual case, following a variety of recommendations and examples. Apart from a set of suitable instruments and correct measures for the extent of tooth shortening (see Section 8.1 in Chapter 8, intraoral diagnostics under anesthesia, and Section 10.3, subtle versus radical trimming of cheek teeth), the individual experience of the practitioner plays a crucial part. Generally, not only is the length of the entire occlusal plane adjusted to the correct height with suitable rotating burs, but there is also a species-specific correction to their normal occlusal angle of approximately 10°.

A correction of the dentition involves shortening of cheek teeth that are either exceptionally long and protruding far beyond the occlusal surface (step mouth), or markedly tilted, or malformed, and removal of pathological tooth spikes (see Figure 3.5 in Chapter 3). The latter, however, must not be confused with slight lingual spurs of the mandibular molars that represent a species-specific, physiologically normal finding (see Figure 3.6 in Chapter 3). An erroneous removal of those kinds of spurs would interfere with the normal physiology of the dentition and can therefore have negative long-term

consequences. Finally, all cheek teeth are trimmed down to normal lengths. The removal of the tooth substance by means of rotating burs is performed as carefully as possible in order to avoid additional iatrogenic injuries to the soft tissue or the dental tissue (see Section 8.2 in Chapter 8).

Pathologically altered teeth (atypical shape, structure, tilting or displacement) basically can be left in occlusion unless they show any signs of periodontal involvement on radiographs. Preferably they are trimmed somewhat further down than the neighboring teeth as they grow back to the level of the occlusal plane and laterally beyond within a very short time. If the molars show signs of periodontal involvement or if they are changed or tilted too severely, then extraction is indicated (Figure 10.57a and b).

A similar approach is adopted in case of a slight loosening of individual cheek teeth. If they do not show any severe intraalveolar pathological changes, an attempt can be made to take the affected teeth out of occlusion by extreme trimming, hoping that immobilization might help to stabilize them over the course of time. Experience has shown, however, that it succeeds very rarely and an extraction of the teeth usually becomes necessary later on.

After completion of the cheek teeth adjustments, the length of the incisors is evaluated and corrected. On contact of the molars (when the mouth is fully closed), the incisors, which are approximately of the same length, should be in a normal position with respect to each other again. In the most favorable case, the cheek teeth are then shortened again so that there is a slight gap in a species-specific way (at rest).

If the incisors are too long compared to the cheek teeth after the cheek teeth shortening, the molars will not occlude properly in the grinding position (abnormal distance of the cheek teeth). Fibrous food will thus not be ground postoperatively (Harcourt-Brown, 2002a). The animals eagerly take up the stalks and try to grind them, only to release them from their mouths largely unchewed. Often this appears to frustrate the animals. Some patients even refuse to eat at all. Such behavior can also be due to painful intraosseous findings that were missed during treatment. Sometimes it can be difficult to differentiate between the two causes. Postoperative radiographs that include a look at the occlusal reference line would reveal a possible need for a length correction of the incisors. If the cause remains

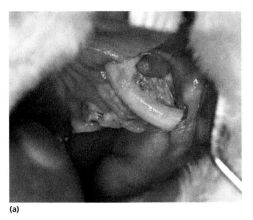 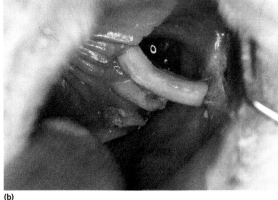

(a)   (b)

Figure 10.57 Advanced malocclusion in a five-year-old rabbit (left maxillary row of cheek teeth). (a) First cheek tooth (P2) markedly elongated intraorally as well as curved buccally, with accumulation of food particles within the dilated tooth socket. (b) Following cleaning of the tooth socket that is markedly dilated buccally: there is intraoral overgrowth and buccal curvature/ deviation of the first cheek tooth (P2); indication for tooth extraction.

The most important steps in dental treatment

- Recent, preoperative, diagnostically conclusive radiographs (including special positionings, if needed)
- Use of reference lines according to Böhmer and Crossley
- Removing tooth spikes and spurs
- Correcting the lengths of individual teeth
- (Excessive Trimming of loose molars)
- Remodeling the occlusal surface in terms of length and angulation
- Extracting individual or several teeth
- Abscess excision
- Periodontal treatment

---

undetected and unresolved, physiological grinding movements will occur again after a while, even without any correction of the incisors, as soon as the cheek teeth have regrown. However, if the molars have already stopped growing in the final stages of an acquired malocclusion, that situation will remain permanently (Harcourt-Brown, 2002a).

Beside tooth extractions, radical abscess excisions may also become necessary during dental treatment (see Chapter 11). Also important is a treatment of concurrent periodontal disorders, as they may lead to deep periodontal pockets and subsequent loosening of teeth as well as periodontal abscesses with all their consequences (see Figure 12.3 in Chapter 12).

Technique

Due to the high risk of splintering of the dental hard tissues, only rotating burs should be used for treatment of the cheek teeth in rabbits (see Figure 8.11 in Chapter 8). Not only can the occlusal surfaces be shortened to physiological lengths without any complications but also smaller tooth spikes as well as more compact tooth spurs can be easily removed (see Section 8.2 in Chapter 8, dental treatment). The necessary intraoral procedures are generally easy to perform in lagomorphs as their mouths can be opened relatively wide and wide-bladed cheek dilators can be used, which greatly improves the view into the oral cavity. Prior to tooth trimming, a rounded metal spatula or a wooden spatula with a suitable width can be inserted between the cheek and cheek dilator. This will help to protect the more caudal area of the cheek. Another spatula serves to protect the tongue.

Alternatively, the plastic part of a one-way syringe can also be used for the protection of soft tissue during burring the mandibular teeth. For this, the cylinder-shaped body of a one-way syringe (10 or 20 ml, depending on the size of the patient) is shortened on both sides and then slit longitudinally. After an additional resection of a narrow longitudinal strip along the slit (roughly corresponding with the width of the molars) and after any sharp edges are smoothed, the "plastic tunnel" can be placed over the row of teeth at an angle of approximately 30°. This will keep the soft tissue away from the teeth in an optimal way.

For the removal of rabbit dental substances in layers, conical or pear-shaped diamond burs with rounded ends have proven to be particularly suitable. This reduces the risk of injuries to the soft tissue, particularly in the caudal area of the oral cavity. The view of the working area is generally better, however, when using instruments with rather pointed ends or narrower burs with a straight end. The entire chewing surface of the cheek teeth, or the occlusal area of individual teeth, is treated preferentially with the long surface of the bur or its rounded tip (trimming of elongated molars). Lingual and palatal or buccal tooth spurs can be removed by guiding the bur across the lateral edges of the teeth. The edges, however, must not be rounded off too much in rabbits as this compromises the physiological interlocking and exact guidance of the cheek teeth (see Figure 2.9 in Chapter 2 and Figure 3.6 in Chapter 3).

When burring the cheek teeth, attention should be paid not to carve out the middle of the occlusal surface by repeatedly moving the instruments in a rostrocaudal direction; there is a tendency to do this owing to the wider chewing surface, particularly in the area of the maxilla. If that happens the results are often very fine palatal and buccal spurs that may facilitate the formation of tooth spurs (secondary enlargement of the occlusal surface) (Figure 10.8). At the same time remodeling of the physiological angle of the molar occlusal surface of approximately 10° is performed.

In the case of a pronounced enamel and dentin hypoplasia, individual, smaller tooth spurs can actually be removed with a fine Luer bone rongeur forceps before treating the entire occlusal surface (Figure 4.18 in Chapter 4). On no account, however, can more compact dental structures or individual elongated teeth simply be "clipped off," not even with special forceps available at specialist retailers. Due to the high risk of tooth splintering, this is an obsolete practice and generally not necessary in rabbits.

10.3.3 Rodentia

In rodents, full anesthesia is also obligatory in order to perform adequate tooth shortening and occlusal correction of the cheek teeth (see Section 7.1 in Chapter 7, anesthesia). Dental treatments without sedation are to be dismissed as deep iatrogenic mucosal lesions in the area of the gingiva of the incisors may be caused simply by introducing the mouth gag, due to the defensive movements of the patients (lateral jaw

movements while the mouth is open). Those lesions tend to be ignored, but it has been proven that they can lead to a progressive periodontopathy and, secondarily, even a loosening and suppuration of incisors. In addition, the more caudal areas of the long and narrow oral cavities of guinea pigs and chinchillas cannot be optimally viewed, let alone reached by instruments. Consequently, many pointed buccal spurs and secondary, deep lesions of the buccal musosa are overlooked, and the last cheek teeth are trimmed to an insufficient extent or not at all (Figure 10.55).

The basic goals of any occlusal correction are to remove sharp dental spurs that may inflict injuries to the soft tissue, to extract individual cheek teeth that are more severely displaced, structurally altered to a high degree or apically infected, and to use general tooth shortening to reconstruct a largely physiological, species-specific occlusal surface and angulation. These measures are supposed to regain the functionality of the dentition. In the long term, however, physiological occlusion will very rarely be kept up in that way because, at the time of first presentation, intraosseous changes of the teeth have usually already progressed too far and are therefore irreversible. The corrective measures are thus merely palliative.

Due to their very long and narrow oral cavity, trimming of cheek teeth is much more difficult in herbivorous rodents than it is in rabbits. Intraoral views can be improved somewhat by using special cheek dilators with narrow, relatively long blades. An additional obstacle is the relatively thick, elongate tongue of guinea pigs, which is attached to the lip commissure on both sides rostrally. Moreover, the oral cavity of guinea pigs, chinchillas and degus cannot be opened as far as in rabbits. All this makes intraoral procedures and the handling of rotating instruments more difficult, particularly when working on the caudal molars (see Figure 8.4 in Chapter 8). Moreover, the soft tissue that is located rostrolaterally from the first lower cheek tooth (P4) is very much exposed in the case of maximal trimming of that tooth. They need to be protected particularly well, using fine spatulae, when shortening (burring) that tooth (Figures 10.33 and 10.43).

Just like incisors, cheek teeth essentially are to be treated only with rotating instruments (see Section 8.2, dental treatment, and Figure 8.10 in Chapter 8). A long, conical bur with a small diameter and a rounded end is best suited for trimming molars. A larger diamond

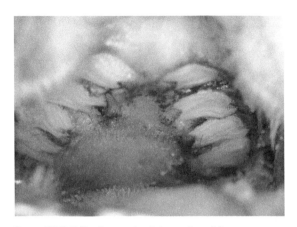

Figure 10.58 Following maximal shortening of the upper cheek teeth in a three-year-old guinea pig (intraoral finding, maxillary row of cheek teeth): the extraalveolar tooth structures have been shortened down to the gum line.

bur impairs the view into the oral cavity and raises the risk of carving out the occlusal surface to a certain degree, particularly if the molars are to be maximally trimmed (Figure 10.58). In order to avoid unnecessary injuries to the gingiva when removing the dental substance, practitioners tend to guide the bur predominantly near the center of the relatively wide occlusal surface of the cheek teeth of guinea pigs. As that rostro-caudal guidance of the instrument is repeated several times, the chewing surface is slightly carved out concavely, which may predispose the formation of new peripheral tooth spurs. Hence the outer dental edges should be checked and reworked, if necessary, after each shortening of the teeth.

The cheek teeth of chinchillas with a severe malocclusion are often markedly altered intraalveolarly due to large areas of tooth resorption. Aditionally, they are which are extremely soft as a result of an enamel and dentin hypoplasia, and mostly loosened due to a severe periodontitis. In such cases, special forceps can be used for an adequate shortening of the cheek teeth (see Figure 8.12a in Chapter 8). This helps to protect the soft tissue during dental treatment. After properly correcting the length of the maxillary premolar (P4), the length of the remaining cheek teeth is adjusted accordingly. The premolar serves as a reference point for the desired length of teeth. If there is an accompanying gingival hypertrophy, the remodeled occlusal surface is now far below the gum line (Figure 10.53b). The redundant tissue of the oral mucosa, which protrudes buccally in the upper jaw,

is simply removed with a scalpel and the resulting slight bleeding stopped with cotton swabs. Most of those kinds of injuries to the soft tissue will heal quickly and easily, but pain management must be provided for at least 48 hours.

The use of forceps will not result in fissures in the tooth when their use is indicated from radiographs (see Figure 8.13b in Chapter 8). The periodontal apparatus of the molars, which is often severely damaged, is strained less by the use of a special forceps. In order to remove enough dental substance with suitable diamond burs, the teeth of those patients must be treated for a relatively long time. If teeth are already loosened, pathology may get worse, and if there are areas of lysis of the tooth structure, the visible tooth crowns may break off (Figure 10.39). The occlusal surface of these molars may appear to be relatively unchanged clinically (intraoral finding). If there is some uncertainty as to the hardness of the tooth substance, the forceps should be avoided and only rotating instruments should be used. In addition, the first mandibular cheek tooth should always be burred as it is triangular in shape and the blades of the forceps will only be able to grasp it unevenly. This would result in splintering of the teeth.

Subsequent to the primary shortening of the cheek teeth by means of forceps, the occlusal surface is reworked with a suitable diamond bur. Occasionally it may even be necessary to additionally remove the coronally elongated alveolar bone. This is done using fine rose-head burs (Crossley & Aiken, 2004). An approximately normal intraoral occlusion may often be reestablished only via radical shortening of the molars. If in doubt about the dental correction, it can be checked by means of a postoperative radiograph and then drawing in the appropriate reference lines (see Figure 5.40b in Chapter 5).

According to Crossley (2003a), gingival proliferations can be prevented by more frequent tooth corrections at regular intervals, with relatively little substance of the cheek teeth being removed each time. In cases with a severe tooth elongation and a very pronounced gingival hypertrophy, only two-thirds of the elongated clinical crown should be removed at the first treatment and then the cheek tooth is trimmed to a normal physiological length two or three weeks later. This permits a regression of the gingiva so that the rest of the redundant dental tissue, which is now visible, can be removed more easily in a second session. The personal view of the author, however, is that the cheek teeth may well be radically trimmed in a single session while the hypertrophic mucosa is simultaneously removed down to the alveolar edge. When choosing the appropriate therapy, the reliability of the animal's owner should also be taken into account.

If any previously unknown structural change of individual teeth is detected while burring or shortening layers of the tooth substance, additional radiographs must be taken before concluding treatment to identify any additional pathology. Those changes can be an abnormal occlusal surface, a split tooth, a rotation of the enamel folds or a discharge of pus from the tooth socket. If only the intraoral finding is recorded and treated (tooth elongation, spurs, bridge formation, etc.), the treatment will not be successful or only short-lived as there may be persistent pain from the "hidden" intraosseous changes – regardless of how professional the dental treatment was performed (Figure 10.34a and b). This especially applies to apical infections.

Because of the pain, herbivorous rodents will put as little pressure as possible on apically altered molars. This manifests itself in a certain asymmetry of the dentition and a dark discoloration of the affected teeth due to missing abrasion (Figure 10.43). If all molars have the same length after treatment and thus receive largely identical amounts of pressure, this might increase the apical pain of teeth with pathology that had previously been out of occlusion. Prolonged anorexia may be the result. If the treatment is not re-evaluated and corrected, the intraosseous pathological processes will progress further until they will no longer be treatable in the terminal stages, due to the severity and multitude of findings. Near the onset of clinical symptoms, a tooth extraction, for example, may even lead to complete healing of the malocclusion in the long term. By contrast, the situation following secondary apical infections (formation of jaw abscesses) and a spread of the changes to neighboring teeth or periapical soft tissue such as the nose, eye socket or masticatory muscles usually becomes much more complicated (Figure 10.59 and see Figure 9.20 in Chapter 9). Sometimes patients have to be euthanized for medical reasons, or more frequently purely financial reasons – and it might only be because some slight finding had been missed and/or proper radiographic examination had not been performed.

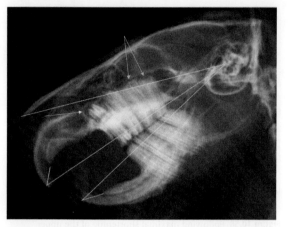

Figure 10.59 Periapical lesion of the first upper cheek tooth (P4) in a three-year-old guinea pig (laterolateral view) with a unilateral epiphora: intraoral elongation of the clinical crowns of all incisors and cheek teeth (yellow reference lines) and retrograde displacement of the apices of the last two upper molars (M2/M3; turquoise arrows).

Most patients refuse to eat by themselves following an inadequate correction of the dentition. It is often assumed in such cases that the jaw muscles that had been overflexed need some time to adjust to the new (physiological) situation following radical tooth shortening. While this may be true in some cases, much more frequent causes of postoperative chewing problems are intraosseous changes that have primarily been overlooked or an insufficient trimming of the last cheek teeth in guinea pigs and chinchillas (Figure 10.56).

Although a secondary overgrowth of the incisors with a rostral displacement of the mandible and a bridge formation in the lower premolars are the dominant findings in clinical examinations of guinea pigs, they must not be misinterpreted as the main findings by any means. If only these two changes are corrected by shortening the incisors and the premolars, a long-term failure is inevitable (see Section 10.1.2). It is vital that all intraorally elongated cheek teeth are trimmed to their physiological lengths. The exact amount of tooth substance that needs to be removed is determined by means of the reference lines according to Böhmer and Crossley. If it is decided to trim the teeth even more, it may well lead to prolonged intervals between dentition corrections in guinea pigs and chinchillas.

Guinea pigs with a malocclusion of cheek teeth are always a particular challenge because severe pathological changes of individual cheek teeth are often the center of attention (Figure 10.31). In most cases those teeth significantly cause the deterioration of an overall situation that would not have been so desperate primarily. The affected molar causes pain-related problems during grinding of food. Secondary changes involve mastication as well as the vertical occlusal pressure as the contralateral row of teeth is preferentially used for chopping up the food. A typical asymmetrical dentition is forming (see Figure 5.32d in Chapter 5 and Figure 9.35b in Chapter 9). Shortening only the "pathologically affected tooth" will not bring success as this does not change the original situation. The tooth needs to be identified and extracted as early as possible (see Section 10.4). This is the only chance for long-term improvement of the overall situation – provided that the generalized pathological changes of the dentition have not already advanced too far. A cure, however, will not be attained in that way either. Most cases follow the rule: "Once a dental patient – forever a dental patient." Hence regular monitoring of the patient is always indicated. The time intervals between individual dental treatments will be significantly longer if whatever causes the overall progression can be identified and treated specifically.

Subsequent to correct shortening of the cheek teeth, the length of the incisors is adjusted. Having finished occlusal correction, the length of the incisors and their position opposed to one another should be correct in a species-specific way, while at the same time the cheek teeth are in immediate contact (when the mouth is closed manually). In addition, the mandible should be free to move in a caudorostral direction and also in a lateterolateral direction to a smaller extent (imitation of the physiological grinding movements). If this fails, the cheek teeth or incisors must be corrected again.

10.4 Extraction of cheek teeth

10.4.1 Indications
Continually growing teeth that keep forming smaller lingual or buccal spurs should not be extracted "prophylactically" – even though that is a frequent wish of owners who hope for a long-term cure (Harcourt-Brown, 2002a). Every extraction of a tooth changes the anatomy as well as the physiology of the entire dentition and can result in some displacements of teeth or

secondary tilting (Figures 10.5 and 10.17). Removing individual teeth from the center of the occlusal row also impairs self-cleaning of the dentition, which may lead to ongoing periodontal problems.

The only indications for a tooth extraction are apical or intraalveolar infections, or individual teeth that protrude far from the row of teeth because they are markedly tilted (Figure 10.57a). Extractions should be performed in the case of intraalveolar transverse fractures of cheek teeth as well as longitudinal splitting of individual premolars (or molars), the latter of which are rather frequent (Figure 10.7). Sometimes the cheek teeth of rabbits have intraalveolar transverse fractures and, additionally, the coronal section of the tooth is split longitudinally. In these cases only the split tooth body is removed and the tooth base is left, as long as there is no apical infection. In most cases the tooth will regrow normally, but regular monitoring of the patient is indicated.

Another indication for tooth extraction can be an individual deformed cheek tooth whose shape (gross thickening) and structure is significantly different from the others. They occur mostly in rabbits, as a result of an enamel and dentin hypoplasia. Although the tooth body of such a deformed molar should be worn down more easily as it is softer than the physiological dental substance in principle, the enormous thickening of the tooth will nonetheless result in an abnormal abrasion by the antagonist. This mainly affects the first mandibular cheek tooth, P3 (Figure 10.60).

Indications for an extraction of cheek teeth
- Apical infection concomitant with a pulpitis
- Intraalveolar, periodontal infection (microabscessation)
- Intraalveolar transverse fracture (check if the apical part can be left there)
- Intraalveolar longitudinal splitting of the tooth (partial or complete)
- Loosening of tooth (periodontitis)
- Intraalveolar splintering of tooth (multiple)
- Carious/resorptive defects (only if corrective shortening is impossible)
- Severe growth disturbances of individual teeth
- Marked tilting of individual teeth
- Severe malformation of teeth with pathologically changed dental substance (thickening of tooth, hypoplasia, dysplasia)

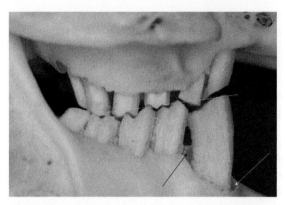

Figure 10.60 Malocclusion in a six-year-old rabbit (specimen, right row of cheek teeth, lateral view) with a thickening of the first mandibular cheek tooth (P3), with a slight mesial, horizontal loss of alveolar bone (white arrow) and a slight rostral tooth deviation, dilation of the approximal area orientated toward the neighboring tooth (black arrow), severe enamel and dentin hypoplasia of the tooth and an abnormal slight inclination of the molar occlusal surface (from the distal toward the rostral end; turquoise line).

10.4.2 General remarks

Prior to any tooth extraction, particularly in the case of teeth that are less severely altered but also in the case of more extensive jaw abscesses, the owner should be informed that even cheek teeth that were completely removed can regrow. This means that sometimes a second surgery might be necessary (Crossley & Aiken, 2004). Especially in the area of more extensive jaw abscesses, a tooth stub or a small dentinoid relatively frequently regrows from mostly completely unstructured existing dental substances (Figure 10.61). This kind of new formation of teeth (pathological tooth substance) will not always be prevented, even if the germinal cells are destroyed and the abscess cavity is curetted most thoroughly intraoperatively. Only a few germinal cells are enough to form dentinoids. During healing, that primitive odontogenic tissue frequently acts as a foreign body (radiolucent fringe) so must be removed (see Figure 9.52 in Chapter 9). It may only be left in situ if there is no inflammation; otherwise the risk of recurring abscesses increases.

Furthermore, the pre-operative radiographs are checked again prior to every planned tooth extraction. If any additional, special images are required, they are taken immediately before surgery. Likewise, the patient is X-rayed again if no recent radiographs are at hand

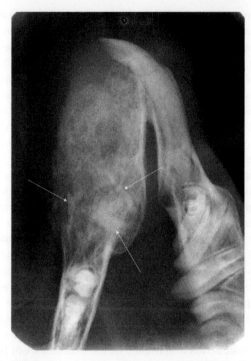

Figure 10.61 Two months postoperative radiograph following excision of an abscess including extraction of the right mandibular incisor and the first two cheek teeth (P3/P4) in a three-year-old rabbit (slightly oblique intraoral view of the mandible); new formation of two small dentinoids (white arrows) in the area of the former abscess; currently nonirritating (inert) as there is no peridental osteolysis visible; dentinoids to be extracted in the case of delayed wound healing; small bone splinters lateral to these structures (yellow arrow) indicate the need for resection.

(e.g. in the case of a postponement of a planned tooth extraction). The current situation of the dentition must be perfectly clear considering that pathological alterations of elodont teeth may change very quickly. This may not only affect the shape and the structure of the individual tooth to be extracted but also the neighboring teeth as well as the jawbone.

Although removing the incisors of herbivorous pets is relatively easy, extracting the hypselodont cheek teeth is significantly more complicated. The view into the narrow oral cavity is poor and the narrow space makes handling of the instruments very difficult. In addition, the alveolar bone in the mandibles of rabbits, guinea pigs, chinchillas and degus is very thin lingually and buccally and tends to break out when instruments are positioned improperly. Furthermore, the molars are often deformed extra- and intraalveolarly and, in rabbits, can also be grotesquely curved in a variety of directions (see Figure 11.9 in Chapter 11). Due to the enamel and dentin hypoplasia, the dental substance is very brittle. Thus the teeth tend to fracture within the tooth socket during mobilization, usually a few millimeters below the gum line in rabbits (Figure 10.62a). The base of the cheek tooth, which has remained intraalveolarly, needs to be removed retrogradely in the lower jaw, accessing it via the area of the abscess or a specific osteotomy of the bone. Incising the gingiva slightly toward the rostral end will help to access the tooth socket of the first cheek tooth (P2) in the maxilla (Figure 10.62b and c).

When removing cheek teeth, there is a general distinction between an intraoral extraction, in other words a complete removal of the dental tissue without surgically exposing the tooth apex, and an extraoral extraction, in which the apical part of the tooth is surgically uncovered in the context of the mobilization of the tooth (apical osteotomy of the jawbone). Since mostly cheek teeth that are more altered intraalveolarly or apically, or infected, are removed in pets, there are hardly any indications for a purely intraoral extraction technique. In rabbits, it is the maxillary molars that only have slight intraalveolar structural changes or infections (Crossley & Aiken, 2004). This also includes individual upper cheek teeth with a severe growth disturbance (Figure 10.57a).

If – following a strict indication – only an intraoral tooth extraction is performed in rabbits, chinchillas or degus, there is generally a certain risk that the intraosseous infection may not subside even though the tooth causing the trouble has been removed. That risk, however, must be weighed against the much more invasive process of a jaw osteotomy. Therefore every case should be carefully evaluated and a tooth extraction should be planned taking into account all advantages and disadvantages and discussing them with the owner.

Often the mobilization that is necessary for an intraoral extraction is not easy to achieve as the molars of rabbits and herbivorous rodents, which are already very long physiologically, are additionally elongated in the case of malocclusions in the apical area. If total removal of the tooth is successful nonetheless, the question remains as to how the tooth socket will be kept clean during the healing process and how it will be checked at regular intervals. That is a problem indeed as a simple gingival suture that seals the alveolus can generally be

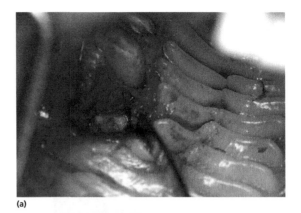

(a)

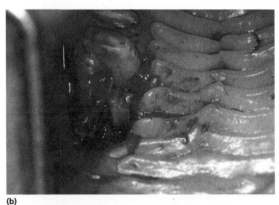

(b)

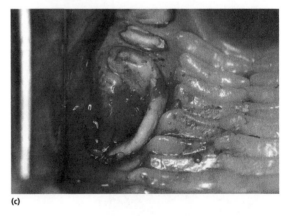

(c)

Figure 10.62 Intraoperative situation during an extraction of the first cheek tooth (P2) of a two-year-old rabbit (left maxillary row of cheek teeth). (a) The P2 is fractured subgingivally; mobilization of the intraalveolar tooth body using a luxator. (b) Extending the access by means of a rostral incision of the gingiva; result is an improved accessibility of the intraalveolar tooth fragment. (c) Following mobilization and partial extraction of the entire tooth body; marked, buccally concave curvature of the P2.

preformed easily in rabbits, but will mostly become dehiscent again within a few days. Alternatively, the tooth socket can be filled with antibiotic beads, a collagenous sponge or a hemostyptic drug (Figure 10.63a to g) (for more possibilities see below).

If the intraoral suture becomes dehiscent or the chosen material does not completely fill the empty tooth socket, saliva and food particles will enter the alveolus. This happens especially frequently after extractions of the cheek teeth of guinea pigs, as their alveoli are

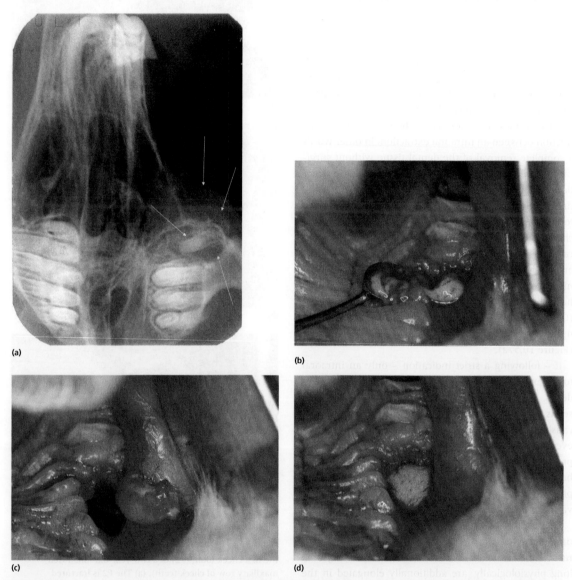

(a)

(b)

(c)

(d)

Figure 10.63 Abscess of the upper jaw (right) in a five-year-old rabbit. (a) Oblique intraoral view of the maxilla: dental tissue (tooth residue) in the area of the widely dilated alveolus of the second cheek tooth (P3; white arrow), partial osteolysis of the facial tuberosity and rostrolateral swelling of soft tissue in the abscess area (yellow arrows). (b) Intraoperative view: curettage of the infected alveolus. (c) Intraoperative view: mobilized and extracted tooth residue (P3). (d) Postoperative view: the empty alveolus is temporarily (approximately 10 days) filled with AIPMMA beads; after that they are removed again. (e) 16 days after tooth extraction: good granulation of the tooth socket. (f) 4 weeks after tooth extraction: the wound area has healed up well. (g) Intraoral radiograph of the maxilla: one month following tooth extraction - the abscess area is healing.

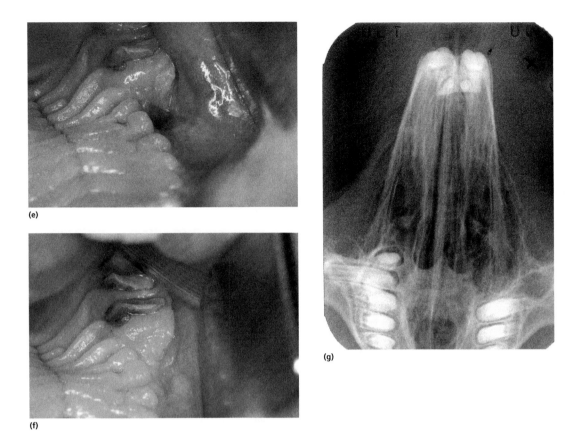

(e)

(f)

(g)

Figure 10.63 (Continued)

extremely spacious and cannot be sutured (Figure 10.64). Hence tooth extractions in guinea pigs should generally never be performed without a jaw osteotomy, neither in the upper nor in the lower jaw; otherwise consequent aftercare of the abscess area will be impossible.

The intraalveolar impaction of foreign material is – independent of species – generally more pronounced in the lower jaw than in the upper jaw and can lead to prolonged wound healing disturbances and even secondary jaw infections or recurring abscesses. It may well take several weeks or months for those infections to clear. Such secondary infections may be misinterpreted as a recurring abscess and are often due to mistakes made with the aftercare.

Sometimes a lateral access involving a buccotomy is recommended for the removal of cheek teeth. Such a procedure, however, generally is too invasive for pets and also involves a very high risk of complications with wound healing as well as secondary infections of soft tissue (Gorrel & Verhaert, 2006).

10.4.3 Intraoral extraction of cheek teeth

Intraoral tooth extractions are surgical procedures and should therefore be performed preferentially in an aseptic environment (Crossley & Aiken, 2004). This requires careful disinfection of the surgery area as well as the use of sterile instruments and surgical gloves. First, the elongated incisors are trimmed to suit the need for a better view into the oral cavity and easier intraoral handling of the instruments. Next, the jaws are opened by means of a mouth gag before the oral cavity is cleaned with fine cotton swabs. This is followed by a disinfection of all teeth, if possible, and the easily accessible oral mucosa with suitable preparations (Chlorhexidine® or Betaisodona® solution). Finally, a cheek dilator is inserted and the tooth to be extracted is locally anesthetized (see Section 7.3.2 in Chapter 7). The patient is laid flat on the operating table, which has been covered with a sterile cloth – without any further restraints – in ventral or lateral

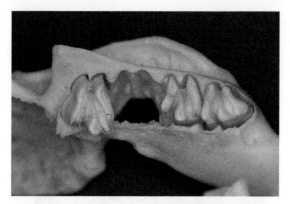

Figure 10.64 Situation after removal of the third cheek tooth (M2) in a guinea pig (specimen, left row of cheek teeth) with an abscess of the lower jaw. Physiologically a very thin alveolar wall can be seen; the wall is extremely thin lingually.

recumbency. An adjustable heat mat prevents the patient from becoming hypothermic; additionally, the animal's body should be covered.

The easiest way to perform an intraoral tooth extraction is when the head of the patient is lying in the left hand of the operating surgeon, firmly immobilized while remaining free to tilt and turn. All steps needed for a mobilization and extraction of the tooth can be performed single-handedly (right hand). An advantage of that method is the fact that the force needed to loosen the periodontal fibers can be immediately estimated by means of the supporting hand, and the desired pressure can be corrected accordingly. Another advantage is the fact that the head can be moved or shifted to suit any stage of the manipulation.

The sharp tip of a luxator or a suitably sized cannula that has been bent in a 90° angle is then used to cut the attached gingival to the level of the alveolar bone on both the buccal as well as lingual/palatal aspects of the tooth. The flat side of the cannula faces toward the cheek tooth (Crossley & Aiken, 2004). A Crossley cheek tooth luxator or a fine Heidemann spatula whose working end has been cut a bit thinner and thus sharper helps destroy the periodontal fibers. It is important that the working ends of all instruments are thin and suitably angled, and that they have sharp edges. Suitable instruments for smaller patients (degus, chinchillas) can be tailormade by bending suitable cannulae. The intraalveolar periodontal fibers are destroyed as the luxator is carefully introduced into the periodontium and the alveolus is continuously expanded (Figure 10.65a).

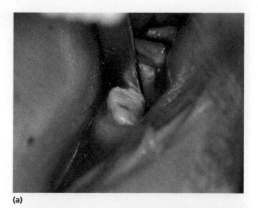

(a)

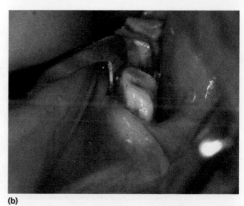

(b)

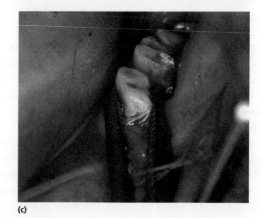

(c)

Figure 10.65 Cheek tooth extraction in a rabbit (intraoperative views, left mandibular row of cheek teeth). (a) The luxator is positioned in the approximal area between the first two cheek teeth (P3/P4); slight discharge of pus from the tooth socket. (b) The approximal area between the anterior two cheek teeth is already dilated (P3/P4). The luxator is positioned in the lingual area of the alveolus. The result is a secondary buccal displacement of the cheek tooth. (c) Grasping the sufficiently mobilized tooth with a blunt Pean clamp and extraction of the tooth by making slight rotating movements.

The luxator is first introduced into the tooth socket along the side of the tooth that faces toward the neighboring tooth (mesial or distal approximal area). That is where the instrument can be guided most easily, preventing accidental slippage and injuries to the soft tissue. The periodontal apparatus is particularly strong mesially and distally, compared to the sides of the teeth (Gorrel & Verhaert, 2006). Both in rabbits and in guinea pigs, it can be difficult to exactly position the instrument in the interdental gap from the occlusal surface as the teeth are very close to one another and the instrument frequently slips from the elevated enamel ridges that touch one another down to the lower-lying dentin columns. In order to prevent this from happening, the tip of the instrument is first inserted between the respective teeth at a 45° angle from laterally (lower jaw) or medially (upper jaw). The luxator can then be turned with respect to the longitudinal axis of the tooth such that it is finally positioned approximally in line with the tooth body (Figure 10.65a). Then it is pushed further and further into the interdental space by means of small, lateral sliding movements. As soon as the final position has been reached, the instrument is left in the tooth socket while applying axial pressure (Crossley & Aiken, 2004). This causes the periodontal ligaments on that side of the tooth socket to be stretched and partially torn. After that, the opposite side of the tooth is loosened accordingly before mobilizing the buccal and lingual or palatal side (Figure 10.65b).

That procedure needs to be repeated three or four times on all four aspects of a tooth. Each time the luxator is reintroduced it is pushed deeper into the periodontium until it finally disappears completely in the tooth socket. No movements involving any outside leverage should be performed – particularly on the sides of the cheek teeth – as this will cause the thin alveolar bone to splinter. In addition, the neighboring tooth must not be accidentally loosened by destroying its periodontal apparatus, which is in close proximity. In order to prevent this, the luxator is ideally inserted in a 15° angle toward the longitudinal axis of the molar to be extracted. Any injury to the germinal zone of the adjacent tooth in particular could have severe consequences. The periodontal infection may also spread more easily to other teeth after an unnecessary severe trauma to the interdental alveolar bone (Figure 10.66).

The repeated application of the luxator causes the periodontal fibers to tear and hematomas are formed on

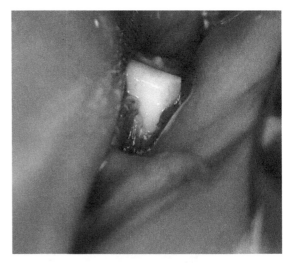

Figure 10.66 Following extraction of the first lower cheek tooth (P3) of a rabbit (left mandibular row of cheek teeth). The mesial alveolar wall of the adjacent cheek tooth is visible.

all sides, which mobilize the tooth further and further, pushing it out of the tooth socket. Finally, the molar can be carefully grasped with special extraction forceps (with the tip of the instrument bent at an angle of 100°) or a smooth, curved Pean clamp and slightly turned in the tooth socket several times (Figure 10.65c). These rotating movements and the simultaneous pull along the longitudinal axis causes all Sharpey fibers that are not yet torn to tear and the tooth to be released from its anchoring.

Normally the "dental sac" (pulp with the germinal cells) adheres to the wide open apex of the extracted tooth. If that is not the case, the germinal cells that still remain within the apical area of the alveolus need to be destroyed by means of a careful curettage (see Section 9.4 in Chapter 9). Alternatively, repeated dental intrusions can be performed just before the tooth is extracted. The tooth that has already been mobilized is pushed into the alveolus a few times, rotating it slightly in the process. The sharp apical edges of the tooth will mechanically destroy the germinal tissue (Crossley & Aiken, 2004). The patient is then repositioned for the subsequent osteotomy of the lower jaw or a cleaning-up of the abscess.

10.4.4 Extraction of cheek teeth including osteotomy of the jaw

Particularly when extracting cheek teeth in the mandible, a concomitant apical osteotomy of the jawbone has been shown to be the best method (Figure 10.67a

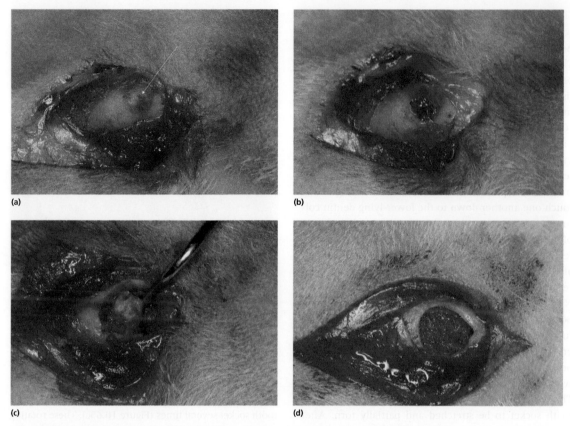

Figure 10.67 Extraction of the first cheek tooth (P3), including ventral osteotomy, in a two-year-old rabbit (right branch of the mandible). (a) Ventral view after skin incision; small, transparent protrusion of the ventral cortical bone of the jaw, with the apex area of the first cheek tooth (P3) shimmering through (white arrow), resulting in an exactly demarcated area of the planned osteotomy. (b) View after opening the tooth socket from the ventral approach. The apex area of the cheek tooth to be extracted (P3) is exposed. (c) Intraoperative view: retrograde mobilization of the cheek tooth by means of a pointed probe. (d) The empty alveolus is retrogradely packed with an iodoform gauze (drainage).

to d). Subsequent to the intraoral removal of the molar, a small ventral opening of the tooth socket is made. In order to avoid accidentally injuring the apices of the neighboring cheek teeth during trepanation of the tooth socket, a pointed explorer probe can be pushed through the tooth socket penetrating the ventral mandibular cortex before positioning the drill. The tip of the instrument will then mark the optimal spot for the osteotomy. Often the apical, infected area of a tooth is already recognizable by a slight protrusion or discoloration of the mandibular bone (Figure 10.67a). After trepanation of the cortical bone, which can be done using a hand drill, the opening is dilated with small rose-head burs or a fine Luer bone rongeur forceps. Many osteotomies are facilitated by the fact that the

apices of the extracted teeth have already perforated the jaw apically.

The osteotomy will allow for the alveolus to be kept clean from the outside so that there will be no complications occurring during healing period of two to three weeks. The empty alveolus is packed almost to the edge of the gingiva, using iodoform gauze soaked in a mixture of granulated sugar and Furacin®-sol ointment (Figure 10.67d). Postoperative care involves regular removal of all foreign material such as food or hairs that may have become impacted in the tooth socket, by means of repeated retrograde flushings of the empty alveolus while changing the drainage. This procedure is regularly performed in time intervals of two to four days until the defect has closed itself against the oral cavity

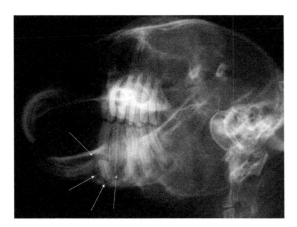

Figure 10.68 Fragment of a tooth root in a seven-year-old rabbit (laterolateral view): apically infected root fragment that has remained in the tooth socket following an intraalveolar transverse fracture of the first cheek tooth (P3); significant, periapical osteolysis (white arrows), dilation of the approximal area toward the distally adjacent neighboring tooth (P4; turquoise arrow). There is a suspected early apical osteolysis of the mandibular incisor (yellow arrow) and therefore an indication for an intraoral view. Note also the mandibular prognathism

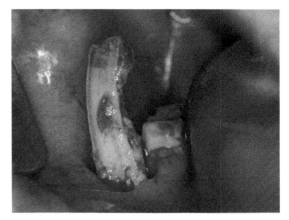

Figure 10.69 Incisor extraction in a four-year-old rabbit (situation during the operation, right mandibular row of cheek teeth): longitudinally split and apically infected first cheek tooth (P3); the distal half of the tooth is mobilized and partially extracted.

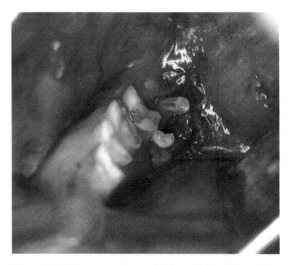

Figure 10.70 The same patient as in Figure 5.4 (in Chapter 5) (row of lower right cheek teeth) with a right-sided abscess of the lower jaw and longitudinal split of the last molar; situation after intraoral mobilization of both tooth halves with the tip of a probe.

after about seven to ten days. A gingival suture that seals the alveolus against the oral cavity (with monofilament material 6/0) can be placed immediately after the tooth extraction. There is, however, the problem of suture dehiscence, which has been mentioned above. If the suture does not dehisce though it will greatly accelerate healing.

An intraalveolar transverse fracture of the tooth body is an absolute indication for a retrograde tooth extraction including an osteotomy of the jawbone. Molars with these fractures often appear to be totally loosened during intraoral examinations, which is incorrect. If merely the coronal tooth fragment that appears to be well-mobilized is removed, the apical, most infected part of the tooth will remain within the alveolus and will thus sustain the purulent local infection (Figure 10.68). By contrast, if the coronal tooth fragment is missing because it has already broken off due to normal chewing pressure, it may be wrongly assumed (if no radiographic examination is performed) that either an earlier, complete tooth extraction had been performed or a complete loss of the tooth had occurred. Any missing or severely mobile cheek teeth should always be an indication for a thorough, preoperative radiographic examination. In contrast to molars with transverse fractures, longitudinally split teeth can mostly be loosened relatively easily in their entire length and extracted in two parts, via the intraoral access – at least in rabbits (Figures 10.69 and 10.70).

An apical osteotomy should be performed in any case where the cheek teeth to be extracted are severely deformed, representing a risk of iatrogenic, intraalveolar fracture, or if those teeth already start to show signs of

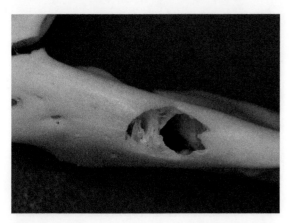

Figure 10.71 Following osteotomy of the lower jaw in a rabbit (specimen, right branch of the mandible, ventral view) in the apical area of the third cheek tooth (M1) with a iatrogenic trauma to the apex of the second cheek tooth (P4).

an apical abscessation. Depending on the location of the (mostly retrogradely displaced) apices, the lower jaw is opened lateroventrally or lateromedially (Figure 10.71; for the technique, see Section 10.4.4, extraction of cheek teeth including osteotomy of the jaw). Following the osteotomy the cheek tooth is carefully mobilized from a ventral approach (Figure 10.67c). The procedure may also be combined with an intraoral mobilization of the tooth. Depending on what will be easier in a particular case, a tooth is either pushed into the oral cavity for extraction (retropulsion) or removed retrogradely.

Extraction of the cheek teeth in guinea pigs is significantly more complicated than in rabbits. Mobilization of the molars, which are more compact overall and larger, is especially difficult and unnerving. Due to the natural curvature of the molar the teeth are usually rooted deeply within the jaw even when they exhibit signs of an apical infection. In order to completely mobilize these molars and to be able to extract them without any complications, both an intraoral and an extraoral access are essentially necessary (Figure 10.72a to f). This is simply because there are no specific luxators suitable for their mobilization, meaning that a tooth can only be loosened approximately 50% from each side (coronally and apically). Whether the cheek tooth is ultimately removed toward the oral cavity or retrogradely to the outside depends on the overall individual situation.

In principle, an apical osteotomy – in other words a direct access to the tooth socket – is also recommended for extractions of apically infected maxillary molars.

The practical implementation of this, compared to the mandibular teeth, is somewhat more difficult due to the species-specific anatomy of the skull, and it may not be possible to perform without more invasive measures (Figure 10.73a to g). Hence an osteotomy of the maxilla is not routinely performed only when there is a case with a specific indication. Whether this surgery is necessary and sensible is decided on a case by case basis.

Thus maxillary cheek teeth that show only slightly pathological periodontal changes are usually extracted by way of primarily intraoral access, with the alveolus left open or sutured closed after being packed with suitable preparations (see Section 11.1.7, alternative methods in treatment, in Chapter 11 and Figure 10.63d). Since the empty alveoli of the upper jaw will usually collect less food, there is reasonable hope for healing without any complications. If any disturbances in wound healing occur or in case of other complications (persistant infection, for example), the required osteotomy can be performed at that time.

In rabbits, the apices of the first two upper cheek teeth (P2/P3) can be reached relatively easily by means of a resection of the cribriform plate or via the base of the zygomatic arch (facial tuberosity) (Figure 10.74). Access is relatively easy and usually heals without any complications. The apical sections of the last four molars (P4–M3), which are located within the orbit, are more difficult to access. If need be, those cheek teeth can be accessed by means of a resection of the zygomatic arch whereby immediate access is gained to the apical part of the molars as well as their entire intraalveolar area (see Figure 11.32 in Chapter 11).

In principle, this also holds true for the last two cheek teeth (M2/M3) of guinea pigs, chinchillas and degus. In all three species, however, the apices are located so far medially within the orbit that they are not really accessible directly without removing the eye (Figure 10.54). If there is an absolute indication for a removal of those molars, the eye will usually have to be sacrificed (Figure 10.34b). An extraction without an enucleation can be attempted, but without any adequate retrograde access, simply mobilizing the affected cheek tooth will pose a problem in guinea pigs. There is also a difficulty of optiaml follow up aftercare of the wound area (see Section 11.2 in Chapter 11).

Indications for an extraction of the first two maxillary cheek teeth (P4–M1) of chinchillas, guinea pigs or degus are rather rare if no apical abscess is present (see

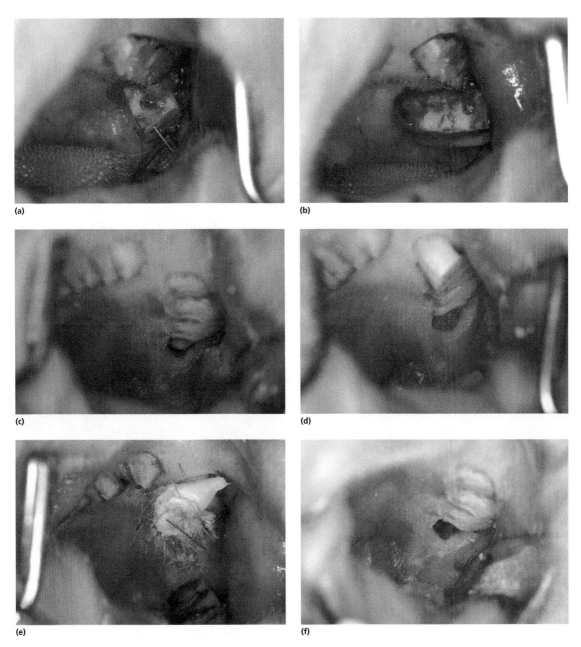

Figure 10.72 Retrobulbar abscess in a four-year-old guinea pig (left maxillary row of cheek teeth). (a) Intraoperative view: partial intraoral extraction of the apically infected last cheek tooth (M3). (b) Following intraoral tooth extraction (M3). (c) Situation 3 weeks after tooth extraction (M3): the alveolus is packed with an iodoform gauze (drainage) almost up to the level of the gingiva. The anterior cheek teeth are trimmed for better accessibility of the tooth socket. (d) Situation 5 weeks after tooth extraction (M3): accumulation of food residue in the empty alveolus. (e) Situation 5 weeks after tooth extraction (M3): hairs removed from the alveolus of the cheek tooth, mixed with pus. (f) Situation 5 weeks after tooth extraction (M3): the tooth socket has been cleaned. No further gauze packet (drainage) is needed.

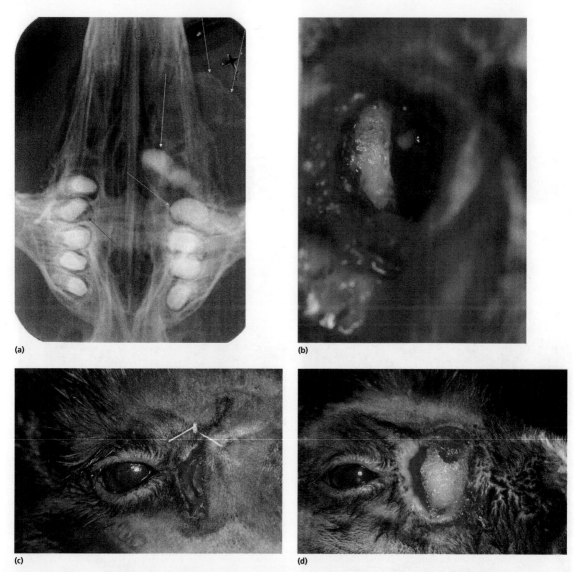

Figure 10.73 Abscess of the upper jaw (right) in a five-year-old rabbit. (a) Intraoral view of the maxilla: structurally altered, severely deformed and rostropalatally displaced first right cheek tooth (P2; white arrow); the alveolus is destroyed; lateral distension of the lamina dura (yellow arrows), structurally altered second right cheek tooth (P3; turquoise arrow) and dilation of the tooth socket of the first two left cheek teeth (P2/P3) with a slight intraalveolar rotation of the second tooth (red arrows). (b) Situation during the operation after osteotomy of the right maxilla in the area of the lamina cribrosa: the altered tooth body of the first cheek tooth is visible in the depth and drops of pus are visible rostrally from there. (c) Following retrograde tooth extraction: the external wound area is closed temporarily. (d) Eight days after tooth extraction: the wound area is repacked, with drainage; good granulation. (e) Situation 2.5 weeks after tooth extraction: the wound is clean and early granulation is visible. An AIPMMA (antibiotic imprenated polymethyl methacrylate) implant is inserted. (f) Six weeks after tooth extraction: the wound area has healed. (g) Intraoral view of the maxilla, follow-up 7 months after abscess excision and tooth extraction: the implants are nonirritating. The desmodontal changes in the area of the left upper cheek teeth have remained the same (red arrows).

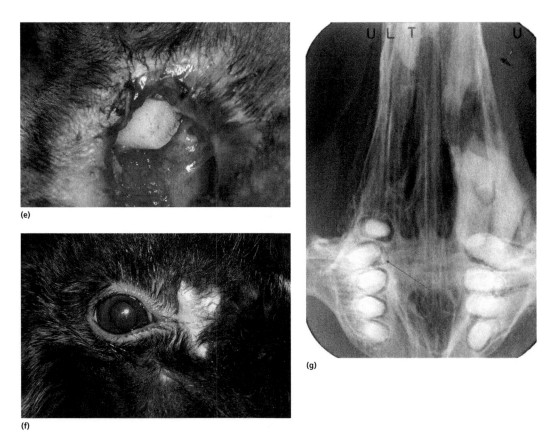

(e)

(f)

(g)

Figure 10.73 (Continued)

Figure 9.20 in Chapter 9 and Figure 10.59). The tooth apices of guinea pigs and degus are concealed and poorly accessible, being located below the lacrimal bone (although that depends on the retrograde displacement of the teeth), whereas they can be accessed better in chinchillas, being located in front of the lacrimal bone bridge. In all three species, the nasolacrimal canal runs in the immediate proximity – in that area, it runs in the rostrum between the apices (Figure 10.75). Routine osteotomy is usually dismissed as an option because of the precarious surgical area, but it is necessary in the case of complications.

10.4.5 Aftercare

There have been many reports of problems caused by elongation of antagonist teeth after extractions of hypselodont premolars and/or molars. Particularly in rabbits, the antagonist is said to grow into the gap resulting from the tooth removal and then become elongated. In extreme cases, this is supposed to cause injuries to the gingiva of the jaw on the opposite side. Hence an antagonist needs to be trimmed regularly or extracted prophylactically (Bieniek & Bieniek, 1993; Wiggs & Lobprise, 1995c; Harcourt-Brown, 2002a; Gorrel & Verhaert, 2006).

Such complications do occur occasionally. Based on the author's experience with cheek tooth extractions in rabbits and guinea pigs, however, there is often a growth retardation or even a halt in growth of the antagonist(s) three to four months after surgery. In rabbits, the maxillary cheek teeth that are not in occlusion tend to tilt slightly buccally in the upper jaw. This has hardly any negative consequences if there is no additional continuous tooth growth. Some patients, however, suffer from a mild inflammation of the gingiva, possibly due to an increase in bacterial colonization as the self-cleaning capacity of the dentition is impaired (Figure 10.76a and b).

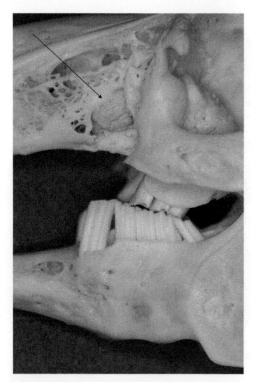

Figure 10.74 Situation 4 months after extraction of the first two maxillary cheek teeth (P2/P3) on both sides in a six-year-old rabbit (specimen, view from the left): the AIPMMA implant is inert (black arrow) and there is no overgrowth of the mandibular antagonists (P3/P4) is visible.

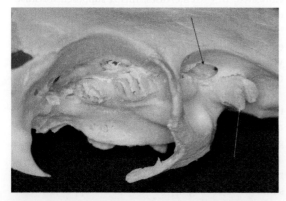

Figure 10.75 Malocclusion in a seven-year-old chinchilla (specimen, right orbital area) with a retrograde displacement of all upper cheek teeth, clearly visible foramen of the bony nasolacrimal canal between the apices of the anterior two cheek teeth (black arrow) and extreme retrograde elongation of the first cheek tooth (P4) with an extensively exposed apical tooth body (turquoise arrow).

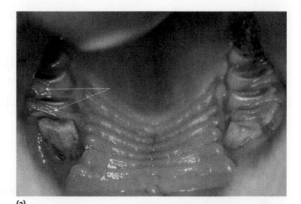

(a)

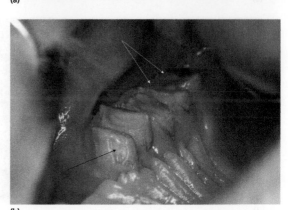

(b)

Figure 10.76 Five months after extraction of all mandibular cheek teeth in the left lower jaw of two different rabbits. (a) Intraoral finding of the maxilla: slight overgrowth of all left maxillary cheek teeth and mild periodontitis with an approximal hyperplasia of the gingiva (white arrows). (b) Left maxillary row of cheek teeth (rostropalatal view): superficial enamel lesion in the area of the mesial surface of the first cheek tooth (P2; black arrow) and slight gingival hyperplasia. The occlusal surfaces of the two distal cheek teeth (M1/M2) are partially covered by a hypertrophic gingiva (white arrows).

When extracting cheek teeth to treat an abscess, the empty alveolar cavity is packed to the gingival margin with a tamponade that is replaced every two to three days (Figure 10.72c). As soon as the alveolar area is clean and starts to heal via granulation, the packing only needs to be replaced once a week (Figure 10.73d). Up to that point in time, the wound should be debrided regularly, with or without anesthesia, depending on the case. In some cases the access to the wound area needs to be enlarged by opening up the skin defect and all deeper necrotic bone tissue or regrown dental tissue (dentinoids) needs to be removed. Nonvital tissue

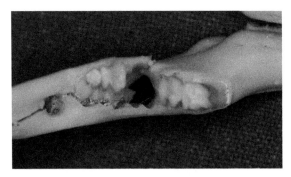

Figure 10.77 Situation after extraction of the third cheek tooth (M1) in a rabbit (specimen, right mandibular row of cheek teeth): fracture of the lingual alveolar wall as well as a fracture of the distal mandible.

Complications of cheek teeth extractions

Possible causes:
- Impatience
- Unsuitable or dirty instruments
- Lever movements

Consequences:
- Intraalveolar tooth fracture
- Excessive trauma to the alveolar bone
- Jaw fracture
- Damage to the germinal cells of the adjacent tooth
- Excessive trauma of soft tissue including hemorrhage (rare)
- Incorrect technique and/or dirty instruments can result in postoperative infection

---

always has a whitish color and does not bleed during curettage. Once the defect has closed orally, the wound can be allowed to heal from the outside (waiving further drainage). In guinea pigs, such wound healings may take several weeks or even months as the alveoli are especially wide due to the large diameter of the teeth.

10.4.6 Complications

Most complications that occur during a tooth extraction are due to a certain amount of impatience on the part of the operating surgeon, the use of unsuitable instruments or as a result of errors in the application of force, e.g. during lever movements. The most common complications are intraalveolar longitudinal or apical transverse fractures of the tooth or excessive trauma to the jawbone, with a fracture of the alveolar wall (Figure 10.77). Uncontrolled use of the instruments may even injure the germinal tissue of the neighboring tooth. That would promote further spread of the infection to the adjacent (pre-)molar or lead to a growth disturbance of the tooth resulting from damage to the germinal cells.

Rarer complications include iatrogenic jaw fractures the prognosis of which would depends of the animal species, as well as the location and the extent of the primary local infection. Accidental fractures that occurred intraoperatively may heal rather well in rabbits when treated conservatively and an operative stabilization often will not be necessary (Figure 10.78c). Favorable prognoses can be given, particularly for all fractures of the caudal mandibular ramus as these are sufficiently immobilized by the strong masseter muscle. If a fracture that is located further rostrally heals even slightly out of

alignment, the slight displacement or angled jaw may lead to a disturbance of normal tooth wear longer term. Surprisingly, the fragments mostly realign in such a favorable way as to ensure physiological wear by contact of the molars at rest (Figure 10.78a to e).

In guinea pigs, however, the prognosis for conservative treatments of jaw fractures is unfavorable as the lower intraoral soft tissue cover entails a significantly increased risk of local abscess formations. Particularly when treating abscesses of the caudal lower jaw, there is a high risk of iatrogenic jaw fractures while extracting teeth as the last molar – even in healthy animals – is merely covered by an extremely thin bone lamella lingually and laterally. If the mandible is additionally weakened by a purulent local infection (osteolysis), the danger of fracturing the jaw intraoperatively will increase (Figure 10.64). Surprisingly, the molars of guinea pigs are always firmly anchored in the alveolus, even in case of an apical infection, which is presumably due to the curvature and length of the cheek teeth. Conservative treatment of the fracture will be unsuccessful as the primarily infected jawbone, which is wide open toward the oral cavity (empty alveolus), is usually not able to heal. Euthanizing the patient is indicated; this scenario should be discussed with the owner prior to any planned tooth extraction.

When attempting to grasp a cheek tooth that has not yet been sufficiently loosened with extraction forceps or a Pean clamp, the tooth tends to break intraalveolarly, close to the tooth apex or near the area of contact with the instrument (Figure 10.62a). Hence only clamps with a smooth working surface should be used in order to

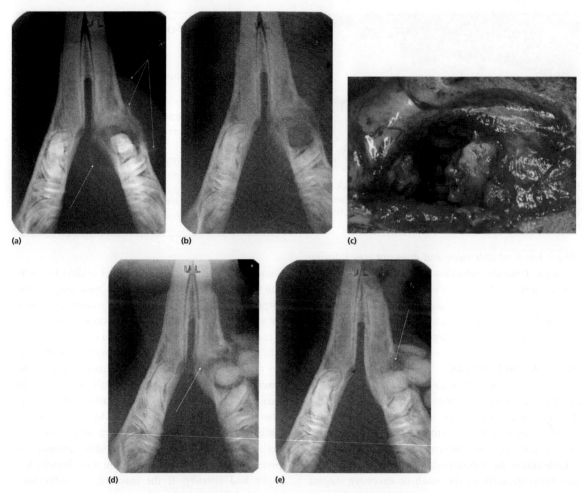

(a)   (b)   (c)

(d)   (e)

Figure 10.78 Abscess (left) in a two-year-old rabbit. (a) Intraoral view of the mandible: significant dilation of the tooth socket in the area of the first left cheek tooth (P3), rostromedial bony distension of the inner cortical bone of the jaw (white arrow) and laterally clear swelling of soft tissue with beginning proliferative bone changes (turquoise arrows), indication for a tooth extraction. (b) Intraoral view of the mandible, after removal of the first cheek tooth (P3): thin, medial and lateral bone lamella in the area of the empty alveolus (P3). (c) Left mandible, ventral view of the area of the excised abscess, 1 week after tooth extraction: transverse fracture of the mandible caused by patient struggling during drainage replacement. (d) Intraoral view of the mandible following placement of several AIPMMA implants in the fracture and the former abscess area with good repositioning of the mandibular fragments (white arrow). (e) Intraoral view of the mandible, 2 months after iatrogenic jaw fracture and implant placement: the fracture area has healed; there is a coronal fracture of the left incisor crown and slightly blurred dental tissue in the apical area (white arrow). There is an indication for frequent follow-up checks of the incisor.

prevent additional damage to the tooth, in other words predetermined breaking points. The removal of the remaining tooth stub, which usually protrudes only slightly beyond the edge of the gingiva or is even hidden intraalveolarly, is usually difficult as the intraalveolar tooth remnant can hardly be grasped with suitable instruments even after complete mobilization. Often the

only way to proceed will be retrograde access via an osteotomy (see Section 10.4.4).

Disturbances caused by bleeding are rare in cheek tooth extractions. However, intraoperative bleeding will occur if the blood vessel in the jaw angle (a branch of the maxillary vein) is injured or if sharp instruments slip off the bone or tooth and into the adjacent soft tissue, such

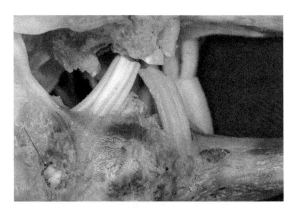

Figure 10.79 Severe malocclusion in a rabbit (specimen, right row of cheek teeth) with an approximal tilting of the first (P3) and next-to-last right cheek tooth (M2) due to a growth disturbance and/or loss of the middle two cheek teeth (P4/M1), retrogradely exposed apex of the next-to-last molar (M2; black arrow) and enamel hypoplasia of all visible maxillary teeth, some of which are fractured (end-stage malocclusion).

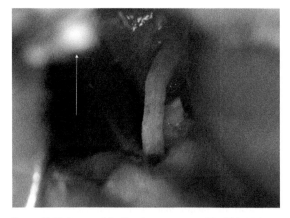

Figure 10.80 Intraoral finding in a two-year-old rabbit (right mandibular row of cheek teeth) with a massively elongated clinical crown of the last cheek tooth (M3) arching from distally to rostrally; food particles and another mandibular cheek tooth are visible below it. For better orientation, the white arrow marks the maxillary incisors, with the cheek dilator underneath them.

as the retrobulbar area, the floor of the oral cavity, the tongue or the cheek. More frequent complications are postoperative infections or wound healing disturbances resulting from the use of dirty instruments or insufficient intraoperative hygiene (surface, gloves, etc.).

A possible complication after a removal of a single mandibular molar in rabbits is a tilting of the adjacent tooth toward the extraction site. The displaced molar may then partly take over the function of the missing tooth and may ensure sufficient, continuous abrasion of the antagonist (Harcourt-Brown, 2002a). Problems start when the tilt of the tooth increases due to constant abnormal pressure conditions, in other words if a really pronounced secondary tilting of the displaced tooth occurs. This, however, usually only happens if a single tooth from the middle of the occlusal plane is removed (Figures 10.5 and 10.79) (Crossley & Aiken, 2004). That will rarely occur with treatment of an abscess and it should be critically evaluated in the case of other indications such as a solitary tooth deformation or tilting.

Regardless of species, there are mostly indications for the extraction of the first or last upper or lower cheek tooth, or two teeth in the abscess area, and the postoperative malalignment of the remaining teeth are rather rare in those cases. However, if a rabbit's anterior three or even four lower cheek teeth on one side (P3–M2) need to be removed, the last, small molar (M3) will proceed to grow rostrally in a shallow arc due to its

physiological direction of growth, which is mesiodorsal (Figure 10.80). As it is progressively pushed downwards by the upper molars, it will ultimately grow over the empty alveoli completely. Even though that elongated molar will serve to wear down the maxillary cheek teeth in a certain way, its length may cause secondary injuries to the soft tissue or a tooth fracture. Hence it is better in the long term to prophylactically remove that molar during primary treatment of the abscess in case there is the need of such extensive tooth extractions later.

Another possible complication after an extraction of an infected cheek tooth is fistula formation. During secondary healing of the wound, a persisting connection between the oral cavity and the outer abscess area develops (Figure 10.81). Those fistulas can be rather resistant to treatment. The wound may eventually heal if food residue is removed from the fistula daily by retrograde flushings with small amounts of NaCl solution (Crossley & Aiken, 2004).

10.5 Alternative possibilities of treatment

All patients with recurring problems involving elongated, regrowing or malaligned cheek teeth can have their lifelong tooth growth stopped in an alternative

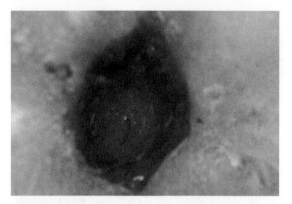

Figure 10.81 Two months following excision of a mandibular abscess in a two-year-old rabbit (ventral view into the empty alveolus with good granulation of the area): there is a small, fistula at the extraction site of the first cheek tooth (P3) and saliva draining into the granulating alveolar area.

way other than tooth extraction (Crossley & Aiken, 2004). There are different methods available for this: apart from cytotoxic substances that kill off the pulp (endodontic application), cryotherapy may also be used (Massler & Schour, 1941; Crossley & Aiken, 2004). With both methods, however, it will be very difficult to confine the destruction of tissue to the desired area, which means that there is a high risk of at least a partial destruction of the local bone (necrosis).

The least extreme method currently is a surgical apicoectomy of individual molars, where the apical dental tissue including the pulp is resected and the wound area is closed without any filling material. In the case of an apical infection, an implant containing antibiotics can also be temporarily inserted. Access to the apical area of the lower cheek teeth is rather simple, whereas exposing the maxillary apices is too complicated and invasive due to the anatomical circumstances.

The result of the surgery is a sudden halt of apical tooth growth, which, surprisingly, leads to continuous tooth eruption nonetheless (Massler & Schour, 1941). The tooth shifts further out of the alveolus until periodontal stabilization is no longer strong enough to keep the tooth – which is relatively short now – in the alveolus; it will then simply fall out (Figure 10.82a and

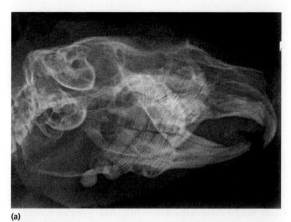
(a)

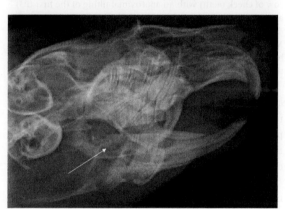
(b)

Figure 10.82 The same patient as in Figure 5.21 (in Chapter 5): apicoectomy in a guinea pig (left oblique view). (a) Following apicectomy of the last left lower molar (M3) in a guinea pig with temporary AIPMMA implants; normal occlusion. (b) Three months after apicectomy of the last left lower molar (M3): the AIPMMA implants were removed 10 days after having been positioned. As a result of the continuous tooth eruption and according wear, only a small part of the tooth body is there (white arrow). Follow up check 2 weeks later showed that the fragment had been lost intraorally.

b). In some cases, however, tooth "eruption" does stop (as had been desired) and the cheek tooth will simply remain in the alveolus until it is worn down at the level of the gingiva and thus is shorter than the neighboring teeth (Crossley & Aiken, 2004).

CHAPTER 11

Abscesses

11.1 Jaw abscesses

11.1.1 Etiology and pathogenesis

In animal species, abscesses in the head/jaw area most frequently are the result of intraalveolarly infected incisors and/or cheek teeth. Odontogenic abscessations are mostly restricted to the periapical area of a tooth in their early stages. Predilection sites for these are always the retrogradely displaced, exposed tooth apices. Infections, however, are rarely recognized at this point because the patients exhibit hardly any clinical symptoms (see Figure 10.59 in Chapter 10). The subtle intraosseous findings can only be verified by means of suitable radiographs. This should be the goal because when dealing with jaw abscesses, there is a general rule:

> The earlier treatment is started, the better the chances of healing.

If, however, a periodontal infection is allowed to spread unrestricted, the result will be a more extensive, purulent osteomyelitis of the adjacent jawbone together with loosening and deformation of the teeth. Progressive, infection-related bone resorption will then lead to a typical jaw abscess, in the center of which there will often be grotesquely deformed incisors or cheek teeth with severe growth disturbances. The size of such an abscess varies greatly between individuals. In extreme cases the entire jaw quadrant can be destroyed.

In principle, abscesses are inflammatory reactions that occur in the presence of pyogenic organisms that resist phagocytosis thanks to their special, capsular polysaccharides (Deeb, 1993; Harcourt-Brown, 2002b).

Neutrophilic granulocytes contain lysosomal granules with special enzymes that play the major part in the destruction of the bacteria. When the neutrophils die after an average lifetime of three to four days, their lysosomal enzymes are released, which not only breakdown the bacteria and the blood cells but also cells from the necrotic tissue in their vicinity (Harcourt-Brown, 2002b). As the purulent infection proceeds further, a sort of cavity is formed, which is increasingly isolated from the surrounding tissue by means of a fibrotic wall (abscess capsule). That wall is made up of connective tissue, collagen fibers and blood vessels on the outside and a layer of degenerated neutrophilic granulocytes on the inside (Chaffee, James & Montale, 1975). The capsule of a jaw abscess is also extensively ossified as it consists mainly of pathologically distended bone tissue (see Figure 11.31 later). Alternatively, the jawbone – and more commonly the mandible – will assume a sponge-like appearance during the bone-remodeling processes (Figure 11.1).

In guinea pigs and chinchillas, primary periodontopathies also seem to play a part in the origin of jaw infections that is not to be underestimated. They are caused by deeper gingival pockets in which food and hair particles may be impacted. An infection develops that spreads and eventually leads to a typical odontogenic abscess (see Figure 12.15 in Chapter 12).

Sometimes the primary cause of an abscess formation is said to be the longitudinal splitting of a cheek tooth, which is relatively frequent. That, however, is not the cause of the apical infection but the result of a periapical microabscessation already present (typical local radiolucency), which leads to a secondary malformation of the tooth substance (see Figure 1.2a in Chapter 1). Another important potential cause of upper jaw abscesses in

Dentistry in Rabbits and Rodents, First Edition. Estella Böhmer.
© 2015 John Wiley & Sons, Ltd. Published 2015 by John Wiley & Sons, Ltd.

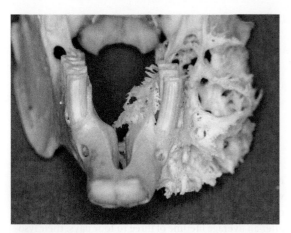

Figure 11.1 Abscess of the left mandible in a two-year-old rabbit (mandible specimen): mandibular abscess originating from the last cheek tooth (M3) with extensive radial proliferation of the jawbone.

rabbits is a chronic infection of the nasolacrimal duct. Since there is mostly a primary retrograde displacement of the apices of the maxillary incisors, which leads to a compression of the nasolacrimal duct, they are – in principle – odontogenic, intranasal or maxillary abscessations. Often the infection will spread to the first upper cheek tooth (P2). In addition, abscesses in the area of the head may be a result of intraoral soft tissue lesions, e.g. diffuse inflammation of the cheek muscles and masticatory muscles caused by buccal tooth spurs, or sometimes a result of external injuries (Figure 11.2).

11.1.2 Diagnosis

While diagnosing larger abscesses of the lower jaw is usually no problem as they can be easily detected by means of examination and palpation, those kinds of changes and their primary causes are much harder to identify in the maxilla. Except for larger abscesses of the facial tuberosity and the cribriform plate (in rabbits), those kinds of changes usually cannot be palpated. They will not become apparent until the surrounding bone tissue has been more severely destroyed and secondary clinical symptoms start to show. The latter are mostly unilateral and affect the upper respiratory pathways or the eye: a dacryocystitis, a purulent nasal discharge or slight protrusion of the eye.

In order to be able to evaluate the overall situation as well as possible, particularly thorough radiographic examinations of the skull are required. As well as the

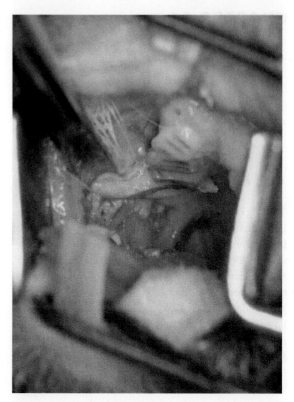

Figure 11.2 Malocclusion in a twelve-year-old chinchilla (right maxillary row of cheek teeth) with a pronounced buccal spur in the last molar (M3) and secondary cheek (muscle) inflammation, and an intraalveolar rotation of the first cheek tooth (P4).

usual radiographs of the head in four views, special positionings such as isolated views of the upper and lower jaws of guinea pigs and chinchillas are taken as described by Böhmer or intraoral images are used to specifically depict various sections of the head or individual teeth. If there are suspicions of changes in the nasolacrimal duct, primary diagnostics should be followed by a dacryocystography, if necessary (see Figures 9.16 and 9.20 in Chapter 9). An alternative is a computed tomographic examination of the head. In the case of intranasal abscessations, endoscopic diagnostics of the nasal cavity may additionally be helpful (Harcourt-Brown, 2002b).

11.1.3 Differential diagnosis

An alternative to jaw abscesses during differential diagnosis can be neoplasias; however, neoplasia of the skull is rather rare in pets (see Section 13.3 in

Chapter 13). In order to differentiate the two find-ings, ultrasonography may be used as well as radio-graphy. If in doubt, an additional fine needle biopsy is undertaken. In addition to teeth or infections of the nasolacrimal duct, foreign bodies in the nose may also be origins of a chronic intranasal abscessation – these are usually small hay stalks. Far more frequent are chronic infections with *Pasteurella multocida* in rabbits, which mostly lead to bilateral problems. Fungal infec-tions (*Mycoses*) of the nasal cavity of small mammals occur only in very few instances. Fractures of the lower jaw may lead to extensive callus formation dur-ing healing. Once the fracture has healed, the area flattens noticeably.

11.1.4 Clinical symptoms

Although dental abscesses have mainly been reported to appear "suddenly," they do in fact develop over a longer period of time so that in most cases it will be chronic abscessations. However, owners often do not notice anything until a typical soft (centrally fluctuating) or harder jaw lump or swelling in the area of the head has developed. They are often firmly attached to the under-lying bone. Sometimes more severe problems during feed intake, or even a complete refusal to eat, eventu-ally prompt the owner to act. In other cases pus will discharge from the oral cavity or the external area of the abscess and the problem becomes apparent for nonpro-fessionals (see Figure 8.2 in Chapter 8). In such cases many people state that the swelling has been present for a while but the animal has not exhibited any symptoms of disease.

In rabbits, abscesses of the mandible are more fre-quent than those of the maxilla or the orbit, whereas in guinea pigs, the locations are approximately equal. Purulent infections in those cases may remain restricted to one of the jaw quadrants (and primarily affect a single tooth), but they may also – more frequently – affect several neighboring cheek teeth. There may also be multicentric abscesses (Figure 11.3). The latter are particularly common in chronically ill animals that have not yet been subjected to any specific examina-tion or surgery. At this stage many abscesses are inop-erable as they infiltrate the bone and the adjacent soft tissue. The infection will always spread to the tissue that offers the least resistance. That is why they prefer-entially perforate the skin or penetrate body cavities (nose).

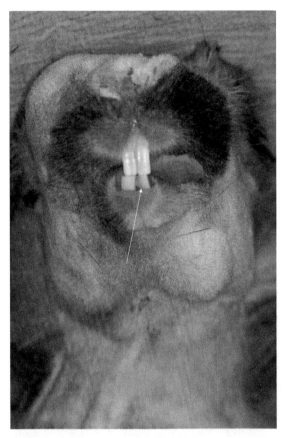

Figure 11.3 Abscess of the right maxilla in a five-year-old rabbit with a unilateral rhinitis (nasal discharge), bilateral abscess of the mandibles and intraalveolar rotation of the left mandibular incisor (white arrow).

A hematogenous or lymphogenous spread of the infection must always be taken considered in patients with jaw abscesses. In rabbits, they usually lead to intra-thoracic and (less frequently) intraabdominal secondary abscesses (Harcourt-Brown, 2002b). Rabbits with intra-thoracic suppurative foci, which are mainly locally con-fined, present with dyspnoea. These abscesses usually remain clinically inapparent and thus undetected for a long time in their early stages. It is only when there is a sudden general weakness of the patient or an inexpli-cable healing complication that secondary complica-tions like this are considered (see Figure 4.4a and b in Chapter 4).

Superficial abscesses are located immediately under-neath the skin and often consist of one single large abscess cavity (Figure 11.4). They are clearly visible and

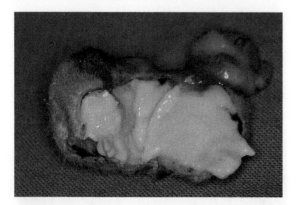

Figure 11.4 Resected soft tissue abscess in a rabbit with a fibrotic capsule and typical, cream-like pus.

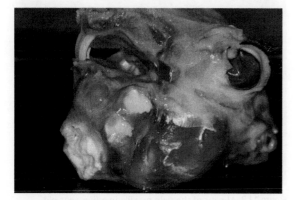

Figure 11.5 Abscess of the mandible in a four-year-old rabbit (specimen): pronounced swelling, comprising several individual chambers, of the left lower jaw. The multiple abscesses were inoperable; hence euthanasia was performed.

can be surgically resected relatively easily. Deeper abscesses, however, often go undetected for a long time, and often pose problems that are hard to solve for an operating surgeon intraoperatively, as they are mostly multichambered and grow infiltratively (Figure 11.5). The primary, deep-lying abscess capsule will fill up with pus until the strained, fibrotic tissue tears in one or several places, causing pus to discharge in the near surroundings (Crossley & Aiken, 2004). This is where new centers of abscessations start to form that are in contact with the original center via a narrow isthmus. After a certain amount of time (possibly several months), the most superficial abscess capsule, which is bursting with pus, will start to leak in one or several places (central skin necrosis), resulting in the contents oozing to the outside.

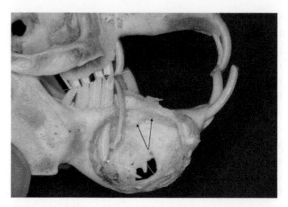

Figure 11.6 Abscess of the lower jaw in a two-year-old rabbit (specimen): bony distension of the right lower jaw and severe elongation of all incisors with abnormal occlusion. The right incisor is displaced rostrally and shows an apical deformation of its tooth structure due to infection (abscess area; black arrows). Longitudinal split of the first cheek tooth (P3), with half of the tooth body already missing (turquoise arrow). Pathological occlusal plane of all cheek teeth with an abnormal distal tilting (turquoise line) and exposed apex of the second mandibular cheek tooth (P4; white arrow) in the abscess area.

11.1.5 Abscesses of the lower jaw

In animal species, purulent infections of the rostral mandible mainly originate from the incisors. Such incisor suppurations are relatively frequent in rabbits and guinea pigs (see Figure 1.1 in Chapter 1 and Figure 9.57 in Chapter 9). They can be the result of improper tooth trimming or a dental trauma. In principle, any irritation of germinal cells that leads to a septic pulpitis may initiate apical abscess formation. In rabbits, the infection tends to spread to the first or the second cheek tooth with time (see Figure 9.32 in Chapter 9). In guinea pigs, the third cheek tooth (M2) is mostly affected because the apex of the incisor is on a level with the second lower cheek tooth (see Figure 9.35c in Chapter 9). This is particularly so the further retrogradely displaced the incisor is, as the apex becomes closer to the premolar. Likewise, apical infections of the premolars may in turn spread to the apices of the incisors secondarily (Figure 11.6).

In rabbits, the apex of the incisor is located just rostral to the row of mandibular cheek teeth, whereas in guinea pigs and chinchillas, it is located medially to it, and caudally in degus. Apical incisor infections in guinea pigs and chinchillas are felt primarily by a swelling that is located on the medial aspect of the lower jaw or

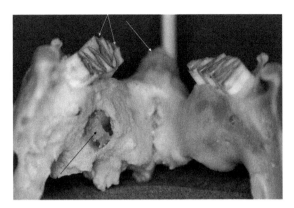

Figure 11.7 Left mandibular abscess in a four-year-old guinea pig (mandible specimen, caudorostral view): osteolysis of the medial mandibular cortical bone; the deformed apex of the left incisor is visible in the area of the medial osseous perforation site (black arrow). Pronounced proliferative changes of the entire medial section of the left lower jawbone; the clinical crown of the left incisor is missing (white arrow); buccal displacement of the first two left cheek teeth (P4/M1; turquoise arrows).

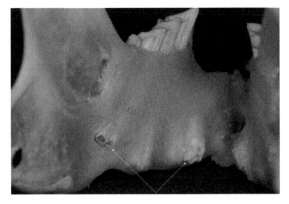

Figure 11.8 Malocclusion in a rabbit (left mandible specimen, caudomedial view) with a retrograde elongation of the first (P3) and next-to-last cheek tooth (M2) with a perforation of the medial cortical bone of the jaw; the pertaining apices are exposed (white arrows).

between the mandibles (Figure 11.7). It is only when the ventrolateral cortical bone has been extensively destroyed that the abscess will progress laterally. If the middle part of the incisor is affected primarily then the intraalveolar abscess will preferentially perforate ventrally and is therefore clinically detected much faster. Surgical treatment of such cases is relatively easy as, there is already immediate access to the tooth socket ("natural" ventral osteotomy), due to the pathological destruction of the alveolar bone, which will greatly facilitate tooth extraction and aftercare (see Figure 9.58 in Chapter 9).

Rabbits

If the abscess has primarily been caused by the first cheek tooth (P3), longitudinal splitting of the tooth will have occurred in many cases – particularly in rabbits. As well as a significant increase in the periodontal space, the most predominant radiographic findings are two tooth parts that are usually elongated but of different lengths. The latter is an important indication of tooth splitting. Clinically, the affected tooth is often mobile, although the split may well be overlooked during an intraoral examination. The apex usually perforates the mandibular cortical bone medially due to the physiological, lingually concave curvature of the premolar (Figure 11.8). Thus smaller periapical abscesses

often originate here too. Without a thorough clinical and radiographic examination those intermandibular abscesses often go undetected in their early stages.

As the premolar (P3) is increasingly tilted and deformed, the abscess spreads further and migrates continuously to the outside. A clinically predominant feature of rabbits is now a ventrolateral jaw swelling of various sizes and consistencies. The remodeling of the bone that is associated with the infection is a clear indicator that the infection is of chronic duration, probably of several months (Figure 11.9). Surgical proceedings are greatly hampered by the osseous changes as it is now necessary to remove rather a lot of bone in order to treat the abscess. Sometimes the mandible is weakened by this to an extent where the risk of a jaw fracture increases.

Larger, periapical abscesses of the middle two lower cheek teeth (P4/M1) of rabbits mostly cause clearly palpable, lateral jaw swellings, while similar infections of the last two molars (M2/M3) may be easily overlooked. The abscess is initially confined to the jaw area below the masseter muscle (see Figure 10.13b in Chapter 10). It is not until the infection starts to spread before the masticatory muscles undergo liquefactive necrosis, allowing the abscess to break out. The retrogradely elongated tooth apices of the last two lower molars tend to perforate the mandibular cortical bone medially and cause abscesses of various sizes there, which will restrict the larynx as well as the pharynx in the late stages (Figure 11.10). The early stages of such changes often

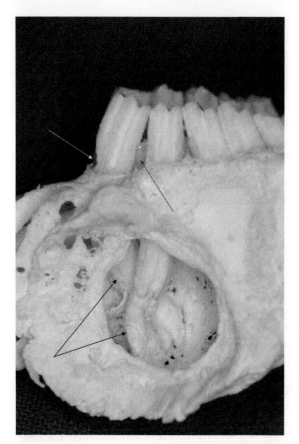

Figure 11.9 Rostral abscess of the lower jaw in a three-year-old rabbit (left mandible specimen, lateral view): markedly displacement and structural change of the anterior two cheek teeth due to an intraalveolar enamel and dentin hypoplasia (P3/P4; black arrows). The apex of the first cheek tooth (P3) perforates the inner cortical bone medially (turquoise arrow); cystic distension of the lateral cortical bone of the jaw, enamel defect near the gingiva on the mesial surface of the first cheek tooth (P3; yellow arrow) and slight expansion of the approximal area orientated toward the neighboring, distal cheek tooth (P4; red arrow).

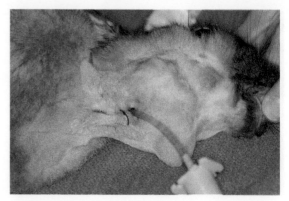

Figure 11.10 Extensive, tooth-associated, intermandibular abscess in a six-year-old rabbit with a narrowing of the pharyngeal area; intubation of the patient by way of a tracheostomy.

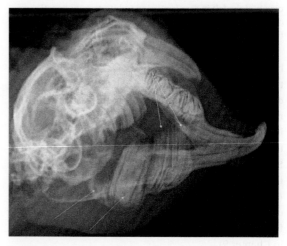

Figure 11.11 Right mandibular abscess in a four-year-old guinea pig (isolated oblique view of the right mandible according to Böhmer): elongation of the clinical crowns of the first two cheek teeth (P4/M1; white arrows) as well as markedly thickened, structurally altered intraalveolar body of the third cheek tooth (M2; yellow arrow). The last tooth is missing (M3). There is a small residual amount of dental tissue in the apical alveolar area (turquoise arrow).

remain undetected. Hence the inner surface of the mandible should also be carefully palpated during all clinical examinations of rabbits. As the infection spreads further, the temporomandibular joint may also secondarily be included in the abscess (see Figure 10.13c in Chapter 10).

Guinea pigs

Although the mandibular cheek teeth of guinea pigs primarily have a lingually concave curvature, their apices usually tend to perforate the jaw ventrally (P4/M1)

or ventrolaterally (M2/M3) during a retrograde displacement (Figure 11.11). If apical abscessations start to develop, a painful, ventrolateral jaw swelling can be palpated in that area. Especially infections of the last two molars (M2/M3) will be hidden underneath the masseter muscle in the early stages (see Figure 8.1b in Chapter 8). If the apical infection remains undetected

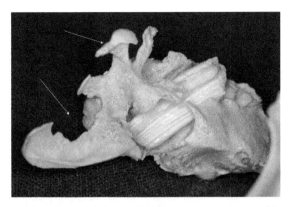

Figure 11.12 Caudal abscess of the lower jaw in a six-year-old guinea pig (specimen, left branch of the mandible, medial view): the tooth body of the last molar (M3) is severely altered structurally; extensive, medial osteolysis of the jawbone in the apical area and marked proliferative changes of the entire mandible with a partial lysis of the caudodorsal mandibular ramus (white arrow). The distal part of the condyle has a pathological shape (yellow arrow).

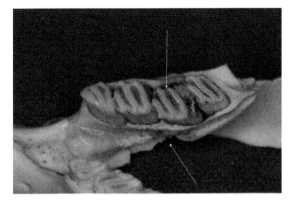

Figure 11.13 Abscess of the lower jaw in a chinchilla (specimen, right mandible, dorsomedial view): fibrous food particles in the approximal area of the last two molars (M2/M3); slight, lingual displacement of the third cheek tooth (M2; yellow arrow); the associated tooth socket is dilated laterally; osteolysis of the ventromedial cortical bone of the jaw (white arrow).

over a longer period, necrosis of the masseter muscle will follow, and the infection will also continue to spread medially. During surgical abscess excision, not only does the affected tooth need to be extracted but all pathologically altered masticatory muscles also need to be resected. This is possible in principle as the animals are able to grind down the food with the aid of the muscles of the contralateral side. Due to a chewing asymmetry that is to be expected postoperatively, however, any long-term normal physiological tooth wear will not be possible. Therefore many patients need tooth corrections at regular time intervals.

In the case of apical abscessations of the last molar (M3) in guinea pigs, the abscess will sometimes break through to the inside primarily, leading to a medial jaw swelling – despite the fact that a major part of the apex is predominantly located in the area of the lateral mandibular wall (Figure 11.12). This is because the inner bone lamella is often thinner than the outer wall of the mandible, which is constantly remodeled during the continuous, retrograde apex displacement. Due to the immediate proximity of the temporomandibular joint to the medial or lateral abscess area (short condylar process), the purulent infection quickly spreads to the temporomandibular joint in some cases.

Chinchillas

Locally confined abscesses of the mandible are rather rare in chinchillas. The predominant features in chinchillas are diffuse, intraalveolar abscessations of several teeth that rarely perforate the mandible (see Figures 10.39 and 10.42 in Chapter 10). If, however, the apices of individual mandibular cheek teeth are infected primarily, lateral jaw swellings of various sizes manifest themselves. Such abscesses usually originate from the last two cheek teeth (M2/M3) (see Figure 10.23 in Chapter 10 and Figure 11.13). Rostral mandibular abscesses that originate primarily from the incisors are more frequent in chinchillas. Initially located between the branches of the mandible, the abscess eventually perforates through ventrolaterally or spreads further intraosseously via the apex area of the nearby first and second mandibular cheek teeth (P4/M1) across the intermandibular area (see Figure 9.26 in Chapter 9).

Degus

The situation in degus is especially confusing. Even though the retrograde displacement of the apices of the mandibular cheek teeth is particularly pronounced here (ventrally in the rostral mandibular area and rather laterally in the caudal area), subsequent abscessations are extremely rare in this species (Figure 11.14). The reasons for this are unknown. In most cases, the cortical jawbone is not just perforated by the apices of the cheek teeth but the apical tooth areas are also exposed by several millimeters.

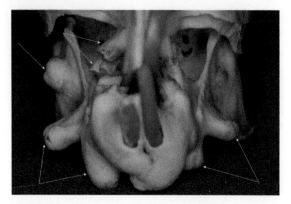

Figure 11.14 Severe malocclusion of cheek teeth in a four-year-old degu (specimen) with a pronounced retrograde displacement and elongation of all cheek teeth. Some of the apices are exposed (white arrows). Step formation, buccal deviation of the intraorally elongated, right maxillary cheek teeth (yellow arrows) and secondary incisor malocclusion.

11.1.6 Abscesses of the upper jaw
Rabbits

In addition to retrobulbar, tooth-related infections (see Section 11.2) as well as apical incisor suppurations with a secondary, palatal abscess formation (see Figure 9.14 in Chapter 9), abscesses in the area of the cribriform plate and the facial tuberosity are relatively frequent in rabbits (see Figure 5.1 in Chapter 5). It is often difficult to distinguish whether their primary origin is an infection of the nasolacrimal duct (retrograde displacement of the apices of the incisors) or whether the first upper cheek tooth (P2) is the cause. Thorough radiographic examinations are necessary for a more precise differentiation of the etiology (see Chapter 5 and Figure 5.3). If a suspected dental cause with an apical infection of the first or the second cheek tooth is confirmed (P2/P3), a tooth extraction via the abscessation area with a radical abscess excision and an osteotomy of the maxilla is necessary. The approach is the same as the procedure described in Section 10.4.4 in Chapter 10 (Figure 10.73a to g).

Guinea pigs, chinchillas and degus
Contrary to rabbits, tooth-associated abscesses of the upper jaw are rare in guinea pigs, chinchillas and degus. If an infection has formed in the area of the apex of the first or second upper cheek tooth (P4/M1), it may penetrate into the nasal cavity and spread further unhindered and often unnoticed. It is often not until a unilateral, purulent nasal discharge occurs that one

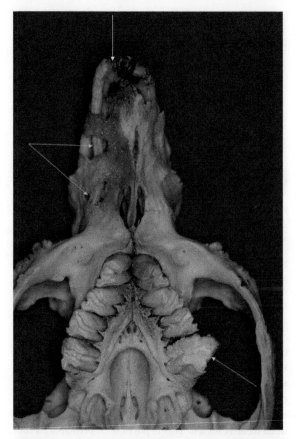

Figure 11.15 Right-sided rhinitis in a three-year-old guinea pig (maxilla specimen, palatal view): incisor malocclusion with a split of the structurally severely altered right incisor (white arrow), right-sided palatal osteolysis of the maxilla (turquoise arrows), structurally altered occlusal surface and buccal spurs in the last left cheek tooth (M3; yellow arrow).

starts to look for the cause of the intranasal infection. Alternatively, the infection may also spread to the nearby nasolacrimal duct (see Figure 9.20 in Chapter 9).

These kinds of abscesses always represent a surgical challenge in that the apices – and thus the abscess area – are located beneath the lacrimal bone and the deep part of the masseter muscle, an area that is difficult to access. As described in Section 10.4.4 in Chapter 10, the infected teeth that are causing this problem are extracted via osteotomy of the maxilla, and radical excision of the abscess. Wound healing is by secondary intention.

Just as in rabbits, apical incisor infections may also lead to palatal or intranasal abscessations (Figures 11.15 and 11.16). In that case the abscess area is also exposed and surgically excised following tooth extraction.

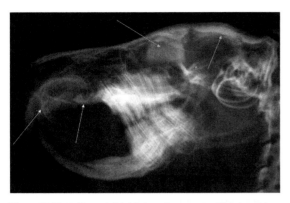

Figure 11.16 Unilateral rhinitis in a three-year-old guinea pig (laterolateral view): intraalveolar deformation of an upper incisor with a retrograde displacement of the apex toward the palatal plate, periapical osteolysis (white arrows), elongation of the mandibular incisors, radiopaque structure in the area of the orbit as well as the roof of the skull (turquoise arrows) and cheek tooth malocclusion with an intraoral elongation of all teeth.

11.1.7 Therapy
General remarks

Whenever treating jaw abscesses, it is critical that the patient is in a stable general condition. If that is not the case and the animal is in a catabolic state, it needs to be stabilized first (see Section 7.1.1, anesthesia – general remarks, in Chapter 7). Otherwise there is a markedly increased anesthetic risk and wound healing may be compromised. In order to gain some time for intensive therapy whilst providing some relief for the patient, larger abscesses can be aspirated or lanced and drained. Radiographic examinations of the head area also easier following drainage however surgical resection of the abscess capsule at a later stage becomes more difficult.

If the animal has a close companion, that other animal can be kept with the patient during the stabilization treatment. It is equally important for the psyche of the patient to treat it in a caring way and to let it roam freely on a lawn at regular intervals, or at least be fed freshly picked grass and herbs. In addition, wound healing can be accelerated by an optimal supply of dietary minerals and vitamins.

Tooth-associated abscesses that are merely lanced without further examination and then treated with a systemic antibiotic cannot heal successfully, even if the abscess is also regularly flushed and kept clean.

In rabbits, abscess treatment is complicated by the fact that the pus – consisting of dead phagocytes

> In order to gain therapeutical success, the cause of the abscess must be removed, which almost always is an infected tooth (or several teeth). The abscess area is radically resected together with obligatory tooth extraction. Experience has shown that this is the only correct procedure.

(predominantly neutrophiles), inflammatory exudate, bacteria and cellular debris – is of a relatively solid consistency similar to pudding or cream. That consistency is the result of a continuous resorption of water (Harcourt-Brown, 2002b). Thus it cannot drain away by itself and even repeated, thorough flushings and curettages mostly do not help to remove it from all hidden recesses of the abscess area. The pus of guinea pigs and chinchillas is similar: it is somewhat less viscous, but still very thick.

While the surgical procedure does not allow many variations as one should follow the respective guidelines, the aftercare as well as the peri- and postoperative antibiotic therapy can be performed in different ways. All that, however, requires a lot of patience both on the part of the practitioner and on the part of the animal's owner – always depending on the extent of the purulent bone infection as well as the number of teeth removed. The primary surgery is usually performed rather quickly, but aftercare can be elaborate and unnerving. Hence, as well as accurate diagnostics, it is most vital to explain things clearly to the owner at the start of any treatment. This is most easily achieved by including individual radiographs that will help to discuss most efficiently the problems concerning the individual situation with all its risks. It is also the time to discuss the estimated costs of treatment, which may be several weeks long. Every owner should be well informed about this. The patients also need to display a certain amount of "fighting spirit" and must be in a stable condition during the entire treatment. Satisfying long-term results will only be achieved if all of these preconditions are met.

Radical abscess excision ("en bloc")

Every single step of the primary surgical treatment is clearly defined and is very similar in all cases. For example, all authors agree that removing the cause is the principal goal of every abscess treatment. That cause is mostly an infected tooth or several of them. Tooth extraction is followed by a radical, surgical resection of the abscess area (Figure 11.17a to h), with the fibrous

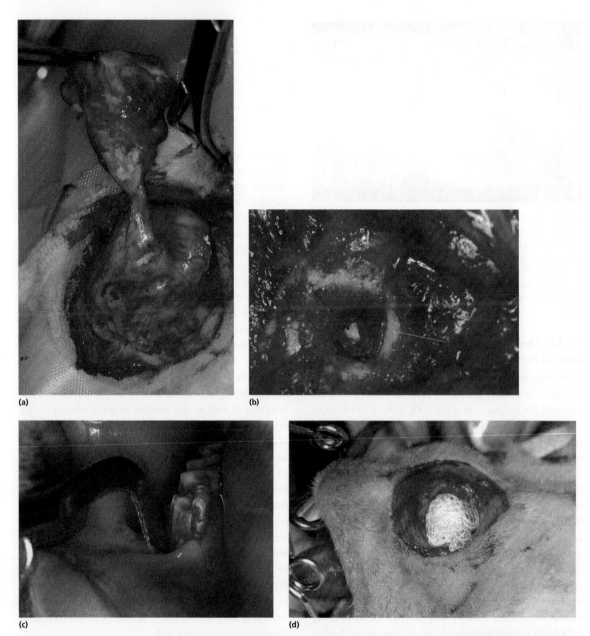

Figure 11.17 Right-sided, tooth-associated abscess of the lower jaw in a rabbit. (a) Intraoperative view after dissection of the fibrotic abscess capsule for an en bloc resection. A small indentation filled with pus is visible in the area of the connection site with the jaw, which corresponds with the apex area of the infected cheek tooth, causing the problem. The slightly elevated circumscribed area is the proliferative change to the jawbone. (b) Following removal of the abscess capsule: cleaned depression of bone located in the area of the pediculated abscess base. Dental tissue is visible in the depth (apex of cheek tooth, black arrow) and the body of another cheek tooth further right (turquoise arrow). (c) Intraoperative view (intraoral view of the right mandibular row of cheek teeth): buccal mobilization of the infected cheek tooth (P3) by means of a Heidemann spatula and discharge of pus from the tooth socket. (d) After excision and retrograde cheek tooth extraction: the alveolus and the wound area are packed with iodoform gauze. (e) Temporary closure of the excision and packed abscess area. (f) One week following excision and cheek tooth extraction: the wound area is contaminated with discharge. There is an indication for a thorough curettage and rinsing. (g) Situation 2.5 weeks after abscess excision: abscess area and tooth socket showing good granulation. (h) Situation 3.5 weeks after abscess excision: the wound area has almost healed and drainage is not necessary any more.

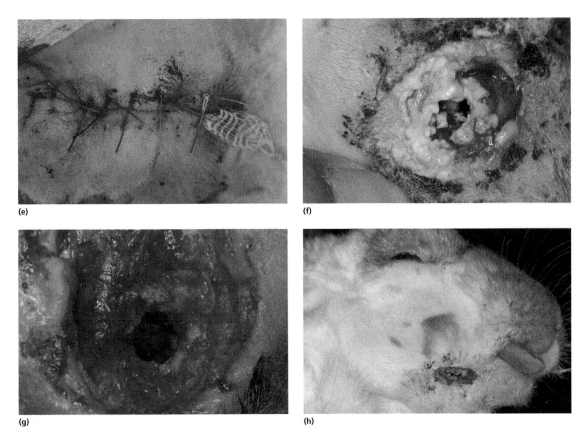

(e)

(f)

(g)

(h)

Figure 11.17 (*Continued*)

abscess capsule being completely removed (Harcourt-Brown, 2002b; Crossley & Aiken, 2004; Bennett, 2008). Further actions can be made in various ways (for alternative methods of treatment see Section 11.1.7).

Depending on the location of the abscess, an extraoral access is preferentially chosen for excision of the purulent infection (Harcourt-Brown, 2002b). That approach also ensures good postoperative accessibility of the wound area and for aftercare. It has proven beneficial to approach all abscesses surgically as if they were neoplastic. First, a spindle shaped area of the overlying skin is resected. Next, the entire abscess capsule is dissected down to its base near the bone carefully, using a fine-tip pair of scissors (Figure 11.17a). The capsule must not be injured during that process. In order to be able to easily move the abscess in any desired direction during the dissection, an arterial clamp is attached to the upper part of the partially exposed capsule, helping to manipulate the tissue. An argument against a simple, straight

incision of the skin is the fact that the view of the surgery area is greatly impaired with a small access, which means that the situation becomes confusing rather quickly. Moreover, excess skin is resected anyway at the end of surgery.

As soon as the capsule has been dissected down to its base, the fibrotic pedicle, which mostly is rather narrow, is totally separated from the underlying bone, making shallow cuts with a scalpel or a pair of scissors. Occasionally the contact surface can be somewhat wider, causing the base of the abscess to be less distinct. Such an en bloc resection minimizes the danger of recurrences as an undamaged capsule will allow the safe removal of large parts of the putrid contents of the abscess without contaminating the wound area with pus. By contrast, if a part of the abscess capsule, which is rather tough and thick, remains in situ, this will predispose the animal to delayed wound healing or to recurrences – due both to an increased local concentration of pyogenic bacteria and the prolonged production of pus.

A subsequent, thorough debridement involves the removal of all infected, necrotic or simply excess soft tissue as far as possible – extending to healthy, well-vascularized tissue. If the abscess capsule is ossified, or if pathological bone proliferations are present, these are also removed thereby smoothing the bony area of infection. Likewise, all nonvital osseous structures (bone sequestra) are removed by means of a fine Luer bone rongeur forceps.

The more extensive the bony involvement due to the infection, the higher the risk of iatrogenic jaw fractures. Special care must be taken in such cases. It can sometimes be a better idea to sacrifice part of the mandible and accept a certain degree of destabilization of the jaw rather than leave necrotic or infected bone tissue in the wound area to reduce the possibility of recurrence (Bennett, 1999). Healing of the surgical wound is by secondary intention.

Surgical en bloc resections can be very difficult or even impossible in the case of multilocular abscesses (Figure 11.18). The fibrotic abscess capsule, which contains various chambers of different shapes, sizes and degrees of maturity, usually cannot be completely dissected and removed as its position and thickness is

constantly changing. In addition, whenever trying to isolate individual cysts, some of which are bursting with pus or extending far into the surrounding soft tissue, pus is likely to exude into the wound area.

If a jaw abscess has already ruptured in a small place, that defect can be clamped using a curved arterial forceps. This will allow the abscess to be resected as a whole. If that fails, the entire putrid contents are carefully removed using a curette with rounded margins, taking care not to contaminate the surrounding tissue of the wound. After that, the radical resection of the remaining abscess capsule follows.

Whilst the tissue is being dissected, hemostasis needs to be performed very meticulously. A small tissue sample – preferably a piece of the capsule with the pus-impregnated inner wall of the abscess – is preserved for an aerobic as well as anaerobic bacterial culture, including a sensitivity test. Pus cannot be used for culture and sensitivity as the bacteria present are already dead. However, many abscess capsules contain different species of bacteria than have been shown to definitely contribute to the abscess formation (Tyrrell et al., 2002).

The bone depression that is usually located in the area of the pediculated resection site (abscess base) is carefully cleared of remaining putrid material by means of a suitable curette. If dental abscesses are present, a part of the tooth causing the local infection will always become visible during this procedure (Figure 11.17b). That tooth may hardly be identifiable (slightly yellowish tissue) or a large part of it is exposed and usually quite deformed– in a bone cavity that is still filled with pus (Figure 11.19).

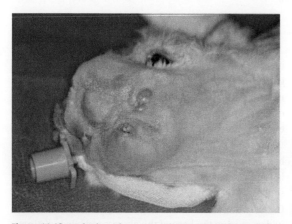

Figure 11.18 Multiple, coherent, tooth-associated abscesses in a six-year-old rabbit, in the area of the left upper and lower jaws.

In such cases, each chamber is treated like an abscess whose capsule is totally resected as far as possible. Otherwise the microorganisms that are enclosed in the walls may lead to a new abscess formation.

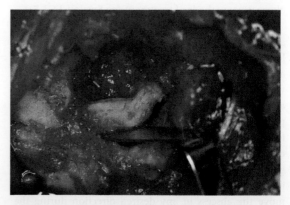

Figure 11.19 Tooth-associated abscess of the lower jaw in a rabbit (situation during the operation): retrograde tooth extraction; partially mobilized, apically deformed cheek tooth (P3) in the abscess area.

Extraction of the tooth (or several teeth) is performed primarily via that extraoral access, in other words retrogradely. However, the tooth can also be extracted intraorally following intraoral mobilization (Figure 11.17c).

In order to remove unwanted pieces of soft tissue and bone tissue (smaller, denuded fragments of the alveolar bone) from the tooth socket, the entire wound area is subsequently flushed with Polyhexanid®. This will help to avoid most recontaminations of the surgical wound with pathogenic bacteria from the primarily infected alveolus.

In the area of an excised abscess cavity or empty alveolar cavity, the lateral surfaces of neighboring molars, some of which are extensively exposed, can often be seen. The cause of this is a generalized bone dysplasia with approximal bone atrophy (loss of the lamina dura). Those teeth do not need to be extracted unless there are any periodontal changes. The molars will need to be monitored at regular time intervals until the abscess has

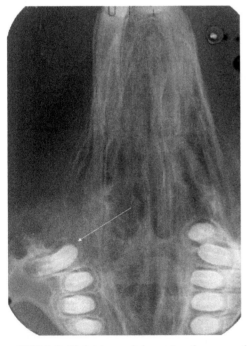

Figure 11.20 Left-sided, intranasal abscess in a three-year-old rabbit (the same patient as in Figure 10.15 in Chapter 10). Intraoral view of the maxilla, situation after extraction of the first cheek tooth: The mesiopalatal alveolar wall of the second cheek tooth is largely destroyed (white arrow). Regular monitoring is necessary and a tooth extraction is indicated in case of further spread of the infection (more severe osteolysis).

healed, as the infection could spread further via that weak spot. Intraoral radiographs are diagnostically very conclusive for a correct evaluation of the periodontium in rabbits. At the same time, they help to find dentinoids that may possibly grow in the excised abscess area which might disturb wound healing (Figure 11.20 and see Section 5.7 in Chapter 5).

After the tooth has been extracted, the empty tooth socket can be packed with a small hemostyptic gelatin sponge (Crossley & Aiken, 2004). The base of the alveolus, as well as the entire adjacent wound area, is subsequently packed with iodoform-soaked gauze (Figure 11.17d). In order to save the tissue from drying out and to facilitate drainage replacements, the gauze is moistened with a small amount of a mixture of granulated sugar and FURACIN®-Nitrofurazon ointment. It is best to place a suture to close the wound temporarily for approximately three days, leaving a small opening where the drainage exits (Figure 11.17e). This allows the traumatized tissue to calm down and the patient to recover without further pain.

Whether the intraoral defect is closed using monofilament suture material (6/0) depends on the individual case, the quality of the soft tissue and the size of the lesion. The intraoral mucosa is mostly easily closed using one or two horizontal mattress sutures after extractions of a single cheek tooth. Experience has shown, however, that the suture will dehisce after three to four days. This means that a gingival suture will often merely lead to additional trauma of the intraoral soft tissue. Therefore it is usually better to let the defect heal intraorally by secondary intention. For this, the empty tooth socket is tightly packed with iodoform gauze via the extraoral access almost up to the gum line (Figure 11.21). This prevents contamination of the alveolus with food during the healing process. At the same time, the intraoral defect may continuously develop a mucosal cover within 10 to 14 days.

The packing and drainage should be replaced on the third postoperative day. For this, all material in the excised wound area is removed with or without sedating the patient, and the wound area is exposed (opened) extensively – depending on its size and the patient's individual situation – by means of a partial or complete removal of the temporary skin sutures. At this point, the abscess area usually looks very "unpleasant." Predominant features include whitish areas of necrotic tissue and many vital structures are also often covered

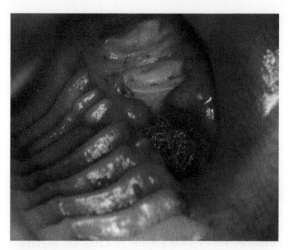

Figure 11.21 Cheek tooth extraction in a rabbit (intraoral view of the right maxillary row of cheek teeth). Situation some days after extraction of the first cheek tooth (P2): the alveolus is packed with gauze almost down to the gingival boundary.

with a layer of slime (Figure 11.17f). Larger pieces of necrotic tissue can be superficially removed with a sterile pair of scissors, if necessary. After another thorough cleaning (curettage) and flushing of the wound as well as the tooth socket, a new drain is inserted. Prior to that, the wound area can be lined directly with the sugar–ointment mix or the drain is moistened with it. That procedure is repeated every two to three days on average, until the empty alveolus and the area of abscess has healed up by means of progressive granulation (Figure 11.17g and h). That will usually occur after approximately three weeks, but it may sometimes take a lot longer. The amount of time depends on the extent of abscess, the number of extracted teeth and possible complications, such as the formation of unwanted dentinoids, a further spread of the infection or findings that went undetected primarily, as well as on the condition of the patient itself. In animals with advanced, chronic abscesses, wound healing is sometimes delayed due to cachexia. A frequent indication of such problems is a typical, whitish discoloration of the wound area. Despite regular debridements, the wound never shows any signs of developing normal pink granulation tissue. If the general condition of the animal deteriorates, there may be no alternative to euthanasia in some cases. Those complications should be discussed with the owner prior to surgery. Unfortunately, there is no guarantee for success in the treatment of most dental abscesses.

Alternative methods of treatment

Especially during the last two decades, many different methods of treatment for dental abscesses have been described whose focus is on the aftercare:

> Possibilities of treating jaw abscesses
> - Local therapy with a mixture of sugar and FURACIN®-SOL ointment
> - Local therapy with honey
> - Inserting drains that are dextrose-soaked into the abscess cavity
> - Marsupialization and flushing
> - Local injection of antibiotics into the abscess wall
> - Implantation of antibiotic impregnated cement bead (AIPMMA beads)
> - Implantation of bioactive ceramics
> - Implantation of gentamicin-soaked collagen fiber plates

Following the radical abscess excision, marsupialization of the wound can be performed (Capello, 2008). For this, the skin is sutured to the outer boundaries of the wound by means of several simple interrupted sutures. This ensures that the abscess cavity remains open and can be flushed with easy postoperative access. Contrary to a fully open wound therapy (as described above), there is a principal risk of a new microabscessation developing unnoticed underneath the sutured skin. Likewise, any long-term insertion of suture material into a wound area that is still infected after radical abscess excision can be unfavorable in individual cases. Every method has certain advantages and disadvantages; it is best to decide according to the individual situation.

About 25 years ago it was recommended that abscess cavities should be completely filled with calcium hydroxide after a tooth extraction and to replace it every week until the wound had healed (Remeeus & Verbeek, 1995). However, that treatment is strongly discouraging for the treatment of jaw abscesses in the opinion of the author. The effect of the calcium hydroxide is based on the extremely alkaline reaction of the preparation with a pH value of 11 to 12. The substance not only has an effect on bacteria (bactericidal) but – secondarily – leads to severe, prolonged necroses and burns to tissue that comes into contact with the preparation, such as alveolar bone, masticatory muscles, subcutis and skin (Eickhoff, 2005; Gorrel & Verhaert,

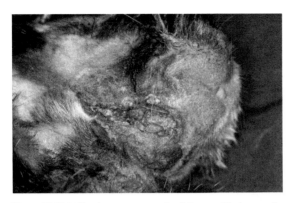

Figure 11.22 Following treatment of a right mandibular, tooth abscess in a six-year-old rabbit with a calcium hydroxide placement: extensive burning and secondary inflammation of soft tissue as a result of the strongly alkaline reaction.

2006). Often the consequences of a local application in the jaw area are fatal (Figure 11.22).

As an alternative to open wound treatment, polymethyl methacrylate beads impregnated with a suitable antibiotic can be inserted both into the abscess area and into the empty alveolus (Bennett, 1999; Crossley & Aiken, 2004). Those AIPMMA (antibiotic impregnated polymethyl methacrylate) beads will release their respective active agent into the surrounding tissue over a longer timespan. This ensures a high local concentration of the antibiotic while the systemic concentration remains very low. Therefore critical antibiotics may principally be used for the respective animal species without having a toxic effect (Tobias, Schneider & Besser, 1996; Ethell et al., 2000; Weisman, Olmstead & Kowalski, 2000). Moreover, it is possible to use preparations that might otherwise cause kidney damage such as amikacin, which has a good effect on purulent infections. Other antibiotics that are heat-resistant and thus suited for bone cement beads are gentamicin, defazolin, ceftiofur, ceftazidime and tobramycin. Enrofloxacin and penicillins are damaged by polymerization heat and can thus not be used. If no pathogens can be found in a bacteriological examination of the tissue sample from the abscess capsule, the use of amikacin or cefazolin is recommended (Bennett, 2008).

In order to find the most effective antibiotic for each individual case, it is best to take a small preoperative tissue sample from the abscess capsule for a bacteriological examination. Alternatively, an antibiotic that has already been approved for the respective animal species

is chosen for the production of the beads and the implant may later be replaced depending on the antibiogram. Experimental studies showed that when using AIPMMA beads, a major part of the antibiotic is released within the first 24 hours. Nonetheless, the local antibiotic concentration remains above the minimal inhibitory concentration of the active agent – and thus within therapeutic range – over the course of the next 7 to 30 days. The variation in timespan is down to different choices of antibiotic as well as the dosages used (Tobias, Schneider & Besser, 1996; Ethell et al., 2000; Weisman, Olmstead & Kowalski, 2000).

As yet, ready-to-use AIPMMA implants that are suited for pets are only available in the United States. They come in small, sterile packs and therefore can be inserted directly into the wound area. Since it is relatively easy to produce the antibiotic beads, it is possible to do it by oneself and then make suitable portions and keep them in a cool place (fridge) for a certain amount of time. For this, a definite amount of the heat-resistant antibiotic powder is thoroughly mixed with 20 g of polymethyl methacrylate powder (radiopaque bone cement – Palacos®) in a plastic bowl (see Table 11.1). After that, the liquid polymer (catalyst) is added to harden the substance. Next, as many beads as possible are molded before the mixture starts to polymerize and harden. The smaller (approximately 5 mm) and rounder (large surface) the implants, the better is the antibiotic diffusion.

In order to facilitate modeling of the mass, which hardens rather quickly, the bone cement can be brought into a 20 ml syringe while still fluid and then

Table 11.1 Production of AIPMMA implants (beads).

Active agent	Per 20 g of PMMA
Amikacin	1.25 g
Cefazolin	2 g
Cephalothin	2 g
Ceftiofur	2 g
Clindamycin	2 g
Gentamicin	1 g
Tobramycin	1 g
Metronidazole	1 g combined with 1 g gentamicin (delayed hardening)

PMMA = polymethyl metacrylate.
Data from Ramos, Howard & Pleasant, 2003.

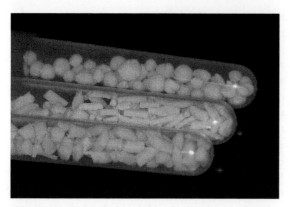

Figure 11.23 Sterile AIPMMA implants of various sizes. They can be stored in the fridge for approximately 4 months without losing their effect.

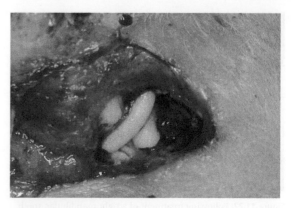

Figure 11.24 Ventral view of the excised mandibular abscess in a two-year-old rabbit, 1 week after insertion of multiple AIPMMA implants: open wound treatment including packing of the abscess area.

emptied on to a sterile, smooth surface (e.g. foil) or sterile cloth as a narrow band. The soft cement strand is cut into suitable pieces with a scalpel and the pieces can be molded into beads or left to remain as small rods (as soon as polymerization has begun). The beads containing antibiotic can be freshly produced intraoperatively, or in advance, and stored in suitable portions (gas sterilization or storage in sterile glass tubes in the fridge) (Figure 11.23). After an abscess excision, the wound cavity is filled with as many beads as possible (Klaus & Bennett, 1999). The smaller the beads the more of them can be implanted, and the larger is the cement surface that releases the antibiotic (Figure 11.24).

Since the cement beads are not ultimately resorbed, they should be removed as soon as the local antibiotic concentration falls below the minimal inhibitory concentration, in other words after approximately three to four weeks, otherwise the implants can be a new center of infection, especially if the antibiotic that was used was not effective. In order to avoid further surgery for implant removal, a risk can be taken to leave the antibiotic beads in situ in certain cases (Figure 11.25). If they had been inserted into the bone in largely sterile conditions, they are biologically inert and in principle should not cause a foreign-body reaction (Bennett, 1999). Long-term monitoring of some patients have shown that they may reside in the tissue without causing any irritation several months after being implanted (Figures 11.26 and 11.27). Any decision about a removal should always depend on the location and extent of the abscess, the local soft tissue and the general condition of

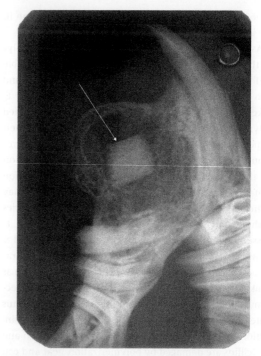

Figure 11.25 Situation 3 months after treatment of a right mandibular abscess in a six-year-old rabbit (mandible, slightly oblique intraoral view) including extraction of the incisor and the first cheek tooth (P3). The AIPMMA implant inserted into the excised abscess area is inert (white arrow).

the patient (suitability for anesthesia). In maxillary abscesses involving the nasal cavity, removal of the AIPMMA beads is strongly recommended due to the increased risk of secondary infections.

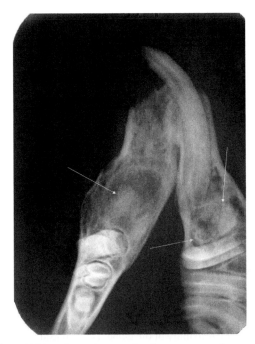

Figure 11.26 Radiograph 6 months after treatment of a bilateral abscess of the lower jaw in a five-year-old rabbit (mandible, slightly oblique intraoral view) including extraction of the incisor and the first cheek tooth (P3) on the right as well as the first left cheek tooth. The bilateral AIPMMA implant is not causing any problems (white arrows). There is a medial dentinoid formation on the left (yellow arrow). It is not currently cause for concern as there is no indication of periodontal lysis, so does not need to be extracted. There is an indication for regular follow-up checks.

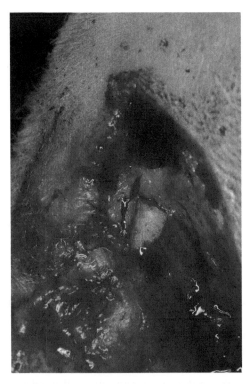

Figure 11.27 Situation 5 weeks after treatment of an abscess of the lower jaw in a rabbit with an AIPMMA implant: visualization of the abscess area from ventrally in order to remove the dentinoid, including exposure of the antibiotic-containing bone cement. The implant has been incorporated into the tissue and is inert.

Antibiotic beads are sometimes recommended in the first instance for the treatment of jaw abscesses in rabbits. The rate of success is reported to be 80–90% (Bennett, 1999). The crucial thing about that method of treatment is that the beads can only be effective locally if the abscess has actually been radically excised and any nonvital or infected bone tissue and soft tissue has been removed. In addition, all infected teeth that have been part of the cause need to be extracted, and the resulting connection to the oral cavity needs to be closed by means of an intraoral mucosal suture. The implants can only be inserted directly into the wound area once all the surgical measures are complete, after which the site is then closed by a skin suture.

Immediate placement of the beads into the freshly excised abscess area has – according to the author's experience – not proven itself as there have been many long-term abscess recurrences (X-ray follow-ups), or wound healing has not been compromised, involving further surgery with removal or replacement of the implant. Moreover, there have hardly been any recent publications on the use of antibiotic beads in pets that have been convincing because they lacked long-term radiographic monitoring. This is not to say that there may not be sustained therapeutical success if the right approach is chosen. According to the author's experience, however, long-term results were much better if AIPMMA implants were not inserted into the abscess area immediately intra- (or actually post-)operatively, but at a later stage when the wound area was relatively clean and no longer required regular debridements. The surgical site should have at least partially healthy granulation tissue that is well-vascularized and bleeds easily during manipulation (Figure 11.17g). There should also not be any remaining connection to the oral cavity. When the antibiotic materials are used at this stage of wound healing, which is highly variable individually and dependent on the general condition of the patient, they will effectively prevent microabscessations and thus recurrences, and will allow healing without complications (Figures 11.25 to 11.27).

As an alternative to the AIPMMA beads, synthetic, bioactive ceramic material (BioGlass®) can be placed into the excised abscess cavity or used to completely fill up the existing osseous defect in the alveolus. After that the wound area is closed. Those ceramic beads already have an antibacterial effect per se, and they are also supposed to stimulate bone and wound healing (Crossley & Aiken, 2004). This bone replacement material is osteoconductive and serves as a guiding frame for the migration of osteoblasts. Just like the bone cement beads, these ceramic ones can also be mixed with an antibiotic that is slowly released locally (Kwanabe, Okada & Matsusue, 1998; Stoor, Soderling & Salonen, 1998; Bellantone, Coleman & Hench, 2000). Long-term effective benzathine penicillin G in powder form should also be usable.

In humans, dogs and cats, bioactive ceramics are primarily used for the treatment of periodontal bone defects as they promote bone regeneration. The material is placed in the cleaned area of the perialveolar bone loss and is then covered with mucosa if possible (Au et al., 2008). Another possible use is the filling of an empty alveolus after tooth extraction as this may induce bone infill (DeForge, 1997). The material is then slowly incorporated into the newly formed bone.

Another possibility to get complete healing of surgically treated abscesses is an implantation of gentamicin-soaked, bovine collagen fiber plates (Sulmycin Implant®) that are available commercially. They can be cut out according to the size of the wound cavity and inserted directly into the abscess area prior to closure of the wound. The carrier substance is dissolved completely. Leukase® N cones can also be used. They contain framycetin sulfate with admixed Lidocaine-HCl. The use of these materials is only indicated if compatible with the antibiogram results.

11.2 Retrobulbar abscesses

11.2.1 Pathogenesis and diagnosis
Rabbits
In an advanced stage of malocclusion, the last four upper cheek teeth (P4–M3) grow – getting continuously longer and at the same time curving concavely

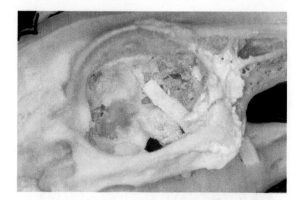

Figure 11.28 Retrobulbar abscess in a three-year-old rabbit (specimen, right orbital area): intraorbitally exposed, retrogradely severely elongated upper cheek tooth (M1).

outwards – further and further into the retroorbital area. This can be clearly seen on radiographs of the head in a laterolateral view, looking at the dorsal reference line. Eventually their vulnerable apices are exposed in immediate proximity of the globe. This can lead to painful local irritations or diffuse discomfort during mastication. Depending on the overall situation concerning pathology of the dentition, individual, intraorbitally exposed cheek teeth may become particularly long and simultaneously develop grotesque malformations (Figure 11.28). They can then be clearly seen, especially on radiographs of the skull in a dorsoventral view, appearing as arc-shaped tooth bodies that protrude far into the orbital cavity (Figure 11.29a).

If the intraosseous tooth changes described above, which may remain clinically nonapparent for a long time despite their extent, are accompanied by an apical or periodontal infection, typical retrobulbar abscesses start to develop (Figure 11.29b to d). The infection in the area of the orbit spreads from the infected apex to the adjacent, retrobulbar soft tissue and the lacrimal glands that are located intraorbitally. The intraorbital or retrobulbar swelling pushes the eyeball out of its orbit, with a prolapse of the nictitating membrane. There is now insufficient closure of the eyelids and a horizontal exposure keratitis develops (see Figure 4.6 in Chapter 4). Depending on the extent of bulb protrusion, an anterior uveitis may follow within a few days, which eventually leads to a panophthalmia or ptysis bulbi. The animals wipe their eyes with their paws due to pain and discomfort, further worsening the local and inflammatory changes. Particularly if a unilateral exophthalmos is present, a

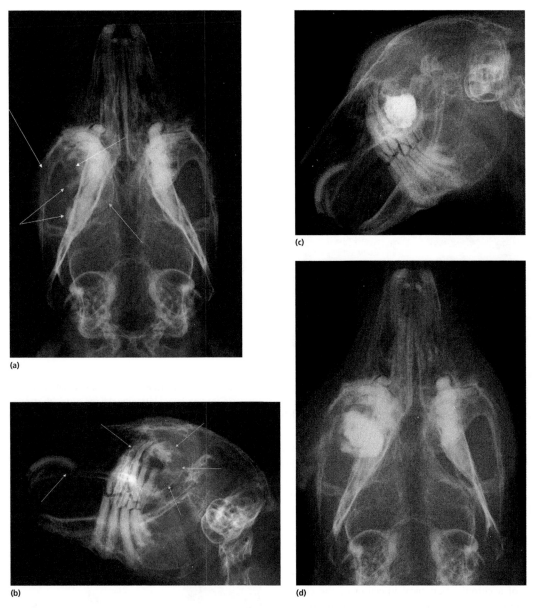

(a)

(b)

(c)

(d)

Figure 11.29 Left-sided, retrobulbar abscess in a two-year-old rabbit. (a) Dorsoventral view: clearly visible, retrogradely displaced dental tissue in the area of the left orbit (yellow arrows) and osteolysis of the zygomatic process as well as the facial tuberosity (white arrows). A crescent-shaped, cystic, bony structure is visible medially from the orbital area (turquoise arrow). (b) Laterolateral view: incisor malocclusion; unilateral, ventral protrusion of the palatal plate (white arrow) and bullous structure in the orbital area (yellow arrows). The third upper cheek tooth (P4) is curved concavely distally, tracing the rostral margin of the bone cyst. Similar deformation of the second maxillary cheek tooth rostrally clinging to the other (P3; turquoise arrow). The last three upper cheek teeth on that side cannot be seen (superimposition of the contralateral jaw); structural change and retrograde elongation of all mandibular cheek teeth and stepped occlusal plane. (c) Laterolateral view: the cherry-sized abscess cavity is largely filled with a contrast agent. (d) Ventrodorsal view, retrobulbar abscess (left); cherry-sized abscess cavity filled up with a contrast agent.

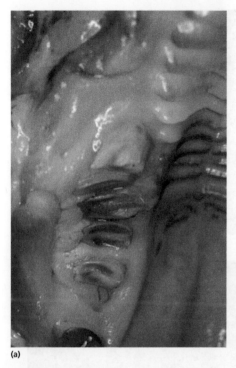
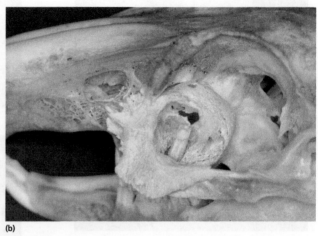

(a) (b)

Figure 11.30 Left-sided retrobulbar abscess in a five-year-old rabbit. (a) Specimen, right maxillary row of cheek teeth: mild malocclusion, slight loosening of the third cheek tooth (P4), no discharge of pus from the alveolus and unphysiological discoloration of the occlusal surfaces of all cheek teeth due to insufficient tooth wear. (b) Specimen: intraorbital bone cyst with strong, proliferative remodeling of the facial tuberosity and retrogradely marked elongated third upper cheek tooth (P4) located near the center of the remodeling.

primary problem concerning the cheek teeth should always be considered and then be excluded or confirmed by means of adequate radiographs. Differential diagnosis could also suggest a primary, purulent suppuration of the lacrimal glands after a hematogenous *Pasteurella* infection or – rather rarely – a retrobulbar neoplasia or an intraorbital hemorrhage.

Unless the eyeball is pushed out of the orbit over the course of a chronic, periapical infection of the cheek teeth (it mostly affects several teeth), there will often be hardly any clinical symptoms even though extensive intraorbital remodeling is taking place (Figure 11.30a and b). Hence many retrobulbar abscessations go completely undetected for a long time. The infected molars, which have exposed alveolar bullae, may again be covered with a bone lamella during the further course of the infection. That cover is equivalent to a new, continuously ossifying, periapical abscess capsule, or the normal, cortical cover of the alveolar bullae, which continues to be displaced further and further into the eye

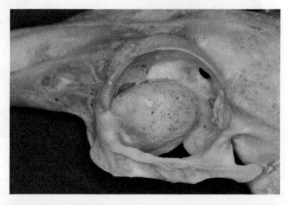

Figure 11.31 Unilateral exophthalmos in a two-year-old rabbit (specimen, left orbital area): solid, retrobulbar bone cyst due to a tooth-associated, apical abscess of three upper tooth (P4–M2), which completely encapsulated toward the orbit.

socket over the course of the chronic infection (Figure 11.31). Such intraorbital bone cysts can be easily verified by means of radiographs of the head in four planes, as can the cheek teeth causing the retrobulbar suppuration, which are often also markedly deformed (Figure 11.29a to d).

Guinea pigs, chinchillas and degus

Retrobulbar abscesses are rather rare in chinchillas and degus. It is easily understood in degus as these animals very rarely suffer from a predisposing retrograde displacement of the apices of the upper cheek teeth (M2/M3). If any, then the last maxillary molar (M3) is affected whose elongated, caudally convexly curved tooth structure penetrates the orbit near the optic canal (see Figure 10.25 in Chapter 10).

It is generally unclear, however, just why retrobulbar infections hardly play a part in chinchillas even though their maxillary molars exhibit the most severe apical changes. When looking at specimens, there is a surprisingly high extent of retrograde tooth elongation and deformation, especially involving the last two molars (M2/M3). Due to the progressive destruction of the lateral alveolar wall, their apical – and often also their middle – section of tooth is often completely and extensively exposed in the orbit (see Figure 10.30a in Chapter 10). However, larger apical abscesses in that area are rather rare.

By contrast, retrobulbar abscesses are very common in guinea pigs. Here, too, the cause is always a pronounced retrograde displacement and infection of the apices of the last two maxillary cheek teeth (M2/ M3) whose occlusal surfaces mostly show typical pathological changes (see Figure 10.34a and b in Chapter 10). Many affected guinea pigs exhibited a preliminary, subtle, uni- or bilateral slight protrusion of the eye that had already occurred several weeks to months prior to the sudden manifestation of the retrobulbar abscess. Pronounced retrobulbar elongations of the maxillary molars that passively push the eye out of the orbit are responsible for those protrusions of the eyeball (see Figure 4.7 in Chapter 4). Despite the irritation or even displacement of the adjacent maxillary nerve, many animals do not exhibit many visible problems in feed intake. Early stages of the process can be identified relatively easily by means of the reference lines.

11.2.2 Therapy
Rabbits

In the case of an intraorbital bone cyst, the accumulation of pus that is below will not become apparent before the bony wall is opened or partially removed with a sharp instrument (Figure 11.31). It is only then that the whole extent of the pathological bone and tooth changes can be accurately evaluated. It is not uncommon that all four cheek teeth (P4–M3) that are exposed intraorbitally need to be extracted during the subsequent, radical excision of the abscess area. If there is also a secondary eye problem caused by the bulb protrusion, the tooth extraction is best achieved via a dorsal access. For this, enucleation should proceed resection of the abscess capsule where possible. That is followed by extraction of the affected cheek teeth. This procedure will allow follow-up aftercare of the wound, which is relatively large and has a wide connection with the oral cavity (healing by secondary intention).

In rabbits with retrobulbar, odontogenic abscesses (P3–M3), it must be decided on an individual basis whether the eye can be preserved or has to be removed in the context of a radical abscess excision. Since most patients suffer from a secondary, irreversible panophthalmia, there is an indication for a enucleation in the majority of cases. This will facilitate the necessary tooth extraction as well as the consequent aftercare through the empty eye socket.

However, if the eye is intact and the periapical jaw changes have not advanced too far (primarily changes of individual teeth), an intraoral cheek tooth extraction without removal of the eye can be attempted. That approach, however, involves a significantly higher long-term rate of complications as intraorbital infections may easily spread to neighboring teeth in the absence of open wound treatment. This is due to the fact that the maxillary jawbone is mostly perforated and extremely thin in the area of the alveolar bullae. The retrobulbar abscess area can be opened ventrally following extraction via the empty alveolus and curetted out as much as possible in order to avoid any further spread of the infection under endoscopic control (Martinez-Jimenez, 2007). Depending on the extent of pathological changes, the infection can heal with concurrent local and systemic antibiotic treatment. A disadvantage of that method is the rather poor intraoperative view of the abscess area (intraoperative bleeding, pus), which means that the full extent of the retrobulbar process (infection) may often not be correctly evaluated. If the abscess capsule is insufficiently resected, recurrences will need treatment, particularly in the long term.

Alternatively, a lateral approach can be chosen for intraorbital abscesses without secondary ocular changes.

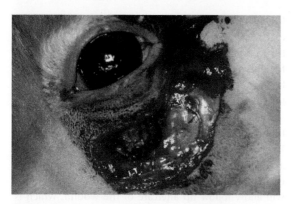

Figure 11.32 Left-sided retrobulbar abscess in a two-year-old rabbit, intraoperative view following resection of the zygomatic process: exposure of the infraorbital abscess area while preserving the eyeball.

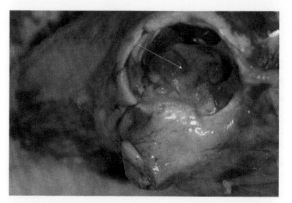

Figure 11.33 Left-sided retrobulbar abscess in a four-year-old rabbit (postmortem specimen): swelling double the size of a cherry in the area of the facial tuberosity as well as the zygomatic process, due to a pronounced retrograde elongation and apical infection of the second to fourth left upper cheek tooth (P3–M1), fibrotic abscess capsule in the rostroventral orbit area (white arrow).

Here, the affected tooth apices are exposed by a lateral approach following resection of the zygomatic process (with or without a resection of the facial tuberosity – depending on the situation). The abscess treatment includes extractions of teeth (P4–M3) while preserving the eye as well as the infraorbital lacrimal gland (Figure 11.32).

However, if there is an indication for enucleation, the whole extent of retrobulbar changes is often not recognized until the eye has been removed. In many cases a single, grotesquely malformed tooth can be clearly seen after this. The tooth may not be immediately visible in the pus-filled orbit or it is hidden underneath a solid, fibrotic abscess capsule that is usually located in the rostroventral orbital area (Figure 11.33). Without additional radiographic examination the abscess capsule may well be mistaken for a normal soft tissue structure and thus be overlooked. It is not until the capsule is opened that the pathologically altered tooth apices become apparent (Figure 11.34).

Subsequent to the eye removal and the retrograde tooth extraction, a radical abscess excision is performed. After the wound area has been thoroughly cleaned, the connection with the oral cavity is closed with monofilament suture material (6/0), if several teeth had been extracted and a suture is principally possible. If only a single molar was extracted, an intraoral suture is not needed and the empty tooth socket is filled with gauze almost up to the gum line. The entire orbital cavity is then packed with moist iodoform gauze (or gauze that is soaked in a mixture of granulated sugar

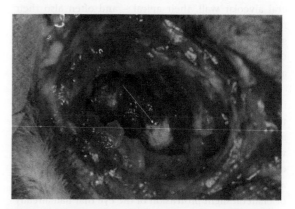

Figure 11.34 Right-sided retrobulbar abscess in a three-year-old rabbit, intraoperative situation, right orbit after removal of the eye: dental tissue is visible in the rostroventral area of the empty eye socket; it is the retrogradely displaced apex of the third upper cheek tooth (P4; white arrow).

and FURACIN®-SOL ointment) before being temporarily closed with a skin suture.

The first drainage replacement is made on the third postoperative day. For this, the suture is largely or completely reopened. Following a careful wound debridement including curettage and flushing of the alveolar and orbital area, the tooth socket and the eye cavity are again packed with gauze; the drainage is then replaced at regular time intervals (Figure 11.35). If all goes well during the healing process, the abscess area will granulate

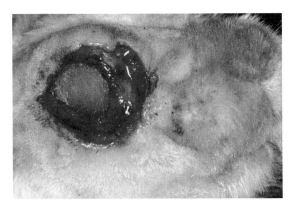

Figure 11.35 Tooth-associated, retrobulbar abscess in a four-year-old rabbit, situation 6 days after enucleation and cheek tooth extraction: The alveolus and the orbit are packed with moist gauze, open wound management is performed.

and close from deep within the defect in approximately three to four weeks. However, if there is a delay in the healing of the oral mucosa, the wound needs to be kept open superficially for as long as it takes the defect to slowly close from within.

Guinea pigs, chinchillas and degus

After specific radiographic examinations (isolated view of the upper molars as described by Böhmer or intraoral images), the primarily infected molar(s) needs to be extracted (Figures 11.36 and 11.37). For this, enucleation needs to be performed even if the eye is unchanged except for a slight bulb protrusion. Contrary to rabbits in which a resection of the zygomatic process can be performed to save the eye, there is hardly an alternative to this in guinea pigs due to the skull anatomy. The apices of the cheek teeth are located too far medially and, the tooth socket, which is markedly curved intraosseously, cannot be kept sufficiently clean postoperatively via a purely intraoral access, not even with repeated debridement and monitoring under general anesthesia. The abscess, which is mostly locally confined primarily (M2 or M3), will spread unhindered in most cases – it is a slow process that may last months. The infection will not only spread to the retroorbital area of soft tissue (lacrimal glands, fat tissue, eye muscles) and the nearby maxillary bone but will also usually involve the adjacent cheek tooth. Since an extraction of two molars (M2/M3), which is now necessary, will create an enormously large connection with the oral cavity, healing of the wound area without any complications will hardly be possible.

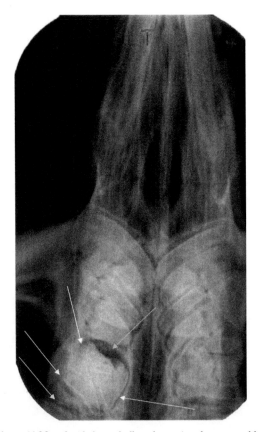

Figure 11.36 Left-sided retrobulbar abscess in a four-year-old guinea pig (intraoral view of the maxilla): pathological occlusal surface of the third left upper molar (M2; intraoral finding), pathologically shaped apical area as well as structurally altered and thickened tooth body of the third left upper molar (M2; white arrows), clearly visible periodontal radiolucency in the area of the mesial tooth surface indicating a periodontitis (turquoise arrow) and less visible change in the distolateral area of the tooth socket (yellow arrow).

In guinea pigs, the situation is aggravated by the fact that the overall robustness of the animals is not as high as that of rabbits, which can be anesthetized once a week for followup aftercare if necessary. Guinea pigs with chronic-purulent infections react more sensitively. They are very demanding anesthetic patients, especially if the source of infection does not resolve and the animals keep refusing to eat by themselves. Hence any surgery that is performed under sedation – such as an intraoral wound flush – should be carefully reconsidered. The better alternative for saving the life of an animal in most cases is the removal of the eye with follow-up aftercare involving an open wound of the

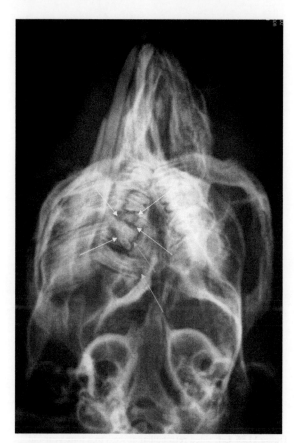

Figure 11.37 Right-sided retrobulbar abscess in a six-year-old guinea pig (isolated view of the maxilla according to Böhmer, slightly oblique view): structural change of the tooth body of the next-to-last right upper cheek tooth (M2; white arrows), which is split longitudinally intraalveolarly, and periapical lysis in its apical intraalveolar area (turquoise arrow), pronounced retrograde elongation of the last right maxillary cheek tooth (M3; yellow arrow) and significant intraalveolar narrowing of the tooth body with a periodontal lysis. There is an indication for the extraction of both molars.

abscess area (Figure 11.38a and b). Even so, wound treatment is always a big challenge as the tooth socket is rather wide and usually takes a very long time to close (Figure 11.39a). Every case needs to be individually considered, based on the general condition of the patient.

After the enucleation, the cheek tooth that has been responsible for the retrobulbar infection can usually be seen well (Figure 11.38a). Subsequent to the retrograde and intraoral mobilization of that tooth, it is extracted either via the open wound or via the oral cavity (see

Figure 10.72a and b in Chapter 10). This is followed by a thorough debridement of the empty alveolus as well as the entire abscess area. Next, the empty alveolus is packed almost up to the gum line with moist gauze that has been soaked in a sugar–FURACIN®-SOL mixture, as is the entire orbital area (Figure 11.39b). The wound is temporarily sutured. The drainage is first replaced after two to three days. Aftercare is the same as described for rabbits above. Should there be insufficient healing despite follow-up care, or should pus keep accumulating deep within the alveolus or the orbit, it is an indication for a radiographic follow-up examination (isolated view of the upper jaw or intraoral image).

11.3 Antibiotic therapy

11.3.1 Herbivorous pets

A day prior to the planned surgery, if possible (if not, then just before the abscess excision and tooth extraction), parenterally administration of a well-tolerated broad spectrum antibiotic, which is suited for the respective species is given (Crossley & Aiken, 2004; Lazarz, 2009, personal communication). This is supposed to restrict a hematogenous spread of bacteria (which is always associated with this kind of invasive surgery) as effectively as possible, by means of achieving good intraoperative serum concentrations of the active agent. Thus, a further spread of the infection and additional damage to other organ systems can be largely prevented. In order to determine the exact bacteria present, a small vital piece of the abscess capsule with the inner coating is sent away for analysis. The pus is mostly sterile and therefore useless. According to the antibiogram, the therapy that has already been started is now continued postoperatively, or antibiosis is changed according to the sensitivity results. Antibacterial treatment should include both aerobic and anaerobic bacteria.

If no bacterial growth is found in the bacteriological examination, a sample of the exudate or pus can be gram-stained in order to be able to choose a suitable antibiotic (Taylor et al., 2008).

Most abscesses in rabbits are polymicrobial infections predominantly caused by anaerobic bacteria (Bennett, 2008; Taylor et al., 2008). The most frequently found bacteria are ones that were also isolated in samples from periodontal diseases in humans (Crossley & Aiken, 2004). For example, a study involving 12 rabbits yielded

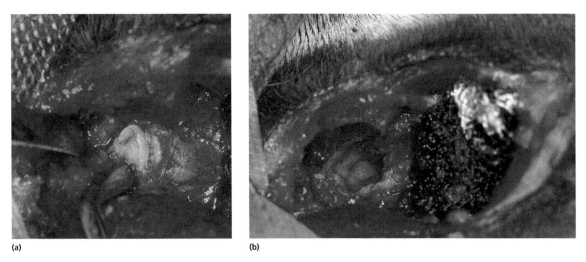

(a)

(b)

Figure 11.38 Retrobulbar abscess in a four-year-old guinea pig. (a) Intraoperative view following enucleation (left): the retrogradely displaced apex of the next-to-last cheek tooth (M2) is exposed intraorbitally. Retrograde mobilization is performed with the aid of a luxator. (b) Following tooth extraction: the empty tooth socket is visible, the dark tissue in the orbital area is gauze-like and resorbable tissue (hemostyptic) covers the stump of the ophthalmic artery (Tabotamp®).

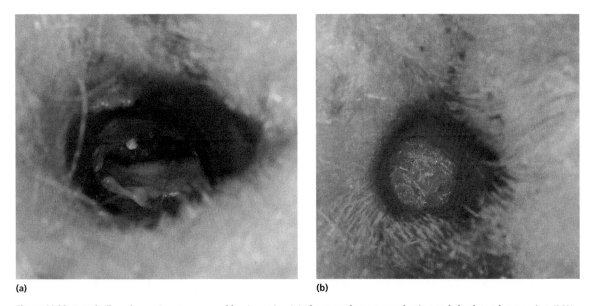

(a)

(b)

Figure 11.39 Retrobulbar abscess in a two-year-old guinea pig. (a) Three weeks post enucleation and cheek tooth extraction (M2). The wound is granulating well; the opening to the oral cavity is just visible (food). (b) Four weeks after enucleation and cheek tooth extraction (M2). The wound area is packed with gauze.

anaerobic, gram-negative bacteria (*Fusobacterium* spp.) and anaerobic, gram-positive, nonsporogenic strains (*Actinomyces* spp.) as well as aerobic, gram-positive cocci (*Streptococcus* spp.) (Tyrrell et al., 2002); 96% of the pathogens were sensitive to penicillins or cefazolin, while 100% of the pyogenic bacteria could be killed off with clindamycin. At least 86% of the bacteria were susceptible to azithromycin and tetracyclines whereas metronidazole were only effective against a mere 54% of the microorganisms. Interestingly, no *Pasteurella* or

Staphylococcus were found. Thus clindamycin, penicillin and cefazolin were shown to be the most suitable antibiotics for the treatment of abscesses. It is just these active agents, however, that may be toxic for rabbits.

Contrary to those studies, other authors found *Pasteurella* in abscesses and also found *Staphylococcus*, *Pseudomonas*, *Bacteroides* spp., *Escherichia coli* and *Proteus* spp. (Chaffee, James & Montali, 1975; Dominguez, Crase & Soave, 1975; Deeb, 1993; Glöckner, 2002; Harcourt-Brown, 2002b, Bennett, 2008, Jenkins, 2008). Even in asymptomatic rabbits, *Pasteurella* bacteria are often a part of the normal intranasal microflora. From there, they may spread to other organ systems when the patient is immunocompromised. There is no detailed information on specific kinds of bacteria in guinea pigs or chinchillas, and there have not been enough of the author's evaluations to sustain a statement.

Thus, both in abscesses and in periodontal disorders, anaerobic bacteria play a part that is not to be underestimated (Crossley & Aiken, 2004; Gorrel & Verhaert, 2006). Hence an additional administration of metronidazole should always be considered. That medication is generally well-tolerated even by small mammals, as long as it is administered in lower dosages (low threshold value) and no longer than two weeks on average (see tables in the Appendix in Chapter 15).

As well as local wound treatment, systemic antibiotic therapy is performed over a limited period of time (approximately 1–3 weeks). Without surgical intervention, however, antibiotics are not effective in abscesses as poor or absent blood flow in the area of a purulent infection does not allow therapeutically effective, local concentrations. The fibrotic abscess capsule isolates the suppurative focus, thus forming an effective barrier. Antibiotics are not used to good effect before a radical wound excision and thus a certain degree of re-vitalization of the infection area. However, they are not a universal remedy, and carry low expectations. In the treatment of jaw abscesses, antibiotics are definitely just one of many components in the context of a complex, mostly prolonged therapy.

It must be borne in mind that, in herbivorous pets, many antibiotics that are recommended especially for a treatment of purulent bone infections in other species – such as lincomycin or clindamycin – must not be administered orally or parenterally, due to known side effects.

Hence no antibiotics should be used that selectively kill off the natural, predominantly gram-positive intestinal bacterial flora, thus promoting a massive increase in pathogenic, gram-negative germs (mainly *Clostridium* spp. and *E. coli*) (Harcourt-Brown, 2002b). Antibiotics administered orally in particular entail that risk, whereas parenteral application usually has a lesser impact on the composition of the intestinal flora. Hence basically all antibiotics that largely or almost entirely have a gram-positive spectrum efficacy, such as penicillins, cephalosporins and lincomycin, are to be avoided. Possible consequences of the wrong choice of antibiotics include an antibiotic-associated enteritis and – in extreme cases – a life-threatening enterotoxemia. Enterotoxins produced fast and in large amounts by the gram-negative bacteria flood the patient and cause damage to vital organs (multiple organ failure).

It is not only the choice of a suitable antibiotic but also species-specifically correct therapeutical dosage that is important as well as the decision about the safest form of application. Penicillins and cephalosporins, for example, usually can easily be administered parenterally in rabbits, whereas oral application can be lethal.

The nephrotoxicity of gentamicin is not a concern in rabbits if it is administered strictly locally (see AIPMMA implants above). As a general rule, clindamycin, lincomycin, azithromycin, amoxicillin, erythromycin, as well as oral ampicillin and penicillins, are dangerous for lagomorphs and rodents, whereas enrofloxacin, chloramphenicol, ciprofloxacin and trimethoprim-sulfamethoxazole combinations are usually well-tolerated when administered orally or systemically, even for longer periods (Harcourt-Brown, 2002b; Donnelly, 2004). In principle, the chosen antibiotic must permeate the tissue well and attain therapeutic concentrations in the infected tissue.

For example, trimethoprim–sulfonamide preparations are often not effective against the pyogenic bacteria that

> Generally, antimicrobial medication must be used very carefully in rabbits, guinea pigs, chinchillas and degus as the sensitive, species-specific balance of microorganisms in the caecum of the animals must not be disturbed by any means.

> Penicillins and cephalosporins must not be used in rodents by any means!

usually occur in rabbits as they are inactivated by the presence of purulent secretions (Harcourt-Brown, 2002b). More favorable are chloramphenicol or cephalexin (Tyrrell et al., 2002; Harcourt-Brown, 2002b). Chloramphenicol has a good effect on aerobic bacteria and some effect on anaerobic ones, and it is a good choice in purulent infections as it is not substantially impaired by pus. Contrary to many reports, the broad spectrum antibiotic enrofloxacin, which can be administered parenterally or orally, has also proven itself in everyday use (Harcourt-Brown, 2002b; author's experience). It does not exhibit any unwanted side effects even when used for longer periods, neither in rabbits nor in other pets. If administered at the correct dosage, high concentrations of the active ingredient are attained in various organ systems (lungs, liver, kidney, skin, bone and lymphatic tissue). However, it appears not to be effective in rabbits with a chronic *Pasteurella* infection of the nasal cavity, the inner ear or the trachea (Mähler et al., 1995). In such cases, cephalosporins should preferentially be used, but only parenterally because oral application is dangerous for rabbits (Harcourt-Brown, 2002b).

The penicillins and azithromycin are recommended particularly for chronic infections. Both of them, however, can only be used in rabbits, and penicillins can only be administered parenterally. Although azithromycin can have a good effect in rabbits, it remains a risky choice as it may cause gastrointestinal problems when administered orally. In summary, there is no one antibiotic of choice for jaw abscesses. However, a chance for a specific therapy will be somewhat less of a problem if the most effective antibiotics are preferentially applied locally (see AIPMMA implants above). The implant, however, must not come in contact with the oral mucosa or the saliva.

In rabbits, there have also been various reports of good long-term results in the case where benzathine penicillin G was used in combination with procaine penicillin G (depot preparation). Animals with a body weight of less than 2.5 kg are given 75 000 IE/animal Bicillin® s.c. every 48 hours (Crossley & Aiken, 2004; Rosenfield, 2009). If the preparation is used in combination with a radical abscess excision and tooth extraction, it can provide very effective support in healing jaw abscesses and preventing recurrences. Alternatively, a mixture of penicillin and streptomycin can also be given (Veracin comp®, 0.1 ml/kg BW s.c.) (Lazarz, 2009).

If surgical treatment of abscesses has become impossible due to advanced changes or extensive infiltrative spread, or if an animal's owner does not want a surgical treatment, penicillins or oxytetracyclines can be used for a long-term "suppression" of the infection. They are able to slow down the further spread of the infection, but they are not able to cure it (Harcourt-Brown, 2002b). When combined with potent analgesics, they may help to improve the patient's quality of life in the short term.

11.3.2 Omnivorous rodents

When choosing a suitable antibiotic for omnivorous rodents, it must be taken into account that both streptomycin and procaine penicillin are toxic for mice and that nitrofurantoin causes neuropathological lesions in rats. Gerbils are also sensitive to streptomycin. Hamsters and guinea pigs even develop life-threatening enterotoxemias after being administered penicillin, erythromycin or lincomycin (Donnelly, 2004).

Since some patients are very small, the practical execution of an antibiotic therapy can also be very difficult, particularly over longer periods. Prior to oral application, even pediatric medication formulations need to be diluted and appropriately prepared for the animal, e.g. with lactulose, syrup or yogurt (Donnelly, 2004). Naturally, a systemic application is easier, although the amounts needed will often be so small that they can hardly be drawn up and administered (Donnelly, 2004). For more detailed information, see the tables in the Appendix in Chapter 15.

11.4 Local wound treatment

During abscess treatment and subsequent wound management, choosing a suitable wound dressing is not as crucial as thoroughly getting rid of the cause (tooth extraction) as well as consequently carrying out wound debridement. Nonetheless, some preparations have proven to be particularly successful here. They include sugar and honey, which is used in human medicine in the form of sterile wound sugar (Debrisorb®) or medical honey (Medihoney®) (Eibl-Eibesfeldt & Kessler, 1997). Both substances have a strong hygroscopic and therefore antioedematous effect. At the same time, they cause infected wounds to become almost sterile as both sugar and honey have been shown to inhibit bacterial growth. Experimental studies with honey found an effect on 200 different isolates, with the most common pus bacteria and antibiotic-resistant bacteria ("problematic pathogens") among them (Molan, 1999).

The antibacterial effect of honey can be attributed to its high sugar content as well as its low pH value. However, other substances in honey, some of which are unknown, are supposed to have an additional bacteriostatic effect. Basically (and just like in the sugar mixture that is used locally), it is the high osmolarity that inhibits bacterial growth, simply by depriving the bacteria of water (Molan, 1999; Dangl, 2009). Alternatively, gauze soaked in dextrose can also be used for local wound tamponades – the mechanism of action is principally identical (Gorrel & Verhaert, 2006).

In an antibacterial environment of honey or sugar, a fast and highly effective autolytic debridement of dirty wounds occurs. Due to their strong osmotic effect, both substances will sustain a moist wound environment by extracting lymph and blood plasma from the wound area. That fluid outflow will provide deep-cleansing of the wound. The osmotic fluid film on the tissue surface also prevents an adhesion of the sensitive granulation tissue to the drain, thereby facilitating pain-free drainage replacements. Moreover, honey has an anti-inflammatory effect and promotes granulation by keeping the wound moist. It also stimulates angiogenesis (as sugar is supposed to), whereby new capillaries are quickly formed that can transport oxygen and nutrients needed for healing into the wound area.

In everyday practice, normal honey or granulated sugar can be used instead of the expensive medical preparations (fresh package). A suitable ointment may be mixed to the latter and the mixture stored in the fridge in a closed container for a while. As an alternative to FURACIN®-SOL ointment, which has a bacteriostatic and anti-inflammatory effect, a variety of other local therapeutics can be used that might have proven themselves individually and have a similar effect, e.g. propolis. As a general rule, only relatively small amounts of the sugar–ointment mixture are applied as the sugar becomes less viscous at body temperature and in association with the normal wound secretion. This may lead to a premature loss of drainage or the surrounding fur may become coated with the sugar–ointment. The sweet taste of the wound liquid encourages animal grooming.

The flushing liquid used during regular wound debridements should generally be of body temperature, should not cause any local irritations and be sterile as well as nonresorbable. If those criteria are met, specialist retailers offer a variety of wound antiseptics that currently represent the drugs of choice for wound flushings. They include octenidin (Octenisept®), polyhexanide (Lavanid®) or povidone–iodine; alternatives can be special dye solutions such as Rivanol®. In principle, all preparations can also be used in pets. The effect of povidone–iodine mixtures, however, is decreased in the presence of blood, pus or exudates (so-called protein error). Moreover, there is an inhibitory effect on wound healing if they are used for longer periods of time (Probst & Vasel-Biergans, 2004).

11.5 Wound healing complications

If wound healing becomes slower for no apparent reason, or if smaller abscessations occur again (pus accumulations in the depth or in smaller niches of soft tissue or bone), another radiographic examination of the abscess area is performed. Since anesthesia is necessary for many isolated views of such problem areas (mostly intraoral views), the procedure should be planned so as to allow a possible follow-up surgery to be performed immediately following radiographic examination. Frequent findings that may cause a retardation or complication of previously inconspicuous wound healing include:
- Nonvital bone sequestra
- Regrown dentinoids
- Impacted foreign bodies from the oral cavity (hay)
- Spread of the infection to adjacent teeth or soft tissue
- Insufficient primary care resulting in renewed abscess formation in nonaccessible niches

Experience has shown that if the cause is removed, the wounds heal up quickly and usually without complications.

11.6 Prognosis

Even with the best efforts, an abscess treatment may sometimes turn out to be a failure. The prognosis depends primarily on the extent of the pathological changes and the general conditions of the patient. However, the accuracy of primary diagnosis, the experience of the practitioner, the specific antibiotic therapy and the chosen treatment method also play a part that is not to be underestimated. Radical surgical treatment of the abscess and a concomitant local and systemic therapy merely represent a precondition for healing. However, the abscesses are often too advanced to be able to stop the osteomyelitis, or the chronic disease has weakened the animal to a degree where it will not survive surgery in the long term despite appropriate therapy. The animal's owner will have to be prepared to carry some of that risk (after having been informed preoperatively). A therapeutical attempt will not be sensible if the owner is not prepared to contribute.

Furthermore, most abscesses are complications that develop from an acquired malocclusion and may not be influenced much, even with a successful therapy of the center of infection. Hence prognoses also depend on those primary changes of the dentition and the possibilities of treating them. When it comes to correct assessments of the long-term prognosis, it must be borne in mind that any tooth extraction can have long-term effects on the antagonist(s) or the overall occlusion. Should it even be necessary to extract several cheek teeth, it is a drastic interference with the normal physiology of the dentition. Lifelong, regular monitoring of the patient is indicated in any case. In that sense, complete cure is rarely achieved. There have always been patients, however, that remained free of complaints for the rest of their lives after an abscess treatment because the antagonists of the teeth that were removed usually cease to grow after about three to four months, meaning that regular tooth trimming had become unnecessary.

Prognoses for retrobulbar abscesses are mostly less favorable. Depending on the extent of the retrobulbar changes of soft tissue and bones as well as the number of cheek teeth to be extracted, they can be good, very cautious or unfavorable. Any chance of long-term healing

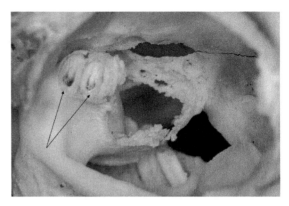

Figure 11.40 Left-sided retrobulbar abscess in an eight-year-old rabbit (specimen, left orbit): osteolysis of the alveolar bulla in the area of the last two missing cheek teeth (M2/M3) with a large communication with the oral cavity. There is an indication for an extraction of the two cheek teeth located mesially (P4/M1; black arrows).

depends primarily on the size of the communication with the oral cavity after radical abscess excision. In many cases all upper cheek teeth need to be removed as the first two premolars (P2/P3), whose apices are located in the area of the lacrimal bone, also exhibit periodontal abscesses. If the bone defects are too extensive, euthanasia of the patient may be indicated (Figure 11.40).

In summary, jaw abscesses should only be treated if the planned therapy has a certain chance of success. If there are findings that have advanced too far, or if patients are too weak, euthanasia of the patient may need to be chosen over an attempt at therapy, for reasons of animal welfare. This is why a discussion of mandibulectomy in rabbits was intentionally omitted here in the context of abscess therapy. While that approach may well be indicated and could be performed in some cases, it must be regarded as being too much of a strain on the animal in the long term.

CHAPTER 12

Periodontal Diseases and Caries

12.1 Periodontal diseases

Periodontal diseases are disorders of the periodontal ligament, in other words the entire tooth socket (desmodontium). There are very many causes of periodontal disorders. As in humans, the diet, the self-cleaning capacity of the dentition, the composition of the saliva, specific bacteria and presumably also the immune system play important roles (Wiggs & Lobprise, 1995b).

12.1.1 Lagomorph and herbivorous Rodents

Inflammatory changes of the periodontium (gingivitis and periodontitis) do indeed occur in herbivorous pets with hypsodont cheek teeth. *In practice* however, they tend to be missed or dismissed (Wiggs & Lobprise, 1995b). This leads to pathological changes often going undetected, and any deterioration of findings that progresses unhindered will sometimes lead to inexplicable, treatment-resistant, recurring problems related to the dentition and mastication (Crossley & Aiken, 2004).

> Disorders of the periodontium can have a crucial influence on the origin and further course of malocclusions.

Especially in chinchillas, for example, primarily periodontal inflammation leads to the typical intraalveolar tooth resorptions. If periodontal diseases responsible for this could be identified in their early stages and treated accordingly, infections with a periodontal origin as well as the concomitant destruction of the periodontal ligament and the tooth substance could presumably be prevented (Figure 12.1). Hence this topic should be dealt with more intensity.

Etiology and pathogenesis

Periodontal diseases rarely affect wild lagomorphs or rodents. They also occur very rarely in herbivorous rodents with a normal occlusion that are fed in a species-appropriate way (mainly grass, herbs and hay), because the intraoral clinical crown of their cheek teeth is relatively short, meaning there really is not enough tooth substance for the attachment of plaque (Crossley & Aiken, 2004). Any reasonable amount of plaque will not adhere to the gingival margin of the tooth as the hypselodont teeth continue to grow. Most importantly, a correct position and structure of the molars ensures that the so-called self-cleaning of the dentition is working. That self-cleaning is particularly important here as hypselodont teeth physiologically have a relatively wide periodontal ligament space, which, in combination with the relatively "loose" structure of the desmodontium promotes an impaction of food and hairs (Figure 12.2).

It is a different situation if a malocclusion is present. Self-cleaning of the dentition is severely hampered by abnormal tooth growth and wear, as well as curving, deformation, rotation or displacement of individual teeth (see Figure 10.28 in Chapter 10). Any abnormal stress and secondary curvature of a tooth will lead to an excessive, asymmetric strain on the periodontium within a very short time. Some of the periodontal fibers will be torn, and as well as a hemorrhage, there will also be an infiltration of leukocytes (Van der Velden, 1980). Thus it is the start of a local inflammation of the periodontium. As a result of various changes of the teeth

Dentistry in Rabbits and Rodents, First Edition. Estella Böhmer.
© 2015 John Wiley & Sons, Ltd. Published 2015 by John Wiley & Sons, Ltd.

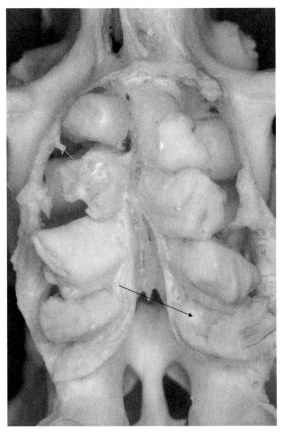

Figure 12.1 Advanced malocclusion in a six-year-old chinchilla (maxilla specimen) with a severe osteolytic expansion of all tooth sockets, complete loss of the lamina dura – and thus the lateral as well as the mutual support of teeth – all cheek teeth are severely altered structurally and curved intraalveolarly concavely buccally, multiple tooth rotations (altered pattern of the chewing surface), osteoclastic resorptions on the palatal surface of the last left molar (M3; black arrow) as well as on the occlusal surface of the second right cheek tooth (turquoise arrow).

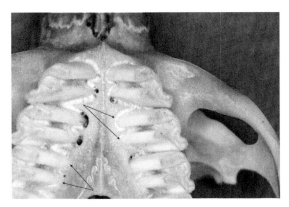

Figure 12.2 Normal occlusion in a two-year-old guinea pig (maxilla specimen) with a normal periodontium of the second left cheek tooth (M1; black arrows) and the third right cheek tooth (M2; black arrows). The rest of the teeth exhibit partial pathological enlargement of the periodontium, with some of the periodontal fibers in the tooth socket of the first right premolar (P4) clearly recognizable.

and the alveolar bone, abnormal peri- and interdental tooth gaps form in which plaque persists and food particles or hairs may become impacted (Crossley, 2003a) (Figure 12.1).

Even in case of a normal occlusion, unsuitable feeding that is not species-appropriate may lead to plaque accumulation, particularly on the crown near the gingiva and continues to accumulate and grows continuously thicker (Wiggs & Lobprise, 1995b; Crossley & Aiken, 2004). In addition, high-carb food will promote the growth of oral pathogenic bacteria (Crossley, 2003a).

These bacteria are always present in lower numbers in the oral cavity. If they proliferate due to thick plaque and/or an improper diet, it may lead to pathological changes of the periodontium in lagomorphs and also in herbivorous rodents.

As described above, a primary formation of plaque is due to a disturbance in the self-cleaning of the dentition, resulting from a cheek tooth malocclusion or improper food high in starch. Softer, sticky plaque represents a breeding ground consisting of glycoproteins from saliva and additional inorganic material from the food as well as bacteria (Baker & Easley, 2003). Whenever bacterial tooth plaque remains attached for longer periods or accumulates to form thicker and thicker layers, free radicals as well as other acidic metabolites and endotoxins are released as a result of bacterial degradation processes; those substances cause irritation to the gingiva and the gingival sulcus. The result is gingivitis, which clinically presents as swollen, hyperemic gingiva. The dominant bacteria in the supragingival areas of inflammation are mainly aerobic species, whereas anaerobic bacteria proliferate in the gingival sulcus (subgingivally) (Baker & Easley, 2003).

Periodontal diseases are primarily predisposed by a generalized, progressive loss of the lamina dura, causing a diffuse dilation of the periodontal space. Several or all teeth can be affected. The teeth are tilted in a typical fashion – buccally in the upper jaw and lingually in the

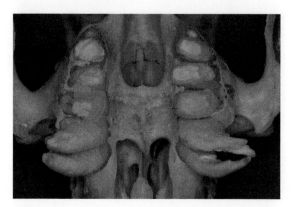

Figure 12.3 Pronounced enamel and dentin hypoplasia of all cheek teeth in a six-year-old rabbit (maxilla specimen, ventral view). The central dentin column is surrounded by a thick, pathologically altered enamel layer. Buccal, bilateral displacement of the anterior two premolars (P2/P3), generalized loss of the lamina dura with a pronounced lateral enlargement of the periodontal space and partially lytic alveolar bones.

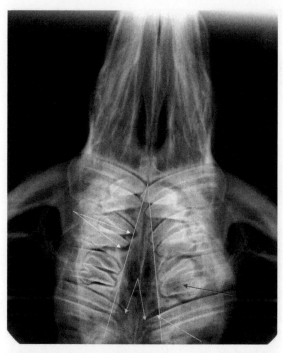

Figure 12.4 Malocclusion in a two-year-old guinea pig (intraoral view of the maxilla) with enlargement of the tooth socket of the second left cheek tooth (M1; white arrows) and the fourth right cheek tooth (M3; yellow arrow), retrograde elongation of the two last molars (M3; turquoise arrows and lines) and structural change of the tooth body of the third right cheek tooth (M2; red arrow).

lower jaw – as a result of a widening of the interdental (approximal) distance between the individual molars, in other words an intraoral dental divergence, as well as a lack of lateral and interior support, respectively, that used to be provided by the now diffusely resorbed alveolar bone (Harcourt-Brown, 2002a) (see Figure 10.8 in Chapter 10 and Figure 12.3).

Malpositioned teeth, in turn, compromise the normal self-cleaning of the dentition, leading to an increase in plaque as well as a secondary infection of the tooth socket. The wide alveoli are subject to impaction of material, usually of fibrous food particles. The food particles mostly remain in the tooth socket for longer periods, secondarily leading to severe periodontal infections (see Figure 2.11 in Chapter 2). If untreated, the inflammation, which is initially confined to the gingiva, will spread further and further, extending apically via the periodontium (periodontitis). The thin, collagenous fibers of the desmodontium and the alveolar bone are destroyed and resorbed more and more due to the inflammation, causing the periodontal space to become wider and wider (radiolucent halo visible on radiographs) (Figure 12.4). The main cause of the destruction of tissue is presumed to be the animal's own immune system, which tries to control the bacterial inflammation by means of granulocytes and enzymes. All those primary and secondary inflammatory processes cause the gingival sulcus to become wider and wider so that even more plaque, food particles and hairs are impacted, causing the periodontal infection to become even worse (Figure 12.5). The extensive loss of dental supportive tissue leads to a secondary loosening of teeth. In the case of more severe bacterial infections, the inflammation will spread along the periodontium (marginal periodontitis) down to the apex (apical periodontitis).

In its early stage, the infection is confined purely to the periodontium before it starts to spread further and further into the bone, along the periodontal ligaments. From this arises a secondary osteolysis of the alveolar bone. Eventually it will result in a loosening of the tooth as well as an extensive apical abscess formation (Gorrel & Verhaert, 2006). Therefore, microabscesses that were locally confined initially will ultimately lead to larger abscesses that cause an extensive disintegration and distension of the jawbone (Baker & Easley, 2003; Crossley & Aiken, 2004; Wiggs & Lobprise, 1995a).

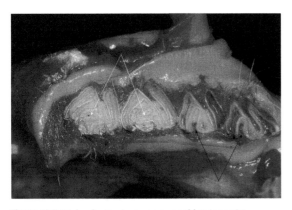

Figure 12.5 Malocclusion in a one-year-old guinea pig (specimen, left mandibular row of cheek teeth): structurally altered occlusal surface of the last two molars (M2/M3; white arrows), partially washed out crown cement of the anterior two cheek teeth (P4/M1; black arrows), dilated gingival pockets filled with hairs and mild caries defects of the lingual occlusal surfaces of all cheek teeth (black discolorations).

The tooth itself will be subject to structural changes of the dental hard tissue, due to an infection-related inflammation of the germinal cells. Thus, the inflammation and infection may not only spread along the tooth socket (periodontal ligament) but also penetrate the pulp cavity via the dentin tubules that are open subgingivally (tubular dentin), causing a purulent pulpitis.

Special findings in guinea pigs and chinchillas

Guinea pigs and chinchillas very often suffer from primary periodontal diseases, when compared with other rodents and rabbits.

Particularly in chinchillas with advanced malocclusions, a diffuse, inflammatory hypertrophy of the gingiva is often present with an elongation and growth disturbance of the teeth. Those changes are mostly restricted to the upper jaw. This often leads to the wrong impression that the cheek teeth are normal in length despite the extensive extraalveolar elongation (see Figure 10.53a and b in Chapter 10). Conversely, intraalveolar, odontoclastic tooth resorptions are the predominant findings in the lower jaw area of chinchillas. Presumably they have their origin primarily in inflammation near the gingival margin (see Figure 10.39 in Chapter 10). It is still unclear just why periodontal disease lead to destructive resorption of the dental hard tissues, especially in the chinchilla. The pathology seems to resemble feline odontoclastic resorption lesion

s (FORLs) in cats (in the author's experience, prepared for publication).

There is some controversy about whether periodontal disease in guinea pigs primarily results from diabetes mellitus or a hypovitaminosis-C. However, deficiency of vitamin C may lead to acute periodontal inflammation with gingival hemorrhage, as well as tooth loosenings or even loss of teeth – similar to scurvy in humans (Howe, 1920; Glickman, 1948; Wiggs & Lobprise, 1995a). Vitamin C has been shown to be essential for collagen synthesis, but guinea pigs are unable to synthesize it. The animals need a daily dose of 10–25 mg/kg of vitamin C (Schaeffer & Donnelly, 1997). During stress situations, pregnancies or in the presence of various diseases, that demand increases up to 30 mg/kg. In order to prevent any short-term deficiency and to support an animal's convalescence, daily therapeutical doses of 50–100 mg/animal p.o. or s.c. are needed (Morrisey & Carpenter, 2004).

An experimental study showed that osteoarthritic changes of the knee joint significantly worsened with a higher vitamin C substitution (Kraus et al., 2004). Likewise, metastatic calcifications are supposedly formed in various soft tissues. Guinea pigs that are fed in a species-appropriate way, receiving high-value green fodder and vegetables (e.g. parsley, broccoli, cauliflower, red peppers or kohlrabi), normally do not need any extra vitamin C.

> Guinea pigs should not be given high doses of Vitamin C parenterally, especially not for long periods without a concrete reason.

A study of various skull specimens of guinea pigs with malocclusions yielded evidence that a widening of the periodontal space that follows severe periodontal disease often occurs in animals whose cheek teeth were severely displaced retrogradely as well as altered in other ways (Figure 12.6). Crown cement, which connects the dentin columns and may also be structurally altered in those kinds of teeth, appears to be washed out more quickly (see Figure 10.35 in Chapter 10). Fibrous food particles and hairs that can secondarily lead to severe periodontopathies may easily be impacted into those "new" cavities or the periodontium, which usually is additionally dilated (Figure 12.7). Hence it is fair to state that a complex tooth structure that leads to a formation of intraoral

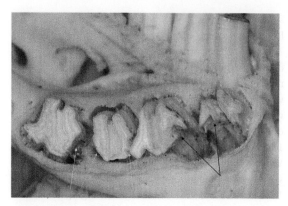

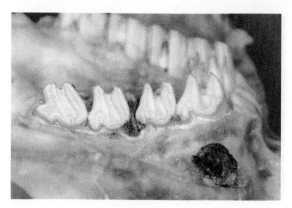

Figure 12.6 Malocclusion in a guinea pig (the same patient as in Figure 9.20 in Chapter 9; specimen, left maxillary row of cheek teeth) and inflammatory resorption of large parts of the buccal tooth structures of the anterior two cheek teeth (P4/M1; black arrows), extensive destruction of the tooth socket with a loss of the lamina dura, pathological occlusal surface of the last cheek tooth (M3) as the mesiobuccal part of the tooth body is missing (white arrow). Secondary enlargement of the tooth socket and mild changes of the occlusal surface of the next-to-last tooth (M2; turquoise arrows).

Figure 12.8 Early malocclusion in a guinea pig (the same patient as in Figure 12.14 later; specimen, left maxillary row of cheek teeth): fibrous food in the approximal area of the second and third cheek teeth (M1/M2) and early, inflammatory loss of the outer alveolar wall.

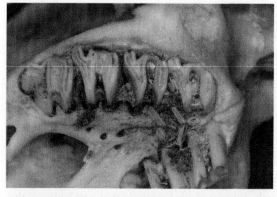

Figure 12.7 Severe periodontitis in a three-year-old guinea pig (specimen, right maxillary row of cheek teeth): washed-out crown cement (decreasing from rostrally to distally), generalized enlargement of the periodontium and impacted, fibrous food parts.

niches predisposes to periodontal disorders if associated with an uptake of mainly fibrous food.

Another study compared the teeth of wild rodents feeding on grass with the teeth of caviomorph rodents that tended to eat fruit (Sone et al., 2005). It transpired that the herbivores did actually become ill with periodontal changes (5.6–8.7% compared to 0.0–1.3%), whereas caries lesions were the most prominent findings

in the fruit-eating animals (10.5–19.8% compared to 1.1–8.7%). The main cause of periodontal disorders in the herbivorous group was fibrous food that had become stuck in the more complexly-structured teeth. Food degradation was followed by a secondary bacterial infection and damage to the gingiva with a subsequent loss of gingiva and bone. Due to the specific etiology of the changes, the interdental area was mainly affected. Thus wild, herbivorous animals do indeed have a relatively high prevalence of periodontal disease. The risk is further increased by malocclusions in individuals that are kept as pets, owing to the fact that they are not able to correctly cut up their food (see Figure 8.8 in Chapter 8 and Figure 12.8).

Due to the continuous tooth growth, supra- and sub-gingival dental calculus is hardly able to form in hypselodont cheek teeth. Calculus was not identified in clinical patients or in a multitude of skull specimens examined.

Diagnosis

Often periodontal pockets are not diagnosed until they have reached a certain size, i.e. above all a considerable depth, and until there are clear signs of an inflammation as well as impacted foreign material (Crossley, 2003a) (Figure 12.9). Fine periodontal probes allow the detection of enlarged periodontal ligament spaces in their early stages. The periodontal ligament of each individual tooth should be carefully checked after an examination of the dentition under anesthesia. The sulcus of each individual tooth is examined with the probe, paying

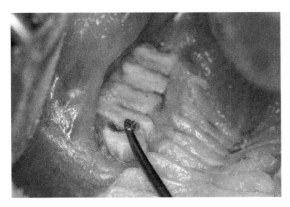

Figure 12.9 Five-year-old rabbit (left maxillary row of cheek teeth): enlarged tooth socket (radiographic finding) of the first cheek tooth (P2) and extended approximal area between the first two cheek teeth (P2/P3); removal of fibrous foreign material with a fine curette.

attention to the depth of any pathological gingival pocket that might be present, as well as signs of concomitant inflammation, such as bleeding or swelling, and impacted foreign material, such as hair or food (see Figure 10.57a in Chapter 10).

In order to measure the depth of a gingival pocket, the periodontal probe, which has a measuring area at the tip, is introduced into the alveolus at an angle of approximately 5–10° to the tooth, applying only slight pressure until some resistance is felt. That resistance depends on the density of the periodontal fibers as well as the solidity of their anchorage on the tooth and the alveolar bone, respectively. Some slight, diffuse pressure applied to the gingiva with a rounded probe helps to check whether pus drains from the suspicious periodontal area, indicating a periodontal microabscessation (Figure 12.10a and b).

Since the cheek teeth of rabbits, chinchillas and degus are very close to one another in a healthy dentition, it is impossible to introduce the probe into the area immediately between the molars. Here diagnostics are rather restricted to the outer and inner surfaces of each individual tooth or any pathologically dilated approximal areas (Figure 12.9). It is a different situation with malocclusions involving tilting or rotation of the teeth. By contrast, at least some of the interproximal areas of guinea pig teeth are accessed rather well with a probe, due to the W-shape of the cheek teeth. Since this is where food particles are usually impacted, it is vital that these areas are examined thoroughly (Figure 12.8).

The tip of the probe is then used to examine the solidity of each individual cheek tooth. If some teeth appear to be mobile or if there are particularly deep gingival pockets detected – indicating a periodontal and/or apical infection – the affected jaw quadrant should be radiographically evaluated very carefully. This is best achieved by means of specific images that will depict the jawbone, including all suspicious cheek teeth without any superimposition, if possible. If there is already a more pronounced vertical bone atrophy with a pathological expansion of the tooth socket, it is decided – depending on the overall situation – whether reconstructive periodontal therapy is feasible (see below) or whether it is best to extract the tooth (Figure 12.10c).

Treatment

If there is evidence indicating periodontitis, teeth and the periodontal pockets are cleaned with scalers, impacted foreign material is removed and a local, occasionally even systemic, treatment is initiated. Individual mobile teeth need to be extracted, which is often impossible as there are mostly multiple changes. Maximal shortening of the teeth for a stabilization of the tooth structure has not proven itself in the long term. An early extraction of the affected tooth is the better alternative to prevent any further spread of the infection.

If a periodontal disorder can be detected early, it may be possible to alleviate or almost heal the inflammation by means of a conventional, conservative periodontal treatment (Crossley & Aiken, 2004). Treatment begins with a thorough supra- and subgingival cleaning of the affected teeth. Although this takes quite some time, it is possible in principle and important in small mammals – just as in cats or dogs. Using anatomical forceps, the finest curettes and scalers, all foreign material is removed from the periodontal pocket (which is usually enlarged) and the approximal areas (which are also often pathologically enlarged) (Figure 12.9). Likewise, persistent tooth plaque is removed (Crossley, 2003a). Finally, lateral surfaces of the cheek teeth that are easily accessible can be worked on with small brushes, giving them additional smoothing.

In most cases, those areas that have been laboriously cleaned will fill up again with new food particles within a short time. In order to restrict or even prevent that, a radical trimming of cheek teeth needs to be performed in addition to cleaning and local treatment of

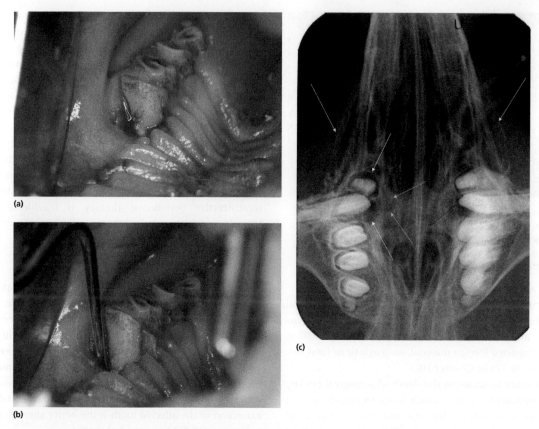

Figure 12.10 Malocclusion in a three-year-old rabbit. (a) Left maxillary row of cheek teeth: discharge of pus from the tooth socket of the first cheek tooth (P2) indicating a chronic periodontitis, intraoral overgrowth of all cheek teeth and gingival hypertrophy. There is an indication for a radiographic examination of the upper jaw (intraoral view). (b) Situation after partial cleaning of the altered tooth socket; probing of the mesial periodontal pocket of the first cheek tooth (P2), foreign material in the palatal approximal area orientated toward the neighboring cheek tooth (P3). (c) Intraoral view of the maxilla: periodontitis of the first left cheek tooth (P2), loss of the lamina dura in the area of the first two left cheek teeth (P2/P3), significant enlargement of the periodontal area (white arrows), osteolysis of the maxilla in the palatodistal area of the second left cheek tooth (P3; turquoise arrows) as an indication for an extraction of both premolars, bilateral lateral distension of the lamina cribrosa (yellow arrows), as well as early enlargement of the tooth socket of the second right cheek tooth (P3; red arrow).

the periodontium, whenever there is intraoral tooth elongation. This will lead to a re-establishment of the self-cleaning capacity of the dentition. Less pronounced periodontal infections will often go into remission merely as a result of these measures.

In addition to the thorough cleaning and treatment of the entire dentition, the intraoral bacterial colonization, which is increased in most cases, is managed. The number of oral pathogenic bacteria can be reduced relatively easily, at least for a short time, by means of special disinfectant solutions. Chlorhexidine digluconate has proven particularly suitable in veterinary medicine for cleaning the oral cavity as well as an application

in the supra- and subgingival area (Eickhoff, 2005). In human medicine, it has been the most effective therapeutic agent in the treatment of periodontal infections for decades, as it is effective on both gram-positive and gram-negative bacteria, as well as aerobic and anaerobic ones, and it also has antiviral and antifungal properties. Experimental studies of small rodents showed that chlorhexidine is also well-tolerated by small mammals and that it sustainably prevents inflammations with its bacteriostatic effect. In addition, it inhibits adhesion, impeding or preventing the formation of new plaque. Since chlorhexidine is well-tolerated by rabbits, guinea pigs and chinchillas, smaller amounts of

1% Chlorhexamed® gel can be easily applied in intra-oral inflammation (according to the author's experience). Chlorhexidine is also suited for the disinfection of the oral cavity prior to surgery or tooth extractions.

A chlorhexidine chip (PeriChip®), which is a biodegradable depot preparation, can be introduced into periodontal pockets that are especially deep and locally confined. It helps to ensure a therapeutically sufficient local concentration of the active agent for longer periods. The implant has a size of a few millimeters (a package contains 20 implants) and consists of a fine membrane that is moistened with chlorhexidine. The introduced chip provides consistent local asepsis for several days. This will help to treat subgingival infections very effectively. The implant is slowly and completely resorbed over a period of 7 to 10 days. After the insert has dissolved, the released chlorhexidine is said to suppress bacterial colonization of the area of application for up to 11 weeks (product information). Since the active agent chlorhexidine is not an antibiotic, there is no need to consider negative side effects. According to experimental studies, the chip can also be used for periodontal therapies of rats and rabbits. A limiting factor, however, is the relative cost of the preparation.

It could be shown in humans that if the chip was applied locally, not only healing of the inflamed gingiva was efficiently promoted but the periodontium was also restabilized and the jawbone was even able to partially regenerate itself. Further study will have to show to what extent such therapies may be a positive influence on severe intraalveolar infections in chinchillas.

It also needs to be evaluated whether it occasionally makes sense to use a variety of bone substitutes in small mammals. Those substitutes may, in theory, lead to a renewed tooth stabilization by remodeling the jawbone (guided bone regeneration) (see also Section 11.1 in Chapter 11). It is proposed, however, that the mobile tooth is unharmed apically and thus worth being preserved in the first place (undisturbed tooth eruption). In addition, antibiotics that are suited for the respective animal species need to be added to the materials (see AIPMMA in Section 11.1.7 in Chapter 11).

All therapeutics mentioned above, however, are merely able to support periodontal treatment; they are not a substitute for thorough cleaning of the affected gingival pockets and an adequate correction of the dentition, possibly including tooth extractions if necessary.

Occasionally a systemic antibiotic therapy is indicated. In addition, a sufficient supply of vitamin C must be ensured in guinea pigs suffering from periodontal diease. If needed, it is administered parenterally in dosages of 25–50 mg/kg BW. The prognosis for periodontal diease generally depends on the overall condition of the dentition and is therefore rather variable individually.

12.1.2 Omnivorous rodents

There is some controversy about periodontal disorders in small, omnivorous rodents that possess brachyodont molars. Some authors report that periodontal diseases are rather rare in these animals (Wiggs & Lobprise, 1995a), whereas others indicate that they may be particularly frequent in pet rodents (Gorrel & Verhaert, 2006) as well as in laboratory animals (Miles & Crigson, 2003). Moreover, periodontal disorders are said to occur more frequently in wild animals, as opposed to caries decay. In a study of skull specimens of wild lemmings in Alaska, 21 out of 100 animals exhibited an inflammatory, horizontal resorption of alveolar bone (Shalla, 1972). In domestic mice, 62.8% of individuals were affected (Sheppe, 1966).

Etiology and pathogenesis

Generally, brachyodont cheek teeth tend to develop inflammation of the periodontium, especially when associated with malnourishment.

Rats are said to be relatively resistant to periodontal disorders by nature. They may only develop a periodontitis under certain conditions, e.g. after having been fed a very sugar-rich diet or in the case of a quite particular, pathogenic intraoral bacteria colonization. The oral mucosa and gingiva of rats is heavily keratinized, which may explain the resistance of the tissue to inflammation (Miles & Crigson, 2003). Yet it seems that relatively many domestic and laboratory rats do suffer from periodontal diease nonetheless, and some of those cases were independent of diet (Rovin, Costich & Gordon, 1966; Taubman et al., 1981; Crossley & Aiken, 2004). The changes predominantly started to occur spontaneously at the age of two (Gottlieb, 1922; Bössmann et al., 1981). However, they may also have been induced experimentally by means of an inoculation with *Actinomyces viscosus* (Baer, 1968).

First, simple and soft plaque is found on the rat's cheek teeth, but this may become mineralized and form true dental calculus. Second, typical periodontal inflammation starts to develop. The periodontitis that is initially confined to the gingival pocket will spread during the further course of the disease. The entire alveolar bone as well as the apical area will be affected, causing the tooth to become mobile. It will then fall out by itself or need to be extracted due to the progressive, purulent root abscess, which is associated with the typical clinical symptoms (see Figure 10.49 in Chapter 10). Often several adjacent molars are affected. Moreover, there is always a danger that the inflammatory process also spreads to the nearby incisor, significantly worsening any prognosis.

Regular cleaning (brushing) of teeth is supposed to remove primary plaque and thus halt the further course of the disease (Crossley & Aiken, 2004). It remains undecided as to whether this can actually be put into practice in domestic rats and it certainly depends on each individual case.

Periodontal disorders were also experimentally triggered in Syrian hamsters that were fed a sugar-rich diet (Keyes, 1968). In the hamsters, the periodontitis progressed significantly faster than in rats. Just as in rats and mice, plaque was initially formed at the tooth surface. The plaque then penetrated further and further into the periodontal pocket, which was enlarged due to the spread of infection. Bone atrophy caused tooth root exposure resulting in the plaque accumulation and sometimes even calculus on the root surface. The alveolar bone was largely resorbed within 100 days and the teeth fell out. Occasionally, such changes may also lead to the formation of a dental abscess (see Figure 10.47 in Chapter 10).

In gerbils, a predisposition for periodontal disorders that was independent of diet was found (Moskow, Wasserman & Rennert, 1968; Vincent, Rodrick & Sodeman, 1979). When fed customary food mixtures for rats and mice, the majority of animals developed a chronic periodontitis. The suspected predisposition, however, may also be due to the fact that the lives of most gerbils under laboratory conditions are somewhat longer than those of other small rodents such as mice or hamsters. The changes increased with age and ranged from plaque to actual dental calculus and the loss of individual teeth (Figure 12.11).

Treatment

Tooth extraction is performed using the sharp tip of small luxators or suitably bent fine cannulae (Wiggs & Lobprise, 1995a; Gorrel & Verhaert, 2006). For the

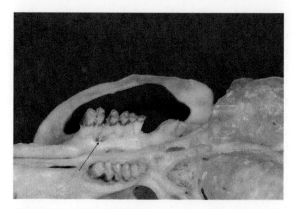

Figure 12.11 Cheek tooth problem in a nine-month-old gerbil (maxilla specimen) with a longitudinal splitting of the first left cheek tooth (M1), early inflammatory loss of the palatal wall of the tooth socket (black arrow), as well as generalized dental calculus.

latter, the tip of the needle is bent at an angle of 90° at a distance that corresponds to the length of the cheek tooth. The further course of action is similar to tooth extraction in dogs or cats (see Figure 10.48b in Chapter 10). The first molar represents some challenge as it has five fine roots that tend to fracture intraalveolarly with rough handling. In addition, there is a certain risk of penetrating the orbit with careless handling of the instruments when extracting the last two maxillary molars (see Figure 10.49 in Chapter 10).

12.2 Caries

12.2.1 Lagomorphs

Caries decay affecting the cheek teeth of rabbits and other species with hypselodont cheek teeth is extremely rare, although there are occasional cases (Wiggs & Lobprise, 1995b; Gorrel & Verhaert, 2006) (Figures 12.12 and 12.14 later). Under normal conditions, caries is prevented by the high pH value of the saliva, the specific intraoral spectrum of bacteria and the diet which – in the case of species-appropriate feeding and keeping – is cariogenic only to a small extent (Eickhoff, 2005). If caries defects do occur, it indicates that tooth growth has either slowed down significantly or ceased completely, due to insufficient physiological abrasion in mostly older rabbits (Harcourt-Brown, 2002a; Mickoleit, 2004). It is only in these conditions, which secondarily lead to a retention of food residue on the tooth surface, that

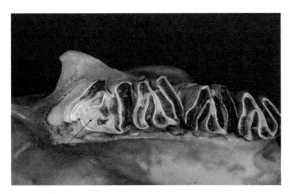

Figure 12.12 Multiple caries lesions in a four-year-old guinea pig, of the occlusal dentin surfaces of all cheek teeth (left mandibular row of cheek teeth), malocclusion and structural change of the distal dentin lamella of the last molar (M3; black arrow).

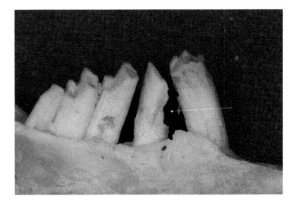

Figure 12.13 Extensive enamel and dentin defect in a three-year-old rabbit (specimen, left mandibular row of cheek teeth) on the mesial surface of the second cheek tooth (P4; white arrow); malocclusion; stepped occlusal surface, extended approximal area between the first three cheek teeth (P3–M1), as well as enamel and dentin hypoplasia of all teeth.

caries is able to establish itself at all in the area of the clinical crown. By contrast, if growth is normal the caries defect is usually simply ground away due to the progressive tooth eruption and rarely causes clinical symptoms (Harcourt-Brown, 2002a). This applies particularly to smaller lesions that wear away with the tooth.

That context confirms experiments in caries research that were performed at the beginning of the last century in rabbits (Mellanby & Killick, 1926). Caries lesions on the occlusal surface of the cheek teeth in the area of the exposed dentin were experimentally induced. Due to the continuous growth, however, the teeth were worn down so fast that the caries defects simply grew out with the continuous tooth eruption. Hence caries generally does not play a crucial part in elodont teeth; the physiological tooth wear is too fast to allow any caries defect to develop (Miles & Crigson, 2003).

If a rabbit's molar is affected by caries, it can be therapeutically trimmed down to a level where the entire caries decay is removed. The elodont tooth will then be able to regrow with a normal structure. There is an increased risk of a caries recurrence, however, until the tooth comes back into occlusion and can then be correctly abraded again. In order to reduce that risk as far as possible, the tooth can be protected after shortening with a preparation containing fluoride. The atubular dentin is thoroughly dried and covered with a thin layer of fluoride varnish (Durophat®) after tooth trimming. Deeper and more extensive caries defects may be more of a problem, especially if they have caused pulp

exposure (lesions near the gingiva). The affected tooth either needs to be treated endodontically (direct pulp capping; see Section 9.3 in Chapter 9) or full extraction is indicated.

If caries changes of the crowns are suspected, the use of intraoral films that are inserted vertically into the oral cavity is indicated for a more precise diagnosis. Those films will help to identify changes of the tooth substance optimally, particularly in the area of the distal tooth surface, and to evaluate the depth and extent of the lesions exactly (see Figure 5.54 in Chapter 5). It is often difficult, however, to differentiate whether there are actual caries lesions (caused by primarily cariogenic bacteria) or resorptive changes of other etiology, e.g. a periodontal inflammation (Figures 12.9 and 12.13). Differential diagnosis may also suggest an enamel and dentin hypoplasia, which likely indicates an apical irritation or infection of the respective tooth.

12.2.2 Herbivorous rodents

Caries changes are rare as they usually will not be able to establish themselves in normal occlusion, with the molars growing throughout life and being continuously worn down (Crossley & Aiken, 2004). The risk of caries is raised, however, if either tooth eruption or wear of individual teeth is reduced due to malocclusion, and there are additional pathological changes of the tooth tissue (dentin and enamel hypoplasia) or the

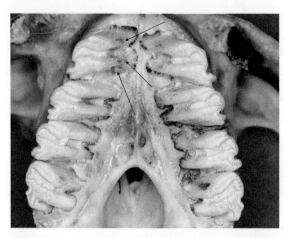

Figure 12.14 Carious or infection related tooth resorptions in a two-year-old guinea pig (maxilla specimen) in the area of the palatal tooth surface near the gingiva of the first right upper cheek tooth (P4; black arrows) with significant widening of the periodontal space, malocclusion and fibrous foreign material between the second and third left cheek teeth (M1/M2).

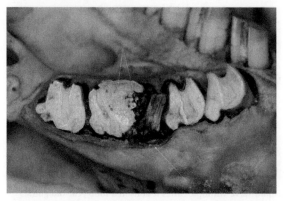

Figure 12.15 Advanced malocclusion in a guinea pig (the same patient as in Figure 12.12; specimen, left maxillary row of cheek teeth): structurally severely altered third cheek tooth (M2) with formation of an abnormal, mesially partially destroyed occlusal surface (turquoise arrows), compact fibrous food particles in the approximal area orientated toward the rostrally adjacent neighboring tooth (M1), secondary dilation of the destroyed tooth socket and horizontal alveolar bone loss (white arrow), generalized widening of the desmodontium and mild caries lesions on the occlusal surfaces of all cheek teeth (brownish discolorations).

periodontium (see Figure 10.41 in Chapter 10 and Figure 12.14). The situation is further aggravated if high-carb food is given. For example, an apple will lower the pH value of the plaque and thus promote the demineralization of a tooth (Sone et al., 2005). As a result of all those processes, the typical caries changes in the occlusal area of the molars are often found in chinchillas and guinea pigs, particularly in stages of advanced malocclusion (Figures 12.12 and 12.15). In many cases all teeth of the affected jaw quadrant are darkly discolored along the enire occlusal surface (insufficient wear). Affected teeth are treated by maximally shortening them down up to the healthy tooth substance.

12.2.3 Omnivorous rodents

Caries tooth changes are rare in wild rodents as the animals take up very little cariogenic food such as sugar or starch in the wild (Mundorff, 1988; Wiggs & Lobprise, 1995a; Crossley & Aiken, 2004). Further reasons are the inhibitory effect of the high intraoral pH value and the natural lack of a cariogenic microflora. Colyer, for example, did not find a single case of caries among 3800 examined skulls of wild rodents (Miles & Crigson, 2003).

However, caries changes of the cheek teeth are more common in domestic animals (Mundorff, 1988; Miles & Crigson, 2003; Crossley & Aiken, 2004).

Etiology

Experimentally, caries can be induced in rats within only 8 to 12 weeks, simply by giving cariogenic food (milk sugar) (McClure & Folk, 1953; Rotilie, 1977). The defects are caused by the intraoral microflora which, as in humans, starts to form acids that damage the teeth. In rats, caries lesions typically occur on the buccal side of the lower molars. It was also shown in hamsters that male animals are more likely to get caries than females (Bivin, Olsen & Murray, 1987).

Thus a diet rich in carbohydrates and sugar generally plays the most important role in the origins of caries in selectively omnivorous, small domestic rodents (Figure 12.16 and see Figure 10.50 in Chapter 10). Another predisposing factor is an insufficient physiological abrasion of the teeth whenever much wet petfood is given; in combination with a reduction in self-cleaning of the dentition, this leads to a retention of food remains (Mickoleit, 2004). It also has an influence on the origins of periodontal disorders.

In rats, for example, the tooth cusps are usually worn down until the age of seven months (Nishijima et al., 2009). This causes the occlusal surface to become smooth first before becoming uneven again as soon as the looplike enamel ridges ("lophs") are all that is left from the

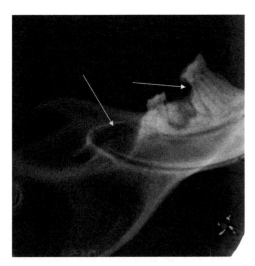

Figure 12.16 Cheek tooth problem in a two-year-old rat (specimen, right branch of the mandible, dental film): the second cheek tooth is partially missing (intraalveolar residue of tooth root); caries defect of the distal surface of the first cheek tooth's crown and neck (M1; white arrow) and clearly visible apex of the incisor ending far behind the cheek teeth (yellow arrow).

worn-down cusps on the occlusal surface, with occlusal dentin exposed in the intermediate spaces (see Figure 2.7 in Chapter 2). This does predispose for caries development, but it is usually no problem if animals are fed in a species-appropriate way, due to the continuous, age-related wear of the tooth substance (in wild animals). The situation will only become critical if additional food rich in carbohydrates and sugar is eaten several times during the course of the day. Caries development is further promoted by a possible intraoral inoculation with specific cariogenic bacteria such as *Streptococcus mutans* (Mundorff, 1988).

Prophylaxis

When applying the experiences laid out above to the feeding of pet rats or other small rodents, it seems advisable to offer the animals no more than very small amounts of high-carb food, and basically no food that contains sugar (cookies, chocolate, yogurt, drops, etc.). The self-cleaning of the dentition can be further improved by offering more vegetables and small live feeder insects, such as crickets and meal worms (from pet shops).

Feeding should be scheduled twice a day and at regular times so that the animals can get used to that rhythm and eat their food relatively quickly and with a healthy appetite. Various kinds of vegetables can be offered *ad libitum*. Fruit contains fruit sugar and is generally a factor predisposing to caries; therefore it is only fed as a rare treat. Apples lower the pH value of the plaque, promoting demineralization of the tooth substance. No food should be offered that has been bitten off by the owner as it may be contaminated with cariogenic bacteria.

Treatment

In principle, tooth-conserving treatment of superficial caries lesions – i.e. an endodontic treatment of the respective tooth – is possible in rats if suitable equipment is used: small instruments and magnifying spectacles. Due to the size of the tooth body, however, this is hardly manageable in practice, meaning that an extraction of the affected tooth is a better alternative (Wiggs & Lobprise, 1995a; Crossley & Aiken, 2004).

Experiments showed that in rats, the use of fluoride and chlorhexidine significantly reduced the formation of plaque and caries, respectively. Hence daily cleaning of an animal's teeth with a brush can be recommended to owners who are interested (whiting with added fluoride). Besides, Na_2HPO_4 can be prophylactically admixed to the food of small rodents as mineral phosphate and fluoride were reported to have a cariostatic effect (McClure & Folk, 1953; McClure, 1959; Rotilie, 1977). There are no precise indications of quantity here.

CHAPTER 13
Other Changes of the Jaw

13.1 Disorders of the temporomandibular joint

Dysplasias and luxations of the temporomandibular joint seem to be very rare in small mammals – no published reports of this occuring. Luxations are thought to be more common in rabbits, mostly caused by iatrogenic damage, i.e. they are caused by opening the jaws too far with a screw type mouth gag (Crossley & Aiken, 2004).

Amongst the author's own patient population over the last 30 years, there has not been a single case of a luxation of the temporomandibular joint, although there were occasional cases of unilateral arthroses as well as dysplasias and two cases of tumors of the temporomandibular joint (sarcomas) (Figures 13.1 and 13.2). Since pathological changes are rather hard to

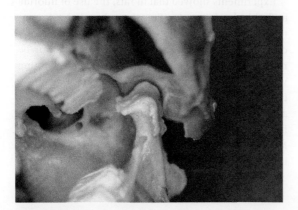

Figure 13.1 Severe osteoarthritis of the temporomandibular joint in a three-year-old guinea pig (specimen, left jaw joint, rostral view) with diffuse osteophytic formation of the mandible condyle.

identify on classic radiographs of the head in four planes, a rostrocaudal view of the head is taken in case of a suspected disorder of the temporomandibular joint (Figure 13.3). If the patient is perfectly positioned, the joints on both sides can be compared and thus evaluated rather well. In addition to that a dorsoventral view of the skull is taken. A lateral displacement of the incisors, which is clearly visible clinically, could theoretically indicate a luxation of the jaw joint, but it is more likely to be the result of an asymmetrical overgrowth of the cheek teeth. In those cases, the occlusion of the incisors will return to normal after proper correction of the dentition.

13.2 Jaw fractures and symphysiolysis

13.2.1 Jaw fractures

Jaw fractures are relatively rare in pets. Animals sometimes fall and hit a hard surface with their heads, injuring either mandibles or the symphysis and the upper jaw. In the case of a rare maxillary fracture, the upper jaw usually fractures immediately caudally to the incisors (diastema), causing the entire rostral maxilla to become unstable. These fractures usually also result in significant trauma to the fine, bony intranasal structures (conchae) and therefore pronounced dyspnoea is usually present, necessitating urgent treatment. In order to avoid long-term complications such as a narrowing of the respiratory pathways, a chronic intranasal infection or a malformation of the upper incisors, a surgical resection of the rostral, completely mobilized part of the jaw including the incisors is indicated. In order to prevent narrowing of the respiratory airways postoperatively, a

Dentistry in Rabbits and Rodents, First Edition. Estella Böhmer.
© 2015 John Wiley & Sons, Ltd. Published 2015 by John Wiley & Sons, Ltd.

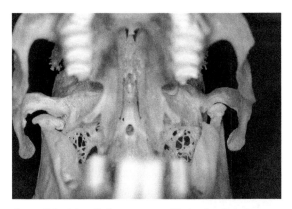

Figure 13.2 Right-sided temporomandibular dysplasia in an eight-year-old rabbit (rostral view); normal occlusion of the cheek teeth.

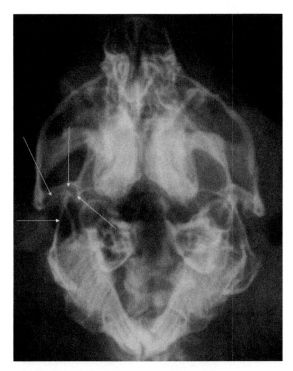

Figure 13.3 Recurring cheek tooth malocclusion in a three-year-old guinea pig (rostrocaudal view) with a suspected pathological change of the right temporomandibular joint including lockjaw (clinical finding). The right joint is structurally altered when compared with the contralateral side; atrophy of the caudal branch of the mandible near the joint (white arrow). The lateral part of the temporomandibular groove (fossa mandibularis maxillae) has been destroyed (turquoise arrow) and the intra-articular space is slightly enlarged (yellow arrows).

small plastic tube can be temporarily placed in each of the respective nasal meatus – in addition to a reconstructing suture for the soft tissue. They can be removed as soon as the local swelling of the wound has subsided. As with all fractures, adequate intra- and postoperative analgesia must be provided. Healing is usually without complications, although it does depend on the extent of local trauma (Figure 13.4a and b).

In the case of fractures of the mandibule, treatment as well as prognosis is largely influenced by whether the injury is located caudally from the last cheek tooth or in the middle or rostral part of the jaw, in other words primarily in the area of the cheek teeth. A fracture of the caudal part of the mandible is usually immobilized rather well by the strong masseter muscle. Most fractures will heal without complications if treated conservatively. The patient is then given soft food for two to three weeks and the teeth are monitored for several weeks. Secondary malocclusions are rare.

If the fracture is located further rostrally, there is always a degree of trauma to the cheek teeth. The teeth are at least partially luxated from their socket often with bony fragments. Mid-body fractures are usually exposed in the oral cavity. The mucosa covering the mandible can either be injured extensively or just very localized thus hardly visible. There is an increased risk of infections (local abscess formation), particularly in guinea pigs. If treated conservatively, those kinds of fractures may heal sufficiently well by suturing the soft tissue and providing systemic antibiotic therapy. A certain degree of secondary malalignment of the cheek teeth may result, in other words a malocclusion that needs to be treated.

The better approach – both for the patient (pain) and for a repositioning of the fragments – would be a surgical stabilization of the mandibular fracture by means of an external fixator, which consists of a relatively thin drill wire and a fine composite bridge. However, it is quite a problem to firmly fix the implants in the bone without causing trauma to the intraalveolar or apical parts of the cheek teeth and incisors as two to three drill wires per each fragment are needed for stabilization. Advantages and disadvantages of a conservative or surgical treatment are considered for every individual case in order to choose the most suitable form of treatment.

If jaw fractures are iatrogenic as a result of severe osteomyelitic damage to the mandible, e.g. having occurred during treatment for an abscess with tooth extraction, the fracture often heals satisfactorily when

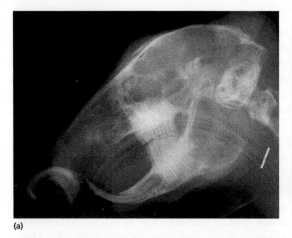

(a)

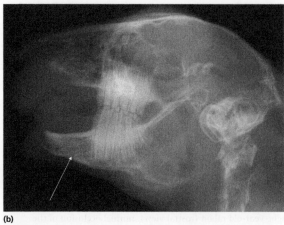

(b)

Figure 13.4 Fracture of the upper jaw in a one-year-old rabbit. (a) Laterolateral view: complete isolation of the rostral jaw area; elongation of all incisors due to congenital maxillary brachygnathia. (b) Postoperative radiograph taken 3 weeks after resection of the rostral part of the upper jaw and extraction of the two mandibular incisors; normal occlusion of the cheek teeth. Inert dentinoid formation (white arrow) present and regular monitoring is indicated.

treated conservatively. Open wound management is very carefully performed and systemic and possibly local application of suitable antibiotics are used, the fragments often heal in a satisfactory way (see Figure 10.78e in Chapter 10). Depending on the overall condition of the teeth as well as the age and general condition of the patient, euthanizing the animal may occasionally be the best alternative.

13.2.2 Symphysiolysis

A common type of injury in herbivorous pets is a trauma-related symphysiolysis, as the two mandibles have a bony link in the area of the symphysis in these animal species. Symphysiolyses may occur in isolation or in combination with an incisor injury. If only the symphysis has been injured, the incisors, which are still firmly attached within the mandible, are tightly connected with each other by means of a composite bridge (Figure 13.5). It is the best way to restore and stabilize the two mandibles.

In order to achieve a solid and exact repositioning of the two mandibles that will facilitate the formation of the composite bridge, a thin cerclage wire is placed around both incisors and then twisted tight labially or buccally by tugging slightly. Prior to repositioning, the fracture area is adequately cleaned (flushing and curettage). In order to avoid the wire slipping off the tip of the teeth as the two lower incisors converge rostrally, a shallow notch is drilled into the lateral surface of each

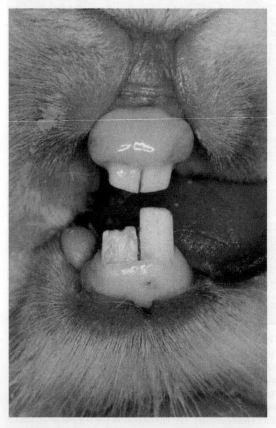

Figure 13.5 Treatment of a mandibular symphysiolysis in a rabbit: composite bridge covering the the upper and lower incisors. The left lower incisor is yet to be trimmed.

incisor. With the wire in position, the mandibles are firmly stabilized and several layers of the composite material are placed immediately on the cerclage wire. Immobilizing the loosened symphysis with only cerclage wire is not sufficient as the shearing forces acting on the symphysis will quickly result in instability of the two mandibles again.

Before the composite material is placed, the tooth surface is thoroughly cleaned (pumice powder and polishing cup or a small toothbrush). After the polishing paste has been thoroughly flushed away, the enamel is etched with 40% phosphoric acid (Figure 13.6). This will roughen the tooth surface and increase the contact area for the composite material, enhancing adhesion to the tooth. The acid is flushed off with water after one or two minutes and the tooth is thoroughly dried with an air jet. Any contact with the tooth is to be avoided now as this may cause the multiple, superficially exposed enamel lamellae to break off.

The next step is to apply a liquid adhesion mediator (bonding material) that is self- or light-cured. That substance fills up the roughened tooth surface, improving adhesion of the composite material on the enamel. In order to form a stable bridge, the material is thinly applied in several separate layers (Figure 13.5). This will allow hardening of every single layer and increase the resilience of the assembly. In order to ensure physiological wear of the incisors, the composite bridge is attached solely on the labial and the buccal surfaces of each lower incisor.

The closer to the gingiva the composite bridge can be positioned, the longer the support will be in place, as it is progressively shifted toward the occlusal surface of the teeth as they continue to grow and erupt. In rabbits and guinea pigs, the composite material will on average, have reached the tips of the teeth after three weeks, which means that it needs to be re-fitted at the gingival margin, as this will usually not have been sufficient time for healing of the symphysis. The following time the composite reaches the tips of the teeth (after approximately 6 weeks in total), the symphysis should be sufficiently stable and the bridge as well as the cerclage wire can be removed.

Long-term prognosis for symphyseal stabilization is generally good, provided both mandibles can be realigned in their physiological position. The smallest deviation from the normal anatomy, however, will inevitably lead to a pathological wear of the incisors and cause secondary incisor malocclusions that will need long term treatment. This will often not become clinically relevant until after

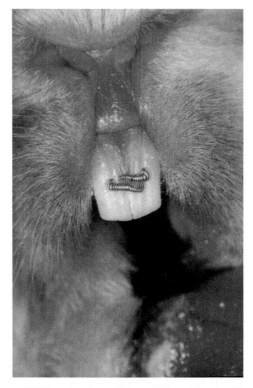

Figure 13.7 Fracture of maxilla in a rabbit, in the area of the palatine suture: parapulpal pins were screwed into both maxillary incisors and bent mesially. After the tooth surface has been etched, it can be covered with composite material.

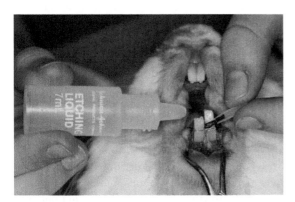

Figure 13.6 Symphseal separation in a rabbit: repositioning of the mandibles by means of a bone forceps as well as a wire cerclage placed around both mandibular incisors and etching of the enamel surface with 40% phosphoric acid (applied for approximately 1–2 minutes).

several months. The prognosis is more guarded if there is severe bacterial contamination of the fracture area. Even with intraoperative wound cleaning, local infections are more likely.

Parapulpar pins can be used instead of the cerclage wire (Figure 13.7). They are screwed into the middle of each incisor and bent in accordance with the tooth surface. The composite bridge is attached above the anchored pins and is able to withstand the shearing forces better. That technique is particularly suited for relatively stable, rostromesial fractures of the upper jaw that are primarily located between the incisors. When used in the lower jaw, it requires temporary repositioning and stabilization of the symphyseal separation with suitable bone rongeur forceps.

13.3 Neoplasia of the jaw

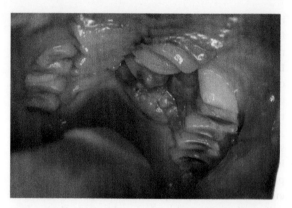

Figure 13.8 Chronic wound in a four-year-old rabbit (left maxillary row of cheek teeth) palatal to the anterior three cheek teeth (P2–P4). The histological examination yielded the diagnosis of a giant cell granuloma.

Classification of neoplasia of the jaw

- Osteogenic tumors (osteomas, osteosarcomas, osteoblastomas)
- Odontogenic tumors
  - epithelial (cementomas, ameloblastomas, odontomas, odontoblastomas)
  - mesenchymal (myxomas, fibromyxomas)
- Soft tissue tumors (fibromas, squamous cell carcinomas, adenocarcinomas)
- Other intraoral proliferations (melanomas, epulides, papillomas)

In small mammals, benign or malignant neoplasms of the oral cavity occur only very occasionally, with the exception being elodontomas (see Section 9.1.4 in Chapter 9) and they are often not detected until the terminal stage of the disease has been reached.

Just like other neoplasms tumors of the teeth and jaw can also be classified according to their origin (tooth, bone or soft tissue) as well as their behavior (benign, malignant, invasive, proliferative or ulcerative) (Baker & Easley, 2003). Hence a distinction can be made between odontogenic, osteogenic and soft tissue tumors.

Osteogenic tumors, which have their origins in the bone, comprise osteomas and osteoblastomas. Both of those are benign neoplasias whereas osteosarcomas are malignant. The latter, which are also called osteogenic sarcomas, are the most common malignant type of neo-

plasia in bones. When compared to the extremely rare odontogenic tumors, osteogenic neoplasias are somewhat more common in small mammals, especially osteo- and chondrosarcomas (Weisbroth & Hurvitz, 1969; Walberg, 1981; Hoover et al., 1986). Among the author's own patient population, osteosarcomas were found particularly in guinea pigs, during the terminal stage of an osteodystrophy (morbus Paget). The patients' temporomandibular joints were completely destroyed (see Figure 5.2 in Chapter 5).

Odontogenic neoplasia, in other words tumors whose origins are in the dental tissue, principally are among the benign tumors. Malignant odontogenic carcinomas and sarcomas are very rare (Eickhoff, 2005). They are caused by proliferations of odontogenic epithelium and connective tissue. According to the tissue of their genetic origin, they are classified as epithelial or mesodermal odontomas (Gorrel & Verhaert, 2006). While those neoplasms are almost always benign, they are usually locally invasively and thus exhibit an aggressive character (Baker & Easley, 2003). Surgical therapy, if it is possible and – above all – sensible in a given case, involves an extensive resection of the tumor tissue. The earlier surgery is performed, the better the prognosis. Complex odontomas contain all elements of a normal tooth, although the clear tooth structure is missing. Compound odontomas have a similar appearance, but their tissue arrangement is more structured like a normal tooth (Baker & Easley, 2003).

Soft tissue tumors can appear as proliferative or ulcerative changes that do not heal (Figure 13.8) (Gorrel & Verhaert, 2006).

Non-neoplastic swellings such as a typical gingival hypertrophy in chinchillas may be confused with neoplasia. Gingival hypertrophy is mostly generalized, diffuse swellings of the gingiva in the upper jaw of chinchillas, which always occurs together with a primary cheek tooth malocclusion. Mild hyperplasia is easily overlooked, especially if one has not had much experience with the respective species, but more pronounced proliferations are usually clearly visible. The consistency of the swellings is usually very hard and there are often relatively deep gingival pockets between the proliferation and a tooth.

If there is any doubt as to the behavior of an intraoral proliferation (i.e. benign versus malignant), a fine needle aspirate including a cytological examination of the obtained cells or a biopsy and/or excision with a subsequent histopathological examination of the tissue should be performed. If a tumor is suspected, radiographs of the head in at least two planes should be taken. It will allow for an accurate evaluation of the bone structures and the growth of the tumor. The further approach is determined by the results of the tissue examination: mandibulectomy or euthanasia.

CHAPTER 14
Follow-up and Prognosis

14.1 Postoperative care

Most patients need a few days before getting back to their normal intake of food following extensive correction of the occlusion, such as radical tooth trimming or even a tooth extraction. The stretched masticatory muscles as well as tendinous structures and temporomandibular joint capsule all need time to readjust to the new positioning. In addition, there is a certain degree of inflammation of the soft tissue caused by procedure itself from the use specific instruments (spatula, mouth gag, cheek dilator, etc.).

For the above reasons as well as the abnormally smooth occlusal surface (missing transverse ridges in lophodont teeth make the grinding of fibrous food very ineffective in the short term), occasionally means that the patients require assisted feeding postoperatively. This should not be continued longer than absolutely necessary to avoid rapid regrowth of the teeth due to insufficient wear. If pellets are soaked and mixed with water to form a slurry, herbivorous pets should be given approximately 30 ml per kg body weight three times a day (Figure 14.1). The mixture is deposited into the cheeks in relatively small portions using an insulin syringe (one-third or half of the syringe each time). The tip of the syringe is cut off and the sharp edges smoothed (with sand paper or the cutting edge of the scissors). The insulin syringes can be re-used for several days if thoroughly rinsed and dried after each feeding session. In order to prevent dysbacteriosis, a probiotic powder is added to the mixture. Guinea pigs should also receive extra vitamin C (approximately 50 mg/kg BW once a day) per os (p.o.) or parenterally.

A simple pellet slurry such as this is enough to maintain a healthy gastrointestinal tract and maintain the weight of the patient – daily weight checks should be performed. If the animals are cachectic or need to gain weight quickly (in preparation for anesthesia), the ideal choice of food is a higher calorie complete feed powder mix which is also more balanced in terms of vitamin and mineral supply (Critical Care® or Rodicare® for herbivores). Feeding 50 ml/kg body weight per day will suffice. Assisted feeding may be necessary for a period of a few days or up to a week.

To encourage autonomous food intake, which is necessary for adequate postoperative tooth wear, food is offered that is both species-appropriate and appetizing, and soft yet abrasive in principle; this includes fresh grass, dandelion, short- and long-leaved plantain as well as other tasty plants and herbs and very fine hay. In order to ensure physiological mastication and thus sufficient dental wear, the food preferably should not be chopped up. However this may be necessary in the short term following painful surgeries such as tooth extractions or if there are any postoperative problems chewing. For these patients finely grated carrots and tender oat flakes can be offered as both of those hardly require any grinding. Dill may be particularly appetizing, especially for rabbits.

Many patients, however, will start eating immediately after correction of the dentition. It is important to monitor and record the weight of these patients over the course of the following weeks. Supplementary feeding is only offered on demand. If the patients have not started eating by themselves again after a week at the most, another clinical and radiographic examination is indicated. Something may have been missed at the time of the previous examination or the correction of the dentition was not correctly performed.

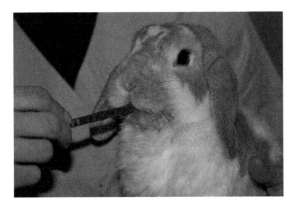

Figure 14.1 Feeding a rabbit with an insulin syringe (the syringe tip is cut off).

14.2 Preventing recurrence

A multitude of factors, some of which are still unknown, is responsible for the continuous wear of hypselodont teeth (see Sections 10.1.1 and 10.1.2 in Chapter 10). Their interaction is very complex. The structure of the food as well as the duration of food intake (chewing) has been proven to play an extremely important role. A regular uptake of only rather meagre food will provide a stable balance between tooth wear and tooth eruption. Guinea pigs living in their natural habitat are particularly undemanding herbivores that do not require any specific food. Wild guinea pigs (*Cavia aperea*) preferentially consume two sorts of grass: *Brachiaria decumbens* (Surinam grass) and *Paspalum notatum* (Bahia grass) (Asher, Spinelli de Oliveira & Sachser, 2004). A lush meadow with various grasses, dandelion, narrow- and broadleaf plantain, clover, etc., actually offers more than enough – and rich – food for that animal species.

The hypselodont cheek teeth of herbivorous small mammals need to be worn down by an average of 1 mm per week (up to three times as much for the incisors) (Crossley & Aiken, 2004). The only way to ensure this is to offer sufficiently abrasive food. By contrast, if mainly pelleted (mixed) food is offered, the cheek teeth are hardly abraded as the pellets can simply be crushed by the molars. Moreover, pellets quickly result in satiety as they are basically high-energy processed food. Hence the teeth are used and worn down even less.

Since an animal's malnutrition is a key factor in the development of an acquired malocclusion, a patient's diet should be critically evaluated after any dental treatment, and optimized if need be. Dietary adjustments, however, are not always easy as many animals refuse to eat species-appropriate food, further upsetting their owners. Many patients are unfamiliar with a natural diet having only eaten tasty processed commercial diets. A certain amount of perseverance will still provide some results here.

It depends on the extent of the pre-existing malocclusion as to whether a dietary adjustment will bring the desired long-term success in management of the dental problem. Changing the diet during the terminal stages of a disorder will rarely lead to an improvement as some patients (particularly chinchillas and rabbits) are unable to grind down raw fiber food such as hay, due to the extremely painful intraosseous changes. Hence even after tooth trimming, sufficient tooth abrasion is not ensured. In these cases, there is often no other option but to offer pellets. The pellets are prehended by the animals and thoroughly mixed and softened with saliva before being worked on by the cheek teeth until they disintegrate and can be swallowed. In principle, feeding is possible in completely edentuolous patients (see Figure 10.40a in Chapter 10). An additional administration of vitamins and minerals may actually improve the bone quality helping to delay the further progression of the disorder (Harcourt-Brown, 2002a).

The primary requisite for a species-appropriate diet of herbivorous small mammals is fresh food with an extremely high fiber content (at least 20%). This is not only important for normal tooth abrasion but also for perfect functioning of the gastrointestinal tract. It also helps to avoid obesity in rabbits and guinea pigs and enhances the mental health of the animals (activity). High-quality hay should be the main food and should be fed *ad libitum*.

In rabbits and guinea pigs hay can largely be replaced with grass (complete grass stalks) and other fresh herbs during the months when plants grow (slow dietary adjustment). It would be best to keep the animals outdoors in the garden during the summer, e.g. in a run area that is fenced and partially roofed, providing opportunities for grazing and browsing as well as exposing them to normal sunlight levels. In an environment like that, fresh or dry foliage from a variety of trees and various other tasty plants are eaten. Gnawing on the bark from twigs of fruit trees or hazelnut allows the animals to wear down their incisors as well as to obtain minerals that are in the germinal layer of the bark.

If there are no possibilities for keeping the animal outdoors, the greenery should be picked on a meadow and fed at home, fresh every day and ideally not chopped up. In cities, however, it can be difficult to find clean grass or other fresh natural food because many meadows are contaminated with the urine or faeces of dogs or wild rabbits (parasites). If this is the case cat grass can be offered, if necessary. Salad rocket (*Eruca sativa*) is accepted as a welcome alternative to dandelion (*beware!* high calcium content). Animals can also be given some additional vegetables and fruits, with the latter being given just occasionally, and in very small amounts due to the fruit sugar. In winter, suitable commercial mixed food with as many long-fiber parts as possible is fed as well as good quality hay and fresh vegetables (green leafy vegetables) in small amounts, to ensure a sufficient supply of minerals, trace elements and vitamins for the animals. It is important not to tolerate selective feeding. One or two tablespoons of the mixed diet per day per animal are enough on average (by no means more than 5–10% of the daily ration). During summer, there is no need for this at all.

In chinchillas and degus, hay is also the main food (approximately 70–80%). It forces the animals to thoroughly chew and grind their food, which automatically results in a sufficient abrasion of the cheek teeth. Vegetables and suitable fresh food is added (at most 10–15%, depending on faecal consistency). In order to ensure a sufficient supply of vitamins, minerals and trace elements, the animals receive one or two teaspoons of pellets every day, or some other suitable mixed food. Fruits are only offered in very small amounts (as treats).

Another basic step in the prevention of more severe, recurrent malocclusions (and, consequently, also a prevention of more extensive abscesses) is to explain to the owner the early symptoms seen that may make one suspicious for a malocclusion requiring treatment. This will ensure that patients are presented for treatment as soon as possible, which can greatly improve long-term prognosis. It is also helpful to weigh an animal once a week (creating a weight curve) as it can be difficult to detect insufficient food uptake, particularly in a group of animals.

A regular dental examination is recommended at least three to four times a year on. If there are any deviations from the norm in terms of intraoral anatomy, or if any known findings have changed, an additional radiograph is taken if need be (overview image). An animal's occlusion should generally also be checked at every opportunity by the practitioner, who should also keep on providing counseling in terms of optimal, species-appropriate diet and keeping.

14.3 Follow-ups

The appropriate time for a follow-up examination after dental treatment depends primarily on the individual clinical and radiographic findings as well as the course of treatment. Regardless, a patient should be free of complaints for at least a few months (3–5 on average) after a straightforward cheek tooth malocclusion has been treated and diet has been adjusted accordingly. If pathological changes can be detected early enough and successfully treated on occasion as well (e.g. a primary dental abscessation), a patient may even be free of complaints for longer periods of time.

By contrast, if a patient keeps being presented for another trimming of cheek teeth every three to five weeks, the treatment should be critically evaluated and the radiographic diagnostics of suspicious areas should be optimized if need be. Occasionally there are exceptions to the rule. End stage disease or advanced changes to the teeth or changes that cannot be specifically treated may require short-term corrections and then, depending on the quality of the patient's life, euthanasia may need to be considered for the longer term welfare of the patient.

14.4 Prognosis

The prognosis of acquired cheek tooth malocclusions as well as secondary incisor disorders depends on a variety of factors. In herbivorous small mammals, a crucial influence is whether husbandry and feeding conditions can successfully be optimized after dental treatment. Regular follow-up appointments are just as important, as many pathological changes can be detected in their early stages and therefore treated early enough (intraoral tooth elongations, apical abscessations, etc.) significantly improving long-term prognosis.

In general, it can be said that both in lagomorphs and in herbivorous rodents with an acquired malocclusion, a long-term prognosis is generally rather unfavorable as many patients are not presented for treatment until they have reached an advanced stage of their respective disorders. If that is the case, any long-term improvement is out of the question, let alone complete resolution of the problem. Pathological processes in the teeth and jaws, which are already mostly generalized, e.g. a retrograde displacement of the tooth apices, will progress further despite being treated, simply because many of them cannot be treated primarily. Hence repeated corrections of the occlusion will only result in a temporary improvement of the clinical symptoms. The more severe and diverse the changes, the less favorable the prognosis will be. Therefore in many cases dental treatment will be merely a palliative treatment (Wiggs & Lobprise, 1995c; Crossley & Aiken, 2004).

Especially in chinchillas and degus, a long-term prognosis is more guarded whenever carious, tooth-resorptive changes are present. If a single tooth is affected, tooth extraction or a long-term antibiotic treatment should be considered. In the case of multiple lesions with extensive exposure of the pulp cavity, euthanasia should be recommended as this is an extremely painful processes.

While pathological changes of the teeth in most animals with a generalized retrograde displacement of the cheek teeth can only be managed for a relatively short time, this can be much longer in some guinea pigs. Time intervals between the required shortening of cheek teeth are longer especially if a particular 'problem tooth' can be identified and specifically treated. Diagnosis is usually challenging, but it can be mastered with the help of special positioning techniques that are described in Section 5.4 in Chapter 5. For an isolated view of the upper or lower cheek teeth of guinea pigs as described by Böhmer, see Section 5.4.2 in Chapter 5. However, if this type of dental problem is not recognized or treated at an early stage, the long-term prognosis is less favorable, because the animals keep refusing to eat despite corrective dental treatment. Tooth shortening may need to be performed again in progressively shorter time intervals, but rarely does this lead to a sustained improvement of the clinical symptoms. Ultimately the upset owner or the exhausted patient will give up, and euthanasia is the only treatment option. In some patients, larger abscesses develop with time, which are often inoperable at the time of diagnosis based on the extent of the concomitant osteomyelitis.

> Long-term prognosis depends mainly on good diagnostics performed as early as possible.

Thus in herbivorous animal species, shortening of cheek teeth should never be performed without anesthesia and without taking appropriate radiographs – for reasons of animal welfare alone. Any short-term saving of expenses in the case where no radiographs are taken is absolutely disproportionate to the costs of treatment that are incurred later and will be much higher.

Contrary to the situation in guinea pigs or degus, malocclusions in rabbits and chinchillas may well settle in the long term, as soon as dental growth ceases during the terminal stage of the dental disease. Many animals have a completely horrendous mouth both intraorally and radiographically, although it is largely asymptomatic (Harcourt-Brown. 2002a; Crossley & Aiken, 2004) (see Figure 10.18 in Chapter 10). Remnants of cheek teeth remain visible in the jawbone, some of which are greatly malformed. Some rabbits are even completely toothless intraorally. Clinical symptoms usually improve around this time and the animals will be able to live without too many problems and without needing constant occlusal correction if they are properly fed, depending on the individual cases. However, not all cheek teeth cease to grow at the same point in time, especially not in rabbits. While some of the structurally altered (pre-)molars fracture at the the gum margin and do not regrow, adjacent teeth that are more tilted and deformed keep on growing unrestricted (see Figure 10.5 in Chapter 10). This may have an adverse influence on the long-term prognosis as secondary abscess formations may occur. Those abscesses are rather rare in the terminal stage of a malocclusion.

As an alternative to lifelong palliative treatment involving regular tooth trimming, euthanizing the patient can be the better option – particularly in the case of severe changes. After all it can be very difficult to exactly assess the pain actually felt by the animals. Being natural prey animals, most small mammals are very adept at hiding illnesses and pain for as long as possible. Even when an animal eats, drinks water, is active, defecates and urinates, huddles up to the owner and exhibits an interest in conspecifics and its surroundings, it cannot be guaranteed that the animal is actually doing well and is pain-free.

> Whenever small mammals suffering from a disease of the teeth or the jaw stop eating due to pain, it is always a serious sign that should prompt anyone to help the animal as soon as possible.

Patients with an isolated abscess or loose tooth have a somewhat better long-term prognosis, especially if the problem is indentified early. If the secondary malocclusion is not too severe, normal occlusion may indeed be attained in the long term or even forever, but may require an additional occlusal correction. Likewise, treatment can be effective in the long term if a diet-related (predominantly intraoral) elongation of cheek teeth is the primary problem and the curvature of the cheek teeth has not yet been pathologically altered. One occlusal correction is usually adequate provided that the feeding conditions of the animals can be optimized at the same time.

Primary incisor malocclusions also have a favorable prognosis as they can usually be treated in a more specific way. This is particularly true for omnivorous rodents with an elongated incisors. Following a single correction of the elongated incisors, husbandry conditions can be improved so as to offer enough material for gnawing. This is usually enough to prevent new malocclusions by way of a physiological tooth wear.

When treating jaw abscesses, the chances of success depend on whether the purulent infection has been identified relatively early (favorable prognosis) or not until a late stage (unfavorable prognosis). If the abscess is confined to a small area of bone and soft tissue and the patient is in a good general condition, the chances of long-term success are significantly better than if a large part of the maxilla or mandible has already been destroyed and several – if not all – teeth in the affected jaw need to be extracted. However, even in such cases, radical surgical debridement, good follow-up aftercare as well as a suitable, local and systemic antibiotic therapy may indeed lead to success. Therefore the prognosis depends very much on the abilities of the practitioner to recognize even the slightest clinical and radiographic findings that indicate very early disease (see Figure1.2a in Chapter 1). High-quality radiographs are required, as well as suitable (special) positionings adequate to requirements. However, more straightforward overview images that might involve suboptimal positioning also often provide important information that can be used in practice.

> Any radiograph is better than none.

It can be said that the veterinary surgeon performing the first examination has a major influence on the further therapeutical approach, as well as the progression of the disease, and ultimately even the long-term prognosis. That responsibility should be fully appreciated and accepted.

In staging prognoses in rabbits, it should be noted that disorders of the teeth and jaws always have a progressive course in rabbits. For a better individual assessment of the likely development of the pathological changes, and therefore a more exact prognosis, malocclusions were classified into five stages by Harcourt-Brown (2002a). Most patients can be assigned to one of those categories if the reference lines are used as an additional tool.

Although such a staging scheme is helpful in principle, it can be somewhat rigid and inflexible. In an everyday veterinary routine, many patients do not fit neatly into one of the categories as most malocclusions are much more complex and a multitude of pathological variations and combinations may occur. For example, it may be that two of the four jaw quadrants are more severely affected (endstage), whereas the other two show hardly any pathological findings at all (Figure 14.2). This may not be taken into account in such a staging system.

In addition, species-specific staging tables are yet to be generated for other animal species (particularly guinea pigs, chinchillas and degus). Therefore it seems

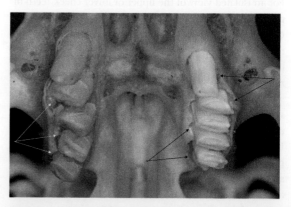

Figure 14.2 Predominantly right-sided cheek tooth malocclusion in a four-year-old rabbit (maxilla specimen): severe enamel and dentin hypoplasia of all intraorally elongated right cheek teeth, expansion of the buccal tooth sockets (white arrows), increased buccal-concave bending of the affected teeth, left-sided slight intraoral overgrowth of the cheek teeth and slight enlargement of the periodontium (black arrows). The structures of the left cheek teeth are largely normal.

Table 14.1 Staging of prognoses.

Stage classification	Clinical finding	Radiographic finding
Stage 1: normal dentition	Intraoral and clinical examination normal	No pathological finding (reference lines)
Stage 2: retrograde apex displacement, deterioration in tooth quality	Often no clinical symptoms (despite early pathological tooth and jaw changes) Horizontal transverse grooves in the incisors (still normal shape and occlusion possible) Nonpainful jaw swellings in the area of the ventral border of the mandible Subtle intraalveolar tooth deformations and displacements Enamel hypoplasia Epiphora (retrograde displacement of the roots of the incisors) Occlusal plane often still even	Clear retrograde tooth displacement, diagnosed by means of the reference lines, (solitary or multiple) Partial or generalized loss of the lamina dura (especially apically) Retrograde displacement of individual or multiple apices (into the cortical bone or beyond) Slightly altered shapes of the cheek teeth (bending) Altered structure of the cheek teeth (enamel and dentin hypoplasia) Periphery of teeth (enamel) and central double fold appearing less dense Smaller, radiolucent bone areas
Stage 3: loss of the lamina dura, changes of tooth position, shape and structure (incisors and cheek teeth), secondary changes (e.g. mucosal lesions)	Usually painful jaw swellings in the area of the ventral border of the mandible Secondary incisor malocclusion (overgrowth, pathological curving of teeth, prognathism) Lingual tilting of the mandibular cheek teeth Buccal tilting of the maxillary cheek teeth Severe enamel and dentin hypoplasia Dilation and secondary inflammation of the periodontium due to impacted food particles Inflammatory loosening of teeth Possible abscess formation	More pronounced retrograde tooth displacement of multiple apices, diagnosed by means of the reference lines Perforation of the cortical bone of the mandible Severely altered structures of the cheek teeth (pronounced enamel and dentin hypoplasia) Central enamel fold missing No differentiation of the two pulpal cavities possible Markedly altered shape of the cheek teeth (severe curving and displacements) Severe retrograde displacement of multiple apices (beyond the mandibular cortical bone) Increased multiple, radiolucent bone areas
Stage 4: tooth growth ceases (as do pathological changes, improvement of clinical symptoms)	Slow uptake of food possible (soft or pelleted food) Usually "improvement" in general condition Longer intervals without tooth treatment Secondary incisor malocclusions of various degrees Multiple, yellowish cheek tooth stubs (dental tissue severely altered pathologically) Hypodontia (missing cheek teeth due to intraalveolar tooth fractures or loss of teeth) Tooth stubs within the jaw, usually asymptomatic completely covered by gingiva Usually no intraoral tooth spikes Largely functional occlusion of cheek teeth (strongly altered occlusal surface) Possible abscess formation (rarer)	More pronounced retrograde tooth displacement of multiple apices, diagnosed by means of the reference lines Clinical tooth crowns missing intraorally or markedly altered Partial or complete dissolution of the intraalveolar parts of teeth Increased radiodensity (abnormal mineralization) of the remaining intraosseous dental tissue Loss of bone detail of the jawbone Indistinct contours of the cheek teeth Poor differentiation between tooth and bone substance Central enamel fold missing

(Continued)

Table 14.1 (*Continued*)

Stage classification	Clinical finding	Radiographic finding
Stage 5: terminal stage: osteomyelitis and abscess formation, increasing calcification of the teeth and the bone	Structure and shape of teeth severely altered pathologically Multiple, painful jaw swellings in the area of the ventral border of the mandible Multiple, yellowish stubs of the cheek teeth (dental tissue severely altered pathologically) Hypodontia (missing cheek teeth due to intraalveolar tooth fractures or loss of teeth) Osteomyelitis and abscess formation in the area of the retrogradely displaced apices (cheek teeth) Intranasal abscesses (incisors)	Severe retrograde tooth displacement of multiple apices, diagnosed by means of the reference lines Severe demineralization of the entire cranial skeleton Clinical tooth crowns missing intraorally or markedly altered Partial or complete dissolution of the intraalveolar parts of teeth Asymptomatic embedded dental fragments within the jawbone Progressive calcification of the tooth stubs (extremely radiodense intraosseous structures) Indicators of a local osteomyelitis (apical infection) Proliferative, mostly periapical changes of the jawbone (enlarged calcifications) Often difficult distinction of dental and bone substance

more reasonable to use purely objective evaluation criteria for stagings and criteria that are applicable to the respective animal species as well as individuals, such as the reference lines (see Section 5.6 in Chapter 5). For rabbits, a combination of those lines with a somewhat modified version of a staging system (Table 14.1) is probably the best way to assess the further course of a disease correctly.

CHAPTER 15
Appendix

Table 15.1 Antibiotic therapy in rabbits.

Active agent	Dosage	Interval	Notes
Amikacin	5–10 mg/kg s.c., i.m., i.v.	Every 24 h (or divided into 3)	Nephrotoxic
Azithromycin	20–30 mg/kg p.o.	Every 24 h	
Cephalexin	11–22 mg/kg p.o.	Every 8 h	
	15 mg/kg s.c.	Every 12 h	
Chloramphenicol	30–50 mg/kg p.o.	Every 12 h	
Chlortetracycline	50 mg/kg p.o.	Every 12 h	
Ciprofloxacin	10–20 mg/kg p.o.	Every 12–24 h	
Doxycycline	2.5 mg/kg p.o.	Every 12 h	
Enrofloxacin	10 mg/kg p.o., s.c., i.m.	Every 24 h	
	5 mg/kg s.c.	Every 12 h	
Gentamicin	4 mg/kg s.c., i.m.	Every 24 h	*Beware*! Nephrotoxic
Metronidazole	10–20 mg/kg p.o.	Every 12 h	In case of infections with anaerobic bacteria
Neomycin	30 mg/kg p.o.	Every 12 h	
Oxytetracycline	10–20 mg/kg s.c., i.m.	Every 12 h	
	50 mg/kg p.o.	Every 12 h	
Procaine penicillin + benzathine penicillin	20 mg/kg PP + 15 mg/kg BP s.c.	Every 7 days	
Penicillin + streptomycin	16 000 IU + 24 000 IU s.c.	Every 14–48 h	
Penicillin G	40 000 IU/kg s.c.	Every 24–48 h	*Beware*! Danger of life-threatening dysbiosis
Tetracycline	50 mg/kg p.o., s.c.	Every 8–12 h	
Trimethoprim sulfonamide	30–40 mg/kg p.o., s.c.	Every 12 h	
Tylosin	10 mg/kg p.o., s.c.	Every 12 h	
Not to be used Amoxicillin, amoxicillin/ clavulanic acid, ampicillin, clindamycin, erythromycin			

Adapted from Harcourt-Brown, 2002b; Morrisey & Carpenter, 2004.

Dentistry in Rabbits and Rodents, First Edition. Estella Böhmer.
© 2015 John Wiley & Sons, Ltd. Published 2015 by John Wiley & Sons, Ltd.

Table 15.2 Antibiotic therapy in guinea pigs.

Active agent	Dosage	Interval	Notes
Amikacin	10–15 mg/kg s.c., i.m., i.v.	Every 24 h (or divided into 3)	
Cephalexin	50 mg/kg p.o.	Every 24 h	
Chloramphenicol	50 mg/kg p.o.	Every 8–12 h	
Ciprofloxacin	10 mg/kg p.o.	Every 12–24 h	
Doxycycline	2.5 mg/kg p.o.	Every 12 h	
Enrofloxacin	10 mg/kg p.o., s.c., i.m.	Every 12 h	
Gentamicin	5–8 mg/kg s.c., i.m.	Every 24 h (or divided into 3)	*Beware!* Nephrotoxic
Metronidazole	10–20 mg/kg p.o.	Every 12 h	In cases of anaerobic infections
Neomycin	15 mg/kg p.o.	Every 12 h	
(Oxytetracycline)	10–20 mg/kg s.c.	Every 24 h	*Beware!*
Tetracycline	10 mg/kg p.o.	Every 8–12 h	*Beware!*
Trimethoprim sulfonamide	15–30 mg/kg p.o., s.c.	Every 12 h	
Tylosin	10 mg/kg p.o., s.c.	Every 12 h	*Beware!*
Not to be used Amoxicillin, amoxicillin/ clavulanic acid, ampicillin, clindamycin, erythromycin, penicillin, lincomycin			

Adapted from Morrisey & Carpenter, 2004. Reproduced with permission of Elsevier.

Table 15.3 Antibiotic therapy in chinchillas.

Active agent	Dosage	Interval	Notes
Amikacin	10–15 mg/kg s.c., i.m., i.v.	Every 24 h (or divided into 3)	
Chloramphenicol	50 mg/kg p.o.	Every 8–12 h	
Chlortetracycline	50 mg/kg p.o.	Every 12 h	
Ciprofloxacin	5–10 mg/kg p.o.	Every 12–24 h	
Doxycycline	2.5 mg/kg p.o.	Every 12 h	
Enrofloxacin	5–15 mg/kg p.o., s.c., i.m.	Every 12 h	
Gentamicin	5–8 mg/kg s.c., i.m.	Every 24 h (or divided into 3)	
Metronidazole	10–20 mg/kg p.o.	Every 12 h	*Beware!*
Neomycin	15 mg/kg p.o.	Every 12 h	
(Oxytetracycline)	10–20 mg/kg s.c.	Every 24 h	*Beware!*
Tetracycline	10–20 mg/kg p.o.	Every 8–12 h	
Trimethoprim sulfonamide	15–30 mg/kg p.o., s.c.	Every 12 h	
Tylosin	10 mg/kg p.o., s.c.	Every 12 h	*Beware!*
Not to be used Amoxicillin, amoxicillin/clavulanic acid, ampicillin, clindamycin, erythromycin, penicillin			

Adapted from Morrisey & Carpenter, 2004. Reproduced with permission of Elsevier.

Table 15.4 Antibiotic therapy in rats and mice.

Active agent	Dosage	Interval	Notes
Amikacin	10 mg/kg s.c., i.m.	Every 12 h	
Ampicillin	20–50 mg/kg p.o., s.c., i.m.	Every 12 h	
Chloramphenicol	30–50 mg/kg p.o.	Every 8–12 h	
Chlortetracycline	10–25 mg/kg p.o., s.c.	Every 12 h	
Ciprofloxacin	10 mg/kg p.o.	Every 12 h	
Doxycycline	5 mg/kg p.o.	Every 12 h	
Enrofloxacin	5–10 mg/kg p.o., s.c., i.m.	Every 12 h	
Erythromycin	20 mg/kg p.o.	Every 12 h	
Gentamicin	5–10 mg/kg s.c., i.m.	Every 24 h (or divided into 3)	
Metronidazole	10–40 mg/kg p.o.	Every 24 h	*Beware!*
Neomycin	25 mg/kg p.o.	Every 12 h	
(Oxytetracycline)	10–20 mg/kg s.c.	Every 24 h	*Beware!*
Penicillin G	22 000 IU/kg s.c., i.m.	Every 24 h	Not in mice!
Tetracycline	10–20 mg/kg p.o.	Every 8–12 h	
Trimethoprim sulfonamide	15–30 mg/kg p.o., s.c.	Every 12 h	
Tylosin	2–8 mg/kg p.o., s.c.	Every 12 h	

Not to be used Streptomycin, nitrofurantoin (in rats)

Adapted from Morrisey & Carpenter, 2004. Reproduced with permission of Elsevier.

Table 15.5 Antibiotic therapy in hamsters.

Active agent	Dosage	Interval	Notes
Amikacin	10 mg/kg s.c., i.m.	Every 12 h	
Chloramphenicol	30–50 mg/kg p.o.	Every 8–12 h	
Chlortetracycline	20 mg/kg p.o., s.c.	Every 12 h	
Ciprofloxacin	10 mg/kg p.o.	Every 12 h	
Doxycycline	2.5 mg/kg p.o.	Every 12 h	
Enrofloxacin	5–10 mg/kg p.o., s.c., i.m.	Every 12 h	
Gentamicin	5–8 mg/kg s.c., i.m.	Every 24 h (or divided into 3)	
Metronidazole	20 mg/kg p.o.	Every 12 h	
Neomycin	30 mg/kg p.o.	Every 12 h	
(Oxytetracycline)	10–20 mg/kg s.c.	Every 24 h	*Beware!*
Tetracycline	10–20 mg/kg p.o.	Every 8–12 h	
Trimethoprim sulfonamide	15–30 mg/kg p.o., s.c.	Every 12 h	
Tylosin	2–8 mg/kg p.o., s.c.	Every 12 h	*Beware!*

Not to be used Amoxicillin, amoxicillin-clavulanic acid, ampicillin, clindamycin, erythromycin, lincomycin, penicillin

Adapted from Morrisey & Carpenter, 2004. Reproduced with permission of Elsevier.

References

Ashcraft, M.D., Southard, K.A. & Tolley, E.A. (1992) The effect of corticosteroidinduced osteoporosis on orthodontic tooth movement. *Am. J. Orthodontic Dentofacial Orthop.*, **102**, 310–19.

Asher, M., Spinelli de Oliveira, E. & Sachser, N. (2004) Social system and spatial organization of wild guinea pigs (*Cavia aperea*) in a natural population. *J. Mammals*, **85**, 788–96.

Au, A.Y., Au, R.Y., Al-Talib, T.K., Eves, B. & Frondoza, C.G. (2008) Consil bioactive glass particles enhance osteoblast proliferation and maintain extracellular matrix production *in vitro*. *J. Biomed. Mater. Res.*, **A 86** (3), 678–84.

Augustin, F. (1937) Form, Wandstarke und tragender Querschnitt des Kaninchennagezahnes bei verschiedenen Leistungszustanden. *Gegenbaurs Morph.*, **80**, 179–200.

Baer, P.N. (1968) Use of laboratory animals for calculus studies. *Ann. NY Acad. Sci.*, **153**, 230–9.

Baer, P.N. & Kilham, L. (1974) Dental defects in hamsters infected with minute virus of mice. *Oral Surg.*, **37** (3), 385–9.

Baker, G.J. & Easley, J. (2003) *Zahnheilkunde in der Pferdepraxis*. Schlütersche, Hannover.

Baum, L.J., Becks, H., Ray, J.C. & Evans, H.M. (1954) Hormonal control of tooth eruption.II. The effects of hypophysectomy on the upper rat incisor following progressively longer intervals. *J. Dent. Res.*, **33**, 91–103.

Becks, H., Collins, D.A., Simpson, M.E. & Evans, H.M. (1946) Changes in the central incisors of hypophysectomised female rats after different periods. *Arch. Path.*, **41**, 457–75.

Bellantone, M., Coleman, N.J. & Hench, L.L. (2000) Bacteriostatic action of a novel four-component bioactive glass. *J. Biomed. Mater. Res.*, **51** (3), 484–90.

Bennett, R.A. (1999) Management of abscesses of the head in rabbits. In: *Vetinary Proceedings of the North American Vetinary Conferance*, Orlando, Florida, pp. 821–3.

Bennett, R.A. (2008) Antibiotic-impregnated PMMA beads – use and misuse. In: *Proceedings of the Western Vetinary Conference*.

Berkovitz, B.K.B. (1972) Ontogeny of tooth replacement in the guinea pig (*Cavia cobya*). *Arch. Oral Biol.*, **17**, 711–18.

Berkovitz, B.K.B. (1976) Theories of tooth eruption. In: *The Eruption and Occlusion of Teeth* (eds Poole, D.F.G. & Stack, M.V.), pp. 193–204. Butterworths, London.

Bieniek, H.J. & Bieniek, K.W. (1993) *Zahnheilkunde fur die Kleintierpraxis*. Enke, Stuttgart.

Bishop, M.A. (1995) Is rabbit dentine innervated? A fine-structural study of the pulpal innervation in the cheek teeth of the rabbit. *J. Anat.*, **186**, 365–72.

Bivin, W.S., Olsen, G.A. & Murray, K.A. (1987) Morphophysiology. In: *Laboratory Hamsters* (eds Van Hoosier, G.L. & McPherson, C.A.W), pp. 9–12. Academy Press, Orlando, Florida.

Böhmer, E. (2001a) Röntgendiagnostik bei Zahn- sowie Kiefererkrankungen der Hasenartigen und Nager. Teil 1: Tierartspezifische Zahn- und Kieferanatomie sowie Pathologie, Indikationen für die Rontgendiagnostik. *Tierärztl Prax.*, **29**, 316–27.

Böhmer, E. (2001b) Röntgendiagnostik bei Zahn- sowie Kiefererkrankungen der Hasenartigen und Nager. Teil 2: Interpretation von Röntgenaufnahmen und tierartspezifische Fallbeispiele. *Tierärztl Prax.*, **29**, 369–83.

Böhmer, E. (2003) Extraktion von Schneidezähnen bei Kaninchen und Nagern – Indikationen und Technik. *Tierärztl Prax.*, **31**, 309–20.

Böhmer, E. (2006) Röntgendiagnostik von Zahnerkrankungen. In: *Proceedings 52, Jahreskongress der DGK-DVG*, Düsseldorf.

Böhmer, E. (2007) Intraoral radiographic technique in lagomorphs and rodents. *EXOTIC DVM*, **9** (3), 27–33.

Böhmer, E., Böttcher, P. & Matis, U. (2002a) Zur Intubation des Kaninchens unter Praxisbedingungen. Teil 1: Literaturübersicht und Anatomie des Larynx beim Kaninchen. *Tierärztl Prax.*, **30**, 295–304.

Böhmer, E., Böttcher, P. & Matis, U. (2002b) Zur Intubation des Kaninchens unter Praxisbedingungen. Teil 2: Eigene Erfahrungen. *Tierärztl Prax.*, **30**, 370–8.

Böhmer, E. & Crossley, D. (2009) Objective interpretation of dental disease in rabbits, guinea pigs and chinchillas: use of anatomical reference lines. *Tierärztl Prax.*, **37** (4), 250–60.

Böhmer, E. & Crossley, D. (2011) Objective interpretation of dental disease in rabbits, guinea pigs and chinchillas: use of anatomical reference lines. *Europ. J. Compan. Animal Pract.*, **21** (1), 47–56.

Bössmann, K.L, Deerberg, F., Preuss, V. & Rehm, S. (1981) Dental and periodontal alterations in ageing Han:WIST rats. *Zeitschr. Versuchstierkd.*, **23**, 305–11.

Boy, S.C. & Steenkamp, G. (2006) Odontoma-like tumours of squirrel elodont incisors – elodontomas. *J. Comp. Path.*, **135**, 56–61.

Dentistry in Rabbits and Rodents, First Edition. Estella Böhmer.
© 2015 John Wiley & Sons, Ltd. Published 2015 by John Wiley & Sons, Ltd.

Boyle, P.E. (1938) The effect of ascorbic acid deficiency on enamel formation in the teeth of guinea pigs. *Am. J. Path.*, **14**, 843–8.

Bradley, T. (2001) Recognizing pain in exotic animals. *EXOTIC DVM*, **3** (3), 21–6.

Brenner, S.Z.G, Hawkins, M.G., Tell, L.A., Hornof, W.J., Plopper, C.G. & Verstraete, F.J.M. (2005) Clinical anatomy, radiography, and computed tomography of the chinchilla skull. *Comp. Contin. Educ. Pract. Vet.*, **27** (12), 933–44.

Brown, S.A. (1992) Surgical removal of incisors in the rabbit. *J. Small Animal Exot. Med.*, **1**, 150–3.

Brown, S.A. & Rosenthal, K.L. (1997) *Self Assessment Colour Review of Small Mammals*. Manson, London.

Burn, C.G., Orten, A.V. & Smith, A.H. (1941) Changes in the structure of the developing tooth in rats maintained on a diet deficient in vitamin A. *Yale J. Biol. Med.*, **13**, 817–30.

Capello, V. (2006) The dental suite: equipment needed for handling small exotic mammals. *J. Exot. Pet Med.*, **15** (2), 106–15.

Capello, V. (2008) Diagnosis and treatment of dental disease in pet rodents. *J. Exot. Pet Med.*, **17** (2), 114–23.

Chaffee, V.W., James, E.A. & Montali, R.J. (1975) Suppurative mandibular osteomyelitis associated with *Pasteurella multocida* in a rabbit. *Vet. Med. Small Animal Clin.*, **70**, 1411–73.

Chai, C.K. (1970) Effect of inbreeding in rabbits. Skeletal variations and malformations. *J. Hered.*, **61**, 2–8.

Chesney, C.J. (1998) CT scanning in chinchillas. *J. Small Animal Pract.*, **39** (11), 550.

Clemm, A. (2008) *Metamizol, Carprofen und Fentanyl bei der Orchiektomie des Kaninchens*. Thesis, Munich.

Cohrs, P., Jaffe, R. & Meessen, H. (1958) *Pathologie der Laboratoriumstiere*. Springer, Berlin.

Crossley, D.A. (1994) Extraction of rabbit incisor teeth. *J. Brit. Vet. Dent. Assoc.*, **2**, 8.

Crossley, D.A. (1995a) Clinical aspects of lagomorph dental anatomy: the rabbit (*Oryctolagus cuniculus*). *J. Vet. Dent.*, **12** (4), 137–40.

Crossley, D.A. (1995b) Clinical aspects of rodent dental anatomy. *J. Vet. Dent.*, **12** (4), 131–5.

Crossley, D.A. (1995c) Dental disease in rabbits. *Vet. Rec.* **137**, 384.

Crossley, D.A. (1996) Diagnosis of malocclusion in rabbits and rodents. *BPT Dental Wet Lab – Small Mammals*, Hamburg.

Crossley, D.A. (2001a) Dental disease in chinchillas in the UK. *J. Small Animal Pract.*, **42** (1), 12–9.

Crossley, D.A. (2001b) The risk of pulp exposure when trimming rabbit incisor teeth. In: *Proceedings of the European Vetinary Dental Society Annual Congress*, Berlin.

Crossley, D.A. (2003a) *Dental disease in chinchillas*. PhD thesis, University Dental Hospital of Manchester.

Crossley, D.A. (2003b) Dental disease in chinchillas in the UK. *Europ. J. Comp. Anim. Pract.*, **13**, 57–65.

Crossley, D.A. & Aiken, S. (2004) Small mammal dentistry. In: *Ferrets, Rabbits and Rodents – Clinical Medicine and Surgery* (eds Quesenberry, K.E. & Carpenter, J.W.), pp. 370–82. Saunders, Philadelphia, Pennsylvania.

Crossley, D.A., Dubielzig, R.R. & Benson, K.G. (1997) Caries and odontoclastic resorptive lesions in a chinchilla (*Chinchilla laniger*). *Vet. Rec.*, **141** (27), 337–9.

Crossley, D.A. & Miguelez, M.M. (2001) Skull size and cheek tooth length in wild-caught and captive-bred chinchillas. *Arch. Oral Biol.*, **46**, 919–28.

Crossley, D.A., Jackson, A., Yates, J. & Boydell, I.P. (1998) Use of computed tomography to investigate cheek tooth abnormalities in chinchillas (*Chinchilla laniger*). *J. Small Animal Pract.*, **39** (8), 385–9.

Dangl, F. (2009) Der Medizinische Honig in der modernen Wundversorgung – Was ist das Geheimnis vom Gold der Biene. *Osterr. Gesellsch. vaskul Pflege*. Thesis, Vienna.

Deeb, B. (1993) Update for veterinary practitioners on pasteurellosis in rabbits. *J. Small Exotic Anim. Med.*, **2**, 112–13.

DeForge, D.H. (1997) Evaluation of bioglass/PerioGlas (Consil) synthetic bone graft particulate in the dog and cat. *J. Vet. Dent.*, **14** (4), 141–5.

Dold, H. (1924) Anaphylaktoide Erscheinungen nach intravenoser Einspritzung geringer Mengen von Formaldehyd. *J. Molec. Med.*, **3** (31), 1405–6.

Dominguez, J., Crase, D. & Soave, O. (1975) A case of pseudomonas osteomyelitis in a rabbit. *Lab. Animal Sci.*, **25**, 506.

Donnelly, T.M. (2004) Disease problems of small rodents. In: *Ferrets, Rabbits and Rodents – Clinical Medicine and Surgery* (eds Quesenberry, K.E. & Carpenter, J.W.), pp. 299–315. Saunders, Philadelphia, Pennsylvania.

Eibl-Eibesfeldt, B. & Kessler, S. (1997) *Verbandlehre*. Urban & Schwarzenberg, Munich.

Eickhoff, M. (2005) *Zahn-, Mund- und Kieferheilkunde bei Klein- und Heimtieren*. Enke, Stuttgart.

Emily, P.P. & Penman, S. (1994) *Handbook of Small Animal Dentistry*. Pergamon, Oxford.

Emmel, L. (1938) Die Herkunft des Schmelzes der erwachsenen Nager mit Untersuchungen uber den Nagezahn von Sciurus vulgaris. *Z. wiss Zool.*, **150**, 358–403.

Erdheim, J. (1906) Tetania parathyreopriva. *Mitteilungen aus den Grenzgebieten der Medizin und Chirurgie*, **16**, 632–744.

Erhardt, W., Henke, J. & Haberstroh, J. (2004) *Anästhesie und Analgesie beim Klein- und Heimtier*. Schattauer, Stuttgart.

Ethell, M.T., Bennett, R.A., Brown, M.P., Merritt, K., Davidson, J.S. & Tran, T. (2000) *In vitro* elution of gentamicin, amikacin, and ceftiofur from polymethylmethacrylate and hydroxyapatite cement. *Vet. Surg.*, **29**, 375–82.

Fakler, O. (2003) Lokalanästhesie und relevante Medikamente in der zahnärztlichen Praxis. In: *Einfuhrung in die zahnarztliche Chirurgie* (eds Gutwald, R., Gellrich, N.C. & Schmelzeisen, R.). Urban & Fischer, Munich.

Fish, E.W. & Harris, L.J. (1935) The effects of vitamin C deficiency on tooth structure in guinea-pigs. *Brit. Dent. J.*, **58**, 3–20.

Flecknell, P. (2009) *Laboratory Animal Anaesthesia*. Elsevier, London.

Fox, R.R. & Crary, D.D. (1971) Mandibular prognathism in the rabbit. Genetic studies. *J. Hered.*, **62**, 23–7.

Fredericia, L.S. & Gudjonsson, S.V. (1936) The effect of vitamin A deficiency on the rate of growth of the incisors of albino rats. *Biol. Med. Kgl. Danske Vidensk Selsk*, **13**, 1–18.

Gabriel, S. (2009) Technical aspects of abrasive dental tools. In: *Proceedings of the 18th European Congress on Vetinary Dentistry*, Zurich.

Gaggermeier, B., Henke, J., Schatzmann, U., Erhard, W. & Korbel, R. (2001) Investigations on analgesia in domestic pigeons. Using buprenorphin and butorphanol. In: *European AAV-DVG-Conference*, Munich.

Gangler, P. & Arnold, W.H. (2005) Struktur und Funktion des Gebisses und der Mundhohle. In: *Konservierende Zahnheilkunde und Parodontologie* (eds Gangler, P., Hoffmann, T., Willershausen, B., Schwenzer, N. & Ehrenfeld, M.). Thieme, Stuttgart.

Ganzer, H. (1908) Über die Bewegungsbahn des Unterkiefers insbesondere beim Menschen und bei den Nagetieren. In: *Sitzungsberichte Gesellschaft Naturforschender Freunde*, Berlin.

Gilsanz, V., Roe, T.F. & Antunes, J. (1991) Effect of dietary calcium on bone density in growing rabbits. *Am. J. Physiol.*, **260**, 471–6.

Glickman, I. (1948) Acute vitamin C deficiency and periodontal disease. I. The periodontal tissue of the guinea pig in acute vitamin C deficiency. *J. Dent. Res.*, **27**, 9–23.

Glöckner, B. (2002) *Untersuchungen zur Atiologie und Behandlung von Zahn- und Kiefererkrankungen beim Heimtierkaninchen*. Thesis, Berlin.

Goodman, S.B., Ma, T., Genovese, M. & Lane Smith, R. (2003) COX-2 selective inhibitors and bone. *Int. J. Immunopathol. Pharmacol.*, **16** (3), 201–5.

Gorell, C. & Verhaert, L. (2006) Zahnerkrankungen bei Hasenartigen (Lagomorpha) und Nagetieren (Rodentia). In: *Zahnmedizin bei Klein- und Heimtieren* (ed. Gorell, C.), pp. 189–212. Urban & Fischer, Munich.

Gottlieb, B. (1922) Die paradentale Pyorrhoe der Rattenmolaren. *Vierteljahrsschrift fur Zahnheilkunde*, **38**, 273–91.

Gracis, M. (2008) Clinical Technique: Normal Dental Radiography of Rabbits, Guinea Pigs, and Chinchillas. *J Exot Pet Med* **17** (2), 78–86.

Habermehl, KH. (1975) *Die Altersbestimmung bei Haus- und Labortieren*. Parey, Berlin.

Hamidur Rahman, A,S,M,, Al-Mahmud, K.A. & Nashiru-Islam, K.M. (1983) Dental malocclusion in New Zealand White rabbit. *Bangladesh Vet. J.*, **16**, 85–8.

Harcourt-Brown, F.M. (1996) Calcium deficiency, diet and dental disease in pet rabbits. *Vet. Rec.*, **139**, 567–71.

Harcourt-Brown, F.M. (1997) Diagnosis, treatment and prognosis of dental disease in pet rabbits. *In Pract.*, **19**, 407–21.

Harcourt-Brown, F.M. (2002a) Dental disease. In: *Textbook of Rabbit Medicine* (ed. Harcourt-Brown, F.M.), pp. 165–205. Butterworth, London.

Harcourt-Brown, F.M. (2002b) Abscesses. In: *Textbook of Rabbit Medicine* (ed. Harcourt-Brown, F.M.), pp. 206–23. Butterworth, London.

Harcourt-Brown, F.M. & Baker, S.J. (2001) Parathyroid hormone, haematological and biochemical parameters in relation to dental disease and husbandry in rabbits. *J. Small Animal Pract.*, **42** (3), 130–6.

Hard, G.C. & Atkinson, F.F.V. (1967a) "Slobbers" in laboratory guinea pigs as a form of chronic fluorosis. *J. Path. Bact.*, **94**, 95–101.

Hard, G.C. & Atkinson, F.F.V. (1967b) The aetiology of "slobbers" (chronic fluorosis) in the guinea-pig. *J. Path. Bact.*, **94**, 103–12.

Harkness, J.E. & Wagner, J.E. (1983) *The Biology and Medicine of Rabbits and Rodents*, pp. 145–6. Lea & Febiger, Philadelphia, Pennsylvania.

Hein, J. & Hartmann, K. (2003a) Labordiagnostische Referenzbereiche bei Kaninchen. *Tierärztl Prax.*, **31**, 321–8.

Hein, J. & Hartmann, K. (2003b) Blutentnahme und labordiagnostische Referenzbereiche beim Meerschweinchen. *Tierärztl Prax.*, **31**, 383–9.

Henke, J. & Erhardt, W. (2001) *Schmerzmanagement bei Klein- und Heimtieren*. Enke, Stuttgart.

Henke, J., Erhardt,W. & Tacke, S. (2008) Analgesieprotokolle vor, wahrend und nach der Anasthesie von Hunden und Katzen mit schmerzhaften Zustanden – Eine Ubersicht. *Tierätztl Prax.*, **36**, 27–34.

Henke, J., Haberstroh, J, Sager, M et al. (2013) *Pain management for laboratory animals – GV-SOLAS Committee on Anaesthesia*.

Henke, J. & Reinert, J. (2006) Anwendung von Medetomidin in der Heimtierpraxis. *Fachpraxis*, **50**, 12–19.

Hernandez-Divers, S.J. (2008) Clinical technique: dental endoscopy of rabbits and rodents. *J. Exot. Pet Med.*, **17** (2), 87–92.

Hill, K.E., Motley, A.K., May, J.M. & Burk, R.F. (2009) Combined selenium and vitamin C deficiency causes cell death in guinea pig skeletal muscle. *Nutr. Res.*, **29** (3), 213–19.

Hillson, S. (2005) *Teeth*. Cambridge University Press, Cambridge.

Hinton, M., Jones, D.R.E. & Festing, M.F.W. (1982) Haematological findings in healthy and diseased rabbits, a multivariate analysis. *Lab. Animals*, **16**, 123–9.

Hirschfield, Z., Weinrab, M.M. & Michaeli, Y. (1973) Incisors of the rabbit: morphology, histology, and development. *J. Dent. Res.* **52** (2), 377–84.

Hochstrasser, G. (2005) Seltene Zahnzahlanomalie bei einem Feldhasen aus dem Banat-Rumanien. *Z. Jagdwiss.*, **15** (4), 162–4.

Hoover, J.P., Paulsen, D.B., Qualls, C.W. & Bahr, R.J. (1986) Osteogenic sarcoma with subcutaneous involvement in a rabbit. *J. Am. Vet. Med. Assoc.*, **189**, 1156–8.

Horowitz, S.L., Weisbroth, S.H. & Scher, S. (1973) Deciduous dentition in the rabbit (*Oryctolagus cuniculus*). A roentgenographic study. *Arch. Oral Biol.*, **18**, 517–23.

Howe, P.R. (1920) The effect of scorbutic diets upon the teeth. *Dent. Cosmos*, **62**, 586–90.

Hunt, A.M. (1959) A description of the molar teeth and investing tissue of normal guinea pigs. *J. Dent. Res.*, **38**, 216–31.

Ida-Yonemochi, H., Noda, T., Shimokawa, H. & Saku, T. (2002) Disturbed tooth eruption in osteopetrotic (op/op) mice: histopathogenesis of tooth malformation and odontomas. *J. Oral Pathol. Med.*, **31**, 361–73.

Imai, A., Eisele, P.H. & Steffey, E.P. (2005) A new airway device for small laboratory animals. *Lab. Animals*, **39**, 111–15.

Jekl, V.,Hauptman, K. & Knotek, Z. (2006) Incidence of dental disease in degus (*Octodon degus*). In: *Proceedings of the British Vetinary and Zoological Society*, Bristol, pp. 45–7.

Jekl, V., Hauptman, K. & Knotek, Z. (2008) Quantitative and qualitative assessments of intraoral lesions in 180 small herbivorous mammals. *Vet. Rec.*, **162**, 442–9.

Jekl, V., Hauptman, K., Skoric, M., Jeklova, E., Fictum, P. & Knotek, Z. (2008) Elodontoma in a degu (*Octodon degus*). *J. Exot. Pet Med.*, **17** (3), 216–20.

Jenkins, J.R. (2008) Rabbit diagnostic testing. *J. Exot. Pet Med.*, **17** (1), 4–15.

Jensen, C. (2008) *Ableitung des Selenbedarfs wachsender Meerschweinchen (Cavia porcellus)*. Thesis, Institut fur Tierernahrung und Ernahrungsphysiologie, Giesen.

Julius, C. (1997) *Untersuchungen zur Knochendichte bei weiblichen ZIKAZuchtkaninchen am Calcaneus sowie am distalen Tibiaende uber einen Zeitraum von mehreren Reproduktionszyklen mittels peripherer Quantitativer Computertomographie (pQCTtm)*. Thesis, Hohenheim.

Kazakos, G.M., Anagnostou, T., Savvas, I., Raptopoulos, D., Psalla, D. & Kazakou, I.M. (2007) Use of laryngeal mask airway in rabbits: placement and efficacy. *Lab. Animals*, **36** (4), 29–34.

Keil, A. (1966) *Grundzüge der Odontologie – Allgemeine und vergleichende Zahnkunde als Organwissenschaft*, pp. 192–8. Gebrüder Borntraeger, Berlin.

Keyes, P.H. (1968) Odontopathic infections. In: *The Golden Hamster, its Biology and its Use in Medical Research* (eds Hoffman, R.A. & Robinson, P.F.). State University Press, Iowa.

Klaus, P. & Bennett, R.A. (1999) Management of abscesses of the head in rabbits. In: *Proceedings of the North American Vetinary Conference*, Orlando, Florida.

Klimm, W. (2003) *Endodontologie: Grundlage und Praxis*. Deutscher Zahnärzteverlag, Köln.

Kotanyi, E. (1927) Die Veranderungen der Zahne und ihrer Umgebung bei experimentellem Skorbut des Meerschweinchens. *Z. Stomat.*, **25**, 655.

Kraus, V.B., Huebner, J.L., Stabler, T., Flahiff, C.M., Setton, L.A., Fink, C., Vilim, V. & Clark, A.G. (2004) Ascorbic acid increases the severity of spontaneous knee osteoarthritis in a guinea pig model. *Arthritis Rheum.*, **50** (6), 1822–31.

Kusner, W., Michaeli, Y. & Weinreb, M.M. (1973) Role of attrition and occlusal contact in the physiology of the rat incisor: V. Impeded and unimpeded eruption in hypophysectomised and magnesium deficient rats. *J. Dent. Res.*, **52**, 65–73.

Kwanabe, K., Okada, Y. & Matsusue, Y. (1998) Treatment of osteomyelitis with antibiotic-soaked porous glass ceramic. *J. Bone Joint Surg. Br.*, **80**, 527–30.

Latour, M.A., Hopkins, D., Kitchens, T., Chen, Z. & Schonfeld, G. (1998) Effects of feeding a liquid diet for one year to New Zealand White rabbits. Lab. Animal Sci., **48**, 81–3.

Lennox, A.M. (2008) Clinical technique: small exotic companion mammal dentistry – anesthetic considerations. *J. Exot. Pet Med.*, **17** (2), 102–6.

Lichtenberger, M. & Ko, J. (2007) Anesthesia and analgesia for small mammals and birds. *Vet. Clin. North Am. Exot. Animal Pract.*, **10** (2), 293–315.

Lindsey, J.R. & Fox, R.R. (1994) Inherited diseases and variations. In: *The Biology of the Laboratory Rabbit* (eds Manning, P.J., Ringler, D.H. & Newcomer, C.E.), 2nd edn, pp. 293–313. Academic Press, San Diego, California.

Lozupone, E. & Favia, A. (1989) Effects of a low calcium maternal and weaning diet on the thickness and microhardness of rat incisor enamel and dentine. *Arch. Oral Biol.*, **34**, 491–8.

Lozupone, E. & Favia, A. (1994) Morphometric analysis of the deposition and mineralization of enamel and dentine from rat incisor during the recovery phase following a low-calcium regimen. *Arch. Oral Biol.*, **39**, 409–16.

McClure, F.J. (1959) Further observations on the cariostatic effect of phosphates. *J. Dent. Res.*, **38**, 776–81.

McClure, F.J. & Folk, J.E. (1953) Skim milk powders and experimental rat caries. *Proc. Soc. Exp. Biol.*, **83**, 21–6.

Mackey, E.B., Hernandez-Divers, S.J., Holland, M. & Frank, P. (2008) Clinical technique: application of computed tomography in zoological medicine. *J. Exot. Pet Med.*, **17** (3), 198–209.

Mähler, M., Stunkel, S., Ziegowski, C. & Kunstryr, I. (1995) Inefficacy of enrofloxacin in the elimination of *Pasteurella multocida* in rabbits. *Lab. Animals*, **29**, 192–9.

Manville, R.H. (1954) Malocclusion in the rat. *J. Mammology*, **35**, 427.

Martinez-Jimenez, D., Hernandez-Divers, S.J., Dietrich, U.M., Williams, C.O., Blasier, M.W., Wilson, H. & Frank, P.M. (2007) Endosurgical treatment of a retrobulbar abscess in a rabbit. *J. Am. Vet. Med. Assoc.*, **230** (15), 868–72.

Massler, M. & Schour, I. (1941) Studies in tooth development: theories of eruption. *Am. J. Ortho. Oral Surg.*, **27** (19),552–76.

Matthews, B. (1972) Continuous recording of tooth eruption in the rabbit. *Arch. Oral Biol.*, **17**, 817–20.

Mellanby, M. & Killick, E.M. (1926) A preliminary study of factors influencing calcification processes in the rabbit. *Biochem. J.*, **20**, 902–26.

Michaeli, Y., Hirschfield, Z. & Weinreb, M.M. (1980) The cheek teeth of the rabbit: Morphology, histology and development. *Acta Anat.*, **106**, 223–39.

Mickoleit, G. (2004) *Phylogenetische Systematik der Wirbeltiere*. Pfeil, Munich.

Miles, A.E.W. & Crigson, C. (2003) *Colyer's Variations and Diseases of the Teeth of Animals*. Cambridge University Press, Cambridge.

Molan, P. (1999) The role of honey in the management of wounds. *J. Wound Care*, **8**, 415–18.

Moriyama, K., Sahara, N., Kageyama, T., Misawa, Y., Hosoya, A. & Ozawa, H. (2006) Scanning electron microscopy of the three different types of cementum in the molar teeth of the guinea pig. *Arch. Oral Biol.*, **51**, 439–48.

Morrisey, J.K. & Carpenter, J.W. (2004) Formulary. In: *Ferrets, Rabbits and Rodents – Clinical Medicine and Surgery* (eds Quesenberry, K.E. & Carpenter, J.W.), pp. 436–44. Saunders, Philadelphia, Pennsylvania.

Moskow, B.S., Wasserman, B.H.& Rennert M.C. (1968). Spontaneous periodontal disease in the Mongolian gerbil. *J. Periodont. Res.*, **3**, 69–83.

Mundorff, S.A. (1988) Dental decay research in animals. *Lab. Animals*, **17**, 19–24.

Ness, A.R. (1956) The response of the rabbit mandibular incisor to experimental shortening and prevention of its eruption. *Proc. Roy. Soc.*, **146**, 129–54.

Nishijima, K., Kuwahara, S., Ohno, T., Miyaishi, O., Ito, Y., Sumi, Y. & Tanaka, S. (2009) Occlusal tooth wear in male F344/N rats with aging. *Arch. Geront. Geriatr.*, **48**, 178–81.

Ohshima, H., Nakasone, N., Hashimoto, E., Sakai, H., Nakakura-Oshima, K. & Harada, H. (2005) The eternal tooth germ is formed at the apical end of continuously growing teeth. *Arch. Oral Biol.*, **50**, 153–7.

O'Malley, B. (2008) *Klinische Anatomie und Physiologie bei kleinen Heimtieren, Vogeln, Reptilien und Amphibien*. Urban & Fischer, Munich.

Otto, K. (2001) *Schmerztherapie bei Klein-, Heim- und Versuchstieren*. Parey, Berlin.

Phalen, D.N., Antinof, N. & Fricke, M.E. (2000) Obstructive respiratory disease in prairie dogs with odontomas. *Vet. Clin. North Am. Exot. Animals Pract.*, **3**, 513–17.

Pohto, M. (1939) The incisor teeth of guinea-pigs in vitamin-A deficiency. *Acta Odontologica Scandinavia*, **1** (2), 147–54.

Probst, W. & Vasel-Biergans, A. (2004) *Arzneimittel zur Keimreduktion*. In: *Wundmanagement* (eds Probst, W. & Vasel-Biergans, A.). Wissensch Verlagsgesellschaft, Stuttgart.

Proffitt, W.R. & Sellers, K.T. (1986) The effect of intermittent forces on eruption of the rabbit incisor. *J. Dent. Res.*, **65**, 118–22.

Ramos, J.R., Howard, R.D. & Pleasant, R.S. (2003) Elution of metronidazole and gentamicin from polymethylmethacrylate beads. *Vet. Surg.*, **32**, 251–61.

Remeeus, P.G.K. & Verbeek, M. (1995) The use of calcium hydroxide in the treatment of abscesses in the cheek of the rabbit resulting from a dental periapical disorder. *J. Vet. Dent.*, **12** (1), 19–22.

Rosenfield, M.E. (2009) *Successful eradication of severe abscesses in rabbits with long-term administration of penicillin G benzathine/penicillin G procaine* (http://bellsouthpwp.net/m/o/morfz/pdf/bicillin.pdf), July 2009.

Rotilie, J.A. (1977) Root surface caries in the molar teeth of rice rats. III. Inhibition of root surface caries by fluoride. *J. Dent. Res.*, **56**, 1408.

Rovin, S., Costich, E.R. & Gordon, H.A. (1966) The influence of bacteria in the initiation of periodontal disease in germfree and conventional rats. *J. Period. Res.*, **1**, 193–203.

Sainsbury, A.W., Kountouri, A., DuBoulay, G. & Kertesz, P. (2004) Oral diease in free-living red squirrels (*Sciurus vulgaris*) in the United Kingdom. *J. Wildlife Dis.*, **40** (2), 185–96.

Santone, P. (1937) Über die Folgen von umschriebenen traumatischen Verletzungen in Gewebe der Zahnanlage. *Dt Zahn-, Mund- und Kieferheilk*, **4**, 323–37.

Schaeffer, D.O. & Donnelly, T.M. (1997) Disease problems in guinea pigs and chinchillas. In: *Ferrets, Rabbits and Rodents: Clinical Medicine and Surgery* (eds Hillyer, E.V. & Quesenberry, K.E.), pp. 260–81. Saunders, Philadelphia, Pennsylvania.

Schour, I. & Massler, M. (1962) The teeth. In: *The Rat in Laboratory Investigation* (eds Farris, E.J. & Griffith, J.Q.), pp. 104–60. Hafner, New York.

Schour, I. & Van Dyke, H.B. (1932) Changes in the teeth following hypophysectomy. 1. Changes in the incisor of the white rat. *Am. J. Anat.*, **50**, 397–433.

Schumacher, M. (2007) Messung der Länge von Backenzahnkronen bei klinisch gesunden Kaninchen. *DFG-Jahrestagung*, Berlin.

Serota, K.S., Jeffcoat M.K. & Kaplan, M.L. (1981) Intraoral radiography of molar teeth in rats. *Lab. Animal Sci.*, **31**, 507–9.

Shadle, A.R. (1936) The attrition and extrusive growth of the four major incisor teeth of domestic rabbits. *J. Mammol.*, **17**, 15–21.

Shadle, A.R., Ploss, W.R. & Marks, E.M. (1944) The extrusive growth and attrition of the incisor teeth of *Erethizon dorsatum*. *Anatom. Rec.*, **90**, 337–41.

Shalla, C.L. (1972) Preliminary evidence of periodontal disease in *Lemmus trimucronatus* skulls from northern Alaska. *J. Dent. Res.*, **51**, 1075–9.

Sheppe, W. (1966) Exploration by the Deer Mouse, *Peromyscus leucopus*. *Am. Midland Natur.*, **76** (2), 257–76.

Smith, J.C., Robertson, L.D., Auhll, A., March, T.J., Deering, C. & Bolon, B. (2004) Rabbit inhalation anesthesia: ease of use and waste gas emissions. *Am. Assoc. Lab. Animal Sci.*, **43** (4), 22–5.

Sone, K., Koyasu, K., Tanaka, S. & Oda, S. (2005) Effects of diet on the incidence of dental pathology in free living caviomorph rodents. *Arch. Oral Biol.*, **50**, 323–31.

Spuzjak, M.I. (1989) Modeling hyperparathyroid osteodystrophy in animals. *Radiol. Diagn.*, **30** (6), 697–702.

Starck, D. & Wehrli, H. (1935) Die Kaumuskulatur von *Marmota marmota* L. *Zeitschr. Säugetierkunde*, **10**, 33–8.

Steedle, J.R., Proffitt, W.R. & Fields, H.W. (1983) The effects of continuously axially-directed intrusive loads on the erupting rabbit mandibular incisor. *Arch. Oral Biol.*, **28** (12), 1149–53.

Steenkamp, G. & Crossley, D.A. (1999) Incisor tooth regrowth in a rabbit following complete extraction. *Vet. Rec.*, **145**, 585–6.

Stoor, P., Soderling, E. & Salonen, J.I. (1998) Antibacterial effects of a bioactive glass paste on oral microorganisms. *Acta Odontol. Scand.*, **56**, 161–5.

Storch, V. & Welsch, U. (2004) *Systematische Zoologie – Rodentia*. Spektrum Akademischer Verlag, Heidelberg.

Sulik, M., Sobolewska, E., Seremak, B., Ey-Chmielewska, H. & Fraczak, B. (2007) Radiological evaluation of chinchilla mastication organs. *Bull. Vet. Inst. Pulawy*, **51**, 121–4.

Taubman, M.A., Buckelew, J.M., Ebersole, J.L. & Smith, D.J. (1981) Periodontal bone loss and immune response to ovalbumin in germ-free rats fed antigen-free diets with ovalbumin. *Inf. and Immunity*, **32**, 145–52.

Taylor, M., Beaufrère, H., Mans, C. & Smith, D.A. (2008) Treatment of odontogenic abscesses in pet rabbits with a wound-packing technique: long-term outcomes. In: *Vetinary Proceedings of the Annual AAV Conference*, Savannah, Georgia, pp. 103–4.

Thenius, E. (1989) Zähne und Gebiß der Säugetiere. In: *Handbuch der Zoologie. Vol. VIII, Mammalia, Teilbd. 56* (eds Niethammer, J., Schliemann, H. & Starck, D.). Walter de Gruyter, Berlin.

Tobias, K.M., Schneider, R.K. & Besser, T.E. (1996) Use of anti-microbial-impregnated polymethylmethacrylate. *J. Am. Vet. Med. Assoc.,* **208** (6), 841–4.

Tomes, C.S. (1882) *A Manual of Dental Anatomy, Human and Comparative.* Churchill, London.

Toth, L.A. & Krueger, J.M. (1989) Haematological effects of exposure to three infective agents in rabbits. *J. Am. Vet. Med. Assoc.,* **195**, 981–5.

Turner, T. (1997) The incidence of dental problems in pet rabbits. In: *Proceedings of the World Vetinary Dental Congress,* Birmingham.

Tyrrell, K.L., Citron, D.M., Jenkins, J.R. & Goldstein, E.J.C. (2002) Periodontal bacteria in rabbit mandibular and maxillary abscesses. *J. Clin. Microbiol.,* **40** (3), 1044–7.

Van der Velden, U. (1980) Influence of periodontal health on probing depth and bleeding tendency. *J. Clin. Periodontol.,* **7**, 129–39.

VanForeest, A.W. (1995) Dentistry in wildlife casualties and exotic animals. In: *BSAVA Manual of Small Animal Dentistry* (eds Crossley, D.A. & Penman, S.), pp. 209–18. BSAVA, Cheltenham.

Vaughan, T.A. (1972) *Mammalogy.* Saunders, Philadelphia, Pennsylvania.

Vincent, A.L., Rodrick, G.E. & Sodeman, W.A. (1979) The pathology of the Mongolian gerbil (*Meriones unguiculatus*) – a review. *Lab. Animal Sci.,* **29**, 645–51.

Vollmerhaus, B., Knospe, C. & Roos, H. (2001) Zur Phylogenie des Equidengebisses. *Anat. Histol. Embryol.,* **30**, 237–48.

Wagner, R.A., Garman, R.H. & Collins, B.M. (1999) Diagnosing odontomas in prairie dogs. *Exotic DVM,* **1** (1), 7–10.

Walberg, J.A. (1981) Osteogenic sarcoma with metastasis in a rabbit (*Oryctolagus cuniculus*). *Lab. Animal Sci.,* **31**, 407–8.

Ward, M.L. (2006) Diagnosis and management of a retrobulbar abscess of periapical origin in a domestic rabbit – case report. *Vet. Clin. Exot. Animal Pract.,* **9**, 657–65.

Washabau, R.J. & Hall, J.A. (1997) Gastrointestinal prokinetic therapy: serotonergic drugs. *Compend. Cont. Educ.,* **19**, 473–9.

Webb, R.A. (1985) Chinchillas. In: *BSAVA Manual of Exotic Pets* (eds Beynon, P.M. & Cooper, J.E.). British Small Animal Association, Cheltenham.

Weinreb, M.M., Kusner, W. & Michaeli, Y. (1973) Role of attrition and occlusal contact in the physiology of the rat incisor. VII. Formation of impeded and unimpeded incisors in magnesium deficient rats. *J. Dent. Res.,* **52**, 498–503.

Weisbroth, S.H. & Hurvitz, A. (1969) Spontaneous osteogenic sarcoma in *Oryctolagus cuniculus* with elevated serum alkaline phosphatase. *Lab. Animal Care,* **19**, 262–6.

Weisman, D.L., Olmstead, M.L. & Kowalski, J.J. (2000) *In vitro* evaluation of antibiotic elution from polymethylmethacrylate (PMMA) and mechanical assessment of antibiotic–PMMA composites. *Vet. Surg.,* **29**, 245–51.

Wiggs, R.B. & Lobprise, H. (1990) Dental disease in rodents. *J. Vet. Dent.,* **7** (3), 6–8.

Wiggs, B. & Lobprise, H. (1995a) Dental anatomy and physiology of pet rodents and lagomorphs. In: *BSAVA Manual of Small Animal Dentistry* (eds Crossley, D.A. & Penman, S.). BSAVA, Cheltenham.

Wiggs, B. & Lobprise, H. (1995b) Oral diagnosis in pet rodents and lagomorphs. In: *BSAVA Manual of Small Animal Dentistry* (eds Crossley, D.A. & Penman, S.). BSAVA, Cheltenham.

Wiggs, B. & Lobprise, H. (1995c) Prevention and treatment of dental problems in rodents and lagomorphs. In: *BSAVA Manual of Small Animal Dentistry* (eds Crossley, D.A. & Penman, S.). BSAVA, Cheltenham.

Williams, C.S.F. (1976) *Practical Guide to Laboratory Animals.* Mosby, St Louis, Minnesota.

Wolf, P. & Kamphues, J. (1995) Probleme der art- und bedarfs-gerechten Ernährung kleiner Nager als Heimtiere. *Prakt. Tierarzt.,* **76** (12), 1088–92.

Wu, D.D., Boyd, R.D., Fix, T.J. & Burr, D.B. (1990) Regional patterns of bone loss and altered bone remodelling in response to calcium deprivation in laboratory rabbits. *Calcif. Tissue Int.,* **47**, 18–23.

Further Reading

Adams, K., Couch, L., Cierny, G., Calhoun, J. & Mader, J. (1992) *In vitro* and *in vivo* evaluation of antibiotic diffusion from antibiotic-impregnated polymethylmethacrylate beads. *Clin. Orthop. Rel. Res.*, **278**, 244–52.

Aiken, S. (2004) Surgical treatment of dental abscesses in rabbits. In: *Ferrets, Rabbits, and Rodents – Clinical Medicine and Surgery* (eds Quesenberry, K. & Carpenter, J.), 2nd edn. Saunders, St Louis, Minnesota.

Alpert, B., Colosi, T., von Fraunhofer, J.A. & Seligson, D. (1989) The *in vivo* behavior of gentamicin–PMMA beads in the maxillofacial region (Abstract). *J. Oral Maxillofac. Surg.*, **47**, 46–9.

Bennett, R.A. (2004) Advances in the treatment of rabbit abscesses. In: *Eastern States Vetinary Association Proceedings of the North American Vetinary Conference*, pp. 1367–9.

Bergman, A., Yanai, J., Weiss, J., Bell, D. & David, M.P. (1983) Acceleration of wound healing by topical application of honey. An animal model. *Am. J. Surg.*, **145**, 374–6.

Blackwell, N.J. (1999) Abscesses in rabbits. *Vet. Rec.*, **144**, 540.

Böhmer, E. & Köstlin, G. (1988) Zahnerkrankungen bzw. -anomalien bei Hasenartigen und Nagern. *Prakt. Tierarzt.*, **69**, 37–50.

Böhmer, E. & Matis, U. (1987) Malokklusion beim Kaninchen – Der klinische Fall. *Tierärztl Praxis*, **15**, 127 and 237–9.

Bordeau, J.E., Schwer-Dymerski, D.A., Stern, P.H. & Langman, C.B. (1986) Calcium and phosphorous metabolism in chronically vitamin D deficient laboratory rabbits. *Mineral and Electrolyte Metabolism*, **12**, 176–85.

Bowyer, G.W. & Cumberland, N. (1994) Antibiotic release from impregnated pellets and beads. *J. Traumatol.*, **36**, 331–5.

Brommage, R., Miller, S.C. & Langman, C.B. (1988) The effect of chronic vitamin D deficiency on the skeleton in the adult rabbit. *Bone*, **9**, 131–9.

Brown, K.M., Saunders, M.M., Kirsch, T., Donahue, H.J. & Reid, J.S. (2004) Effect of COX-2-specific inhibition on fracture-healing in the rat femur. *J. Bone Joint Surg. – American*, **86**-A (1), 116–23.

Burling, K., Murphy, C.J. & DaSilva, C.J. (1991) Anatomy of the rabbit nasolacrimal duct and its clinical implications. *Prog. Vet. Comp. Ophthalmol.*, **1**, 33–40.

Butson, R.J., Schramme, M.C., Garlick, M.H. & Davies, J.V. (1996) Treatment of intrasynovial infection with gentamicin-impregnated polymethylmethacrylate beads. *Vet. Rec.*, **138**, 460–4.

Calhoun, J.H. & Mader, J.T. (1989) Antibiotic beads in the management of surgical infections. *Am. J. Surg.*, **157**, 443–9.

Capello, V. (2002) Incisor extraction to resolve clinical signs of odontoma in a prairie dog. *Exotic DVM*, **4** (1), 9.

Capello, V. (2003) Dental diseases and surgical treatment in pet rodents. *Exotic DVM*, **5** (3), 21–7.

Capello, V. (2004) Endoscopic assessment and treatment of cheek teeth malocclusion in pet rabbits. *Exotic DVM*, **6** (2), 37–40.

Capello, V. (2008) Clinical technique: treatment of periapical infections in pet rabbits and rodents. *J. Exot. Pet Med.*, **17** (29), 124–31.

Capello, V. & Cauduro, A. (2008) Clinical technique: application of computed tomography for diagnosis of dental disease in the rabbit, guinea pig, and chinchilla. *J. Exot. Pet Med.*, **17** (2), 93–101.

Capello, V., Gracis, M. & Lennox, A.M. (2005) *Rabbit and Rodent Dentistry Handbook*. Zoological Education Network, Lake Worth, Florida.

Chapin, R.E. & Smith, S.E. (1967) Calcium requirement of growing rabbits. *J. Animal Sci.*, **26**, 67–71.

Chapman, M.W. & Hadley, K. (1976) The effect of polymethylmethacrylate and antibiotic combinations on bacterial viability. *J. Bone Joint Surg.*, **58**, 76–81.

Colmery, B. & Frost, P. (1986) Periodontal disease: etiology and pathologenesis. *Vet. Clin. North Am. Small Animal Pract.*, **16**, 817–33.

Cornell, C.N., Tyndall, D., Waller, S., Lane, J.M. & Brause, B.D. (1993) Treatment of experimental osteomyelitis with antibiotic-impregnated bone graft substitute (Abstract). *J. Orthop. Res.*, **11**, 619–26.

Crossley, D.A. (2000) Rabbit and rodent radiology. In: *An Atlas of Veterinary Dental Radiology* (eds DeForge, D.H. & Colmery III, B.H.), pp. 247–59. Iowa State University Press, Ames, Iowa.

Dentistry in Rabbits and Rodents, First Edition. Estella Böhmer.
© 2015 John Wiley & Sons, Ltd. Published 2015 by John Wiley & Sons, Ltd.

Crossley, D.A. (2001) Pathophysiology of continuously growing teeth in small pets. In: *DVG-Jahreskongress 47*, Berlin.

Crossley, D.A. (2003) Oral biology and disorders of lagomorphs. *Vet. Clin. North Am. Exot. Animal Pract.*, **6** (3), 629–59.

Crossley, D.A. & Roxburgh, G. (1999) The site of obstruction of the lacrimal drainage system in chinchillas (*Chinchilla laniger*) with "wet eye". In: *Proceedings of the British Small Animal Vetinary Association Congress*, Cheltenham.

Derrell, C.J. (1987) Historical perspectives and taxonomy. In: *Laboratory Hamsters* (eds VanHoosier, J.R. & McPherson, C.A.W.). Academic Press, Orlando, Florida.

DeVree, F. (1977) Mastication in guinea pigs (*Cavia porcellus*). *Am. Soc. Zool.*, **17**, 886.

Dhasmana, K.M., Prakash, O. & Saxena, P.R. (1982) Effects of fentanyl and the antagonism by naloxone on regional blood flow and biochemical variables in conscious rabbits. *Arch. Int. Pharmacodyn.*, **260**, 115–29.

Divers, S.J. (1997) Incisor malocclusion in the rabbit (*Oryctolagus cuniculus*). *Vet Times*, **27**, 12–15.

Divers, S.J. (2000) Mandibular abscess treatment using antibiotic-impregnated beads. *Exotic DVM*, **2** (5), 15–18.

Doff, R.S. & Rosen, S. (1977) Root surface caries in the molar teeth of rice rats – 1. A method of quantitative scoring. *J. Dent. Res.*, **56**, 1013–16.

Doff, R.S. & Rosen, S. (1977) Root surface caries in the molar teeth of rice rats – 2. Quantitation of lesions induced by a high sucrose diet. *J. Dent. Res.*, **56**, 1011–12.

Eisenmenger, E. & Zetner, K. (1982) *Tierärztliche Zahnheilkunde*. Parey, Berlin.

Emily, P. (1991) Problems peculiar to continually erupting teeth. *J. Small Exot. Animal Med.*, **1**, 56–9.

Engstrom, C. & Noren, J.G. (1986) Effects of orthodontic force on enamel formation in normal and hypocalcaemic rats (Abstract). *J. Oral Pathol.*, **15**, 78–82.

Evans, R.P. & Nelson, C.L. (1993) Gentamycin impregnated polymethylmethacrylate beads compared with systemic antibiotic therapy in the treatment of chronic osteomyelitis. *Clin. Orthop. Rel. Res.*, **295**, 37–42.

Fairham, J. & Harcourt-Brown, F.M. (1999) Preliminary investigation of the vitamin D status of pet rabbits. *Vet. Rec.*, **145**, 452–4.

Firestone, A.R., Graves, C.N. & Feagin, F.F. (1988) The effects of different levels of dietary sucrose on root caries subsequent to gingivectomy in conventional rats infected with *Actinomyces viscosus* M-100. *J. Dent. Res.*, **67** (19), 1342–5.

Fitzgerald, R.L. & Keyes, P.H. (1960) Demonstration of the etiologic role of *Streptococci* in experimental caries in the hamster. *J. Am. Dent. Assoc.*, **61**, 9–19.

Flick, A.B., Herbert, J.C., Goodell, J. & Kritiansen, T. (1987) Noncommercial fabrication of antibiotic impregnated polymethylmethacrylate beads. *Clin. Orthop.*, **223**, 282–6.

Gabriel, S. (2008) *Zahnerkrankungen bei Kaninchen – Diagnostik und praxisgerechte Behandlungen*. Spektrum Tiermedizin.

Glickman, I. & Shklar, G. (1954) The effect of systemic disturbances on the pulp of experimental animals. *Oral Surg. Oral Med. Oral Pathol.*, **7** (5), 550–8.

Greenberg, T. (2000) Premolar extraction in the domestic rabbit. *Exotic DVM*, **2** (4), 11.

Harcourt-Brown, F.M. (1995) A review of clinical conditions in pet rabbits associated with their teeth. *Vet. Rec.*, **137**, 341–6.

Harcourt-Brown, F.M. (1999) Treatment of facial abscesses in rabbits. *Exotic DVM*, **1**, 83–8.

Harcourt-Brown, F.M. (2002) Anorexia in rabbits. Causes and effects. *In Pract.*, **24**, 358–67.

Harcourt-Brown, F.M. (2002) Anorexia in rabbits. Diagnosis and treatment. *In Pract.*, **24**, 450–67.

Harcourt-Brown, F.M. (2005) *Metabolic bone disease as a possible cause of dental disease in pet rabbits*. PhD Thesis, Royal College of Veterinary Surgeons, London.

Harcourt-Brown, F.M. (2007) The progressive syndrome of acquired dental disease in rabbits. *J. Exot. Pet Med.*, **16** (3), 146–57.

Harcourt-Brown, F.M. (2009) Dental disease in pet rabbits 1. Normal dentition, pathogenesis and aetiology. *In Pract.*, **31**, 370–9.

Harkness, J.E. (1987) Rabbit husbandry and medicine. *Vet, Clin, North Am, – Small Animal Pract.*, **17** (5), 1019–44.

Harris, S.S. & Naviy, J.M. (1980) Vitamin A deficiency and caries susceptibility of rat molars. *Arch. Oral Biol.*, **25**, 415–21.

Hebel, R. & Stromberg, M.W. (1986) *Anatomy and Embryology of the Laboratory Rat*. Biomed Verlag, Wörthsee.

Heikkila, J.T., Aro, H.J., Yli-Urpo, A., Happonen, R.P. & Aho, A.J. (1995) Bone formation in rabbit cancellous bone defects filled with bioactive glass granules. *Acta Orthop. Scand.*, **66** (5), 463–7.

Henke, J. & Erhardt, W. (1999) Kaninchen und Nager: Möglichkeiten zur Injektionsnarkose. *Kleintier Konkret (Poster)*.

Henry, S.L. & Galloway, K.P. (1995) Local antibacterial therapy for the management of orthopaedic infections – pharmacokinetic considerations. *Clin. Pharmacokin.*, **29**, 36–45.

Hernandez-Divers, S.J. (2001) Molar diseases and abscesses in rabbits. *Exotic DVM*, **3** (3), 65–9.

Hinton, M. (1979) Mandibular osteomyelitis in the rabbit. *Vet. Rec.*, **103**, 263–4.

Hoefer, H.L. (1994) Chinchillas. *Vet. Clin. North Am. – Small Animal Pract.*, **24** (1), 103–11.

Huang, C.M. (1987) Morphometric relationships between skull traits and malocclusion in the domestic rabbit. *Bull. Inst. Zool. Acad. Sin.*, **26**, 123–31.

Hupf, K.D., Askaka, Y., Griffin, A.L., Berg, W.P., Seager, M.A. & Berry, S.D. (2004) Differential mastication kinematics of the rabbit in response to food and water: implications for conditioned movement. *Integr. Physiol. Behav. Sci.*, **39** (1), 16–23.

Ireson, H. (1968) A preliminary report on an abnormal dental condition in rabbits. J. Inst. Animal Tech., **19**, 36–9.

Jacob, E., Setterstrom, J.A., Bach, D.E., Heath, J.R., McNiesh, L.M. & Cierny, G. (1991) Evaluation of biodegradeable ampicillin anhydrate microcapsules for local treatment of experimental staphylococcal osteomyelitis (Abstract). *Clin. Orthop.*, **267**, 237–44.

Johnson-Delaney, C.A. (2005) *Practical Rabbit and Rodent Anesthesia and Analgesia*. Rabbit and Rodent Dentistry Wet Lab, Ft Lauderdale, Florida.

Jordan, H.V. & Keyes, P.H. (1964) Aerobic, grampositive, filamentory bacteria as etiological agents of experimental periodontal disease in hamsters. *Arch. Oral Biol.*, **9**, 401–8.

Kenneth, E.B. (1982) Mandibular movement and muscle activity during mastication in the guinea pig (*Cavia porcellus*). *J. Morphol.*, **170**, 147–69.

Keogh, B.S., Triplett, R.G., Aufdemorte, T.B. & Boyan, B.D. (1989) The effect of local antibiotics in treating chronic osseous *Staphylococcus aureus* infection (Abstract). *J. Oral Maxillofac. Surg.*, **47**, 940–5.

Keyes, P.H. & Fitzgerald, R.J. (1962) Dental caries in the Syrian hamster – IX. *Arch. Oral Biol.*, **7**, 267–78.

Khaliq, Y., Rouse, M., Piper, K.E., Steckelberg, J.M. & Patel, R. (2001) Amikacin or clindamycin release kinetics from polymethylmethacrylate or Matrix III beads in a continuous flow chamber. *Abstr. Intersci. Conf. Antimicrob. Agents & Chemotherapeutics*, **41**, 37.

King, G.M. & Custance, D.R. (1982) *Colour Atlas of Vertebrate Anatomy*. Blackwell Scientific, Oxford.

Klugh, D.O. (2005) Intraoral radiology in equine dental disease. *Clin. Tech. Equine Pract.*, **4**, 162–70.

Knight, H.D., Hietala, S.K. & Jang, S. (1980) Antibacterial treatment of abscesses. *J. Am. Vet. Med. Assoc.*, **176**, 1095–8.

Könighaus, H. (2007) *Anästhesiologische und sonographische Evaluierung des Einflusses von Metamizol/Propofol und Fentanyl/ Propofol auf die Vasoaktivität und Hämodynamik beim Kaninchen.* Thesis, Munich.

Kotanyi, E. (1927) Veränderungen der Zähne und ihrer Umgebung bei experimentellem Skorbut des Meerschweinchens. *Zschr. Stomat.*, **25**, 655–719.

Krasse, B. & Carlsson, J. (1970) Various types of *Streptococci* and experimental caries in hamsters. *Arch. Oral Biol.*, **15**, 25–32.

Landry, S.O. (1957) Factors affecting the procumbency of rodent upper incisors. *J. Mammology*, **38**, 223–34.

Langenbach, G.E., Weijs, W.A. & Koolstra, J.H. (1991) Biomechanical changes in the rabbit's masticatory system during postnatal development. *Anat. Rec.*, **230**, 406–16.

Legendre, L.F.J. (2002) Malocclusions in guinea pigs, chinchillas and rabbits. *Can. Vet. J.*, **43**, 385–90.

Legendre, L.F.J. (2003) Oral disorders of exotic rodents. *Vet. Clin. North Am. Exot. Animal Pract.*, **6** (3), 601–28.

Levine, B.S. (2003) Review of antibiotic-impregnated polymethylmethacrylate beads in avian and exotic pets. *Exotic DVM*, **5** (4),11–14.

Lipman, N.S., Weischedel, A.K., Connors, M.J., Olsen, D.A. & Taylor, N.S. (1992) Utilization of cholestyramine resin as a preventive treatment for antibiotic (clindamycin) induced enterotoxaemia in the rabbit. *Lab. Animals*, **26**, 1–8.

Listgarten, M.M. & Kamin, A. (1969) The development of a cementum layer over the enamel surface of rabbit molars – a light and electron microscopic study. *Arch. Oral Biol.*, **14**, 961–85.

Lobprise, H.B. & Wiggs, R.B. (1991) Dental and oral disease in lagomorphs. *J. Vet. Dent.*, **8** (2), 11–17.

Longmore, B. (1969) Coronal cementum in the rabbit, guinea pig and the horse. *J. Dent. Res.*, **47**, 997–8.

McClure, F.J. & McCann, H.G. (1960) Dental caries and composition of bones and teeth of white rats: effect of dietary mineral supplements. *Arch. Oral Biol.*, **2**, 151–61.

Mackey, D., Varlet, A. & Debeaumont, D. (1982) Antibiotic loaded plaster of Paris pellets; an *in vitro* study of a possible method of local antibiotic therapy in bone infection. *Clin. Orthop.*, **167**, 263–8.

Martinez-Jimenez, D., Hernández-Divers, S.J., Dietrich, U.M., Williams, C.O., Blasier, M.W., Wilson, H. & Frank, P.M. (2007) Endosurgical treatment of a retrobulbar abscess in a rabbit. *J. Am. Vet. Med. Assoc.*, **230** (6), 868–72.

Mathews, K.A. & Binnington, A.G. (2002) Wound management using sugar. *Compend. Contin. Educ. Vet. Pract.*, **24** (1), 41–50.

Meredith, A. (2007) Rabbit dentistry. *Europ. J. Comp. Animal Pract.*, **17** (1), 55–62.

Miclau, T., Dahners, L.E. & Lindsey, R.W. (1993) *In vitro* pharmacokinetics of antibiotic release from locally implantable materials (Abstract). *J. Orthop. Res.*, **11**, 627–32.

Miwa, Y. (2006) Mandibulectomy for treatment of oral tumors (cementome and chondrosarcoma) in two rabbits. *Exotic DVM*, **8** (3), 18–22.

Morimoto, T., Inoue, T., Nakamura, T. et al. (1985) Characteristics of rhythmic jaw movements of the rabbit. *Arch. Oral Biol.*, **30**, 673–7.

Murray, M.J. (2000) Application of rigid endoscopy in small exotic mammals. *Exotic DVM*, **2** (3), 13–18.

Nelson, W.B. (2000) Rabbit and dental care: protocols for rabbit incisor extraction. *Exotic DVM*, **2** (4), 12.

Okada, S., Ohta, Y., Nishimura, K., Matsushita, J. & Nakamura, M. (1990) Microvascular architecture of the enamel organ of the upper major incisor in the rabbit (Abstract). *Okajimas Folia Anat. Jpn*, **67**, 231–41.

Okuda, A., Hori, Y., Ichihara, N., Asari, M. & Wiggs, R.B. (2007) Comparative observation of skeletal-dental abnormalities in wild, domestic, and laboratory rabbits (Abstract). *J. Vet. Dent.*, **24** (4), 224–9.

Omeroglu, H., Ates, Y., Akkus, O. & Korkusuz, F. (1997) Biomechanical analysis of the effects of single high-dose vitamin D3 on fracture healing in a healthy rabbit model. *Arch. Orthop. Trauma Surg.*, **116**, 271–4.

O'Rourke, D.P. (2004) Disease Problems of Guinea Pigs. In: Ferrets, Rabbits and Rodents – Clinical Medicine and Surgery. (eds. Quesenberry, K.E. & Carpenter, J.W.), 2nd ed., Saunders, Philadelphia.

Orten, A.U., Burn, C.G. & Smith, A.H. (1937) Effects of prolonged chronic vitamin A deficiency in the rat with special reference to odontomas. *Proc. Soc. Exp. Biol. Med.*, **36**, 82–4.

Phillips, H., Boothe, D.M., Shofer, F., Davidson, J.S. & Bennett, R.A. (2007) *In vitro* elution studies of amikacin and cefazolin from polymethylmethacrylate. *Vet. Surg.*, **36** (3), 227–78.

Pindborg, J.W. (1953) The pigmentation of the rat incisor as an index of metabolic disturbances. *Oral Surg.*, **6**, 780–9.

Pollock, S. (1951) Slobbers in the rabbit. *J. Am. Vet. Med. Assoc.*, **119**, 443–4.

Popesko, P., Rajtova, V. & Horak, J. (1990) *A Colour Atlas of Anatomy of Small Laboratory Animals*, Vols 1 and 2. Wolfe, Aylesbury.

Ranta, R., Ylippavalniemi, P., Altonen, M. & Calonius, P.E.B. (1981) Transplantation of free tibial periosteal graft on alveolar bone defect in adult rabbit. *Int. J. Oral Surg.*, **10**, 122–7.

Redrobe, S. (2000) Surgical procedures and dental disorders. In: *Manual of Rabbit Medicine and Surgery* (ed. Flecknell, P.). BSAVA, Cheltenham.

Redrobe, S. (2001) Imaging techniques in small mammals. *Sem. Avian Exot. Pet Med.*, **10** (4), 187–97.

Reiter, A.M. (2008) Pathophysiology of dental disease in the rabbit, guinea pig, and chinchilla. *J. Exot. Pet Med.*, **17** (2), 70–7.

Rosskopf, W.J. & Woerpel, R.W. (1982) Malocclusion in pet rabbits. *Mod. Vet Pract.*, **63**, 482.

Roux, F.Ph. (2005) Extraction of the incisors in a dwarf rabbit. *Schweiz. Arch. Tierheilkd.*, **147** (7), 311–13.

Russell, A.P. (1998) The mammalian masticatory apparatus: an introductory comparative exercise. Chapter 17 in: *Tested Studies for Laboratory Teaching*, Vol. 19 (ed. Karcher, S.J.), Proceedings of the 19th Workshop/Conference of the Association of Biology Lab Education, pp. 271–86.

Salomon, F.V., Geyer, H. & Gille, U. (2008) *Anatomie fur die Tiermedizin*. Enke, Stuttgart.

Sasnau, R. (1994) Perforation einer Wange infolge exzessiven Zahnwachstums eines Prämolaren beim Meerschweinchen (*Cavia aspera* f: *porcellus*). *Prakt. Tierarzt.*, **7**, 618–19.

Schour, I., Bhaskar, S.N., Greep, R.O. & Weinmann, J.P. (1949) Odontom-like formations in a mutant strain of rats. *Am. J. Anat.*, **85**, 73–112.

Schour, I., Hoffmann, M.M. & Smith, M.C. (1941) Changes in the incisor teeth of albino rats with vitamin A deficiency and the effects of replacement therapy. *Am. J. Pathol.*, **17**, 529–51.

Schwartz, G., Enomoto, S., Valiquette, C. & Lund, J.P. (1989) Mastication in the rabbit: a description of movement and muscle activity. *J. Neurophysiol.*, **62**, 273–87.

Seligson, D., Mehta, S. & Voos, K. (1992) The use of antibiotic polymethylmethacrylate beads to prevent the evolution of localised infection. *J. Orthop. Traumatol.*, **6**, 401–6.

Silverman, S. & Tell, L.A. (2005) *Radiology of Rodents, Rabbits and Ferrets. An Atlas of Normal Anatomy and Positioning*. Saunders, St Louis, Missouri.

Slootweg, P.J., Kuijpers, M.H.M. & Van de Kooij, A.J. (1996) Rat odontogenic tumors associated with disturbed tooth eruption. *J. Oral Pathol. Med.*, **25**, 481–3.

Souza, M.J., Greenacre, C.B., Avenell, J.S. ,Wall, J.S. & Daniel, G.B. (2006) Diagnosing a tooth root abscess in a guinea pig (*Cavia porcellus*) using micro computed tomography imaging. *J. Exot. Pet Med.*, **15** (4), 274–7.

Stanford, M. (2002) Use of DOXIROBE GelR. *Exotic DVM*, **4** (5), 11.

Storch, V. & Welsch, U. (2004) *Systematische Zoologie – Lagomorpha*, 6th edn. Spektrum Akademischer Verlag, Heidelberg.

Taglinger, K. & König, H.E. (1999) Makroskopisch-anatomische Untersuchungen der Zähne des Kaninchens (*Oryctolagus cuniculus*). *Wiener Tierärztliche Monatsschrift*, **86**, 129–35.

Taylor, M. (1999) Endoscopy as an aid to the examination and treatment of the oropharyngeal disease of small herbivorous mammals. *Semin. Avian Exot. Pet Med.*, **8** (3), 139–41.

Taylor, M. (2003) A wound packing technique for rabbit dental abscesses. *Proc. ICE Exotic DVM*, **5** (3), 28–31.

Teaford, M.F. & Byrd, K.E. (1989) Differences in tooth wear as an indicator of changes in jaw movement in the guinea pig – *Cavia porcellus*. *Arch. Oral Biol.*, **34** (12), 929–36.

Tell, L.A., Silverman, S. & Wisner, E. (2003) Imaging techniques for evaluating the head of birds, reptiles and small exotic mammals. *Exotic DVM*, **5** (2), 31–7.

Verstreate, F.J.M. (2003) Advances in diagnosis and treatment of small exotic mammal dental disease. *Semin. Avian Exot. Pet Med.*, **12** (1), 37–48.

Verstraete, F. & Osofsky, A. (2005) Dentistry in pet rabbits. *Comp. Cont. Educ. Pract. Vet.*, **27** (9), 671–85.

Vlaminck, L., Verhaert, L., Steenhaut, M. & Gasthuys, F. (2007) Tooth extraction techniques in horses, pet animals and man. *Vlaams Diergeneeskundig Tijdschrift*, **76**, 249–61.

Wagner, R. & Johnson, D. (2001) Rhinotomy for treatment of odontoma in prairie dogs. *Exotic DVM*, **3** (5), 29–34.

Weisbroth, S.H. & Ehrman, L. (1967) Malocclusion in the rabbit: a model for the study of the development, pathology and inheritance of malocclusion. *J. Hered.*, **58**, 245–6.

Westerhof, I. & Lumeij, S.J. (1987) Dental problems in rabbits, guinea pigs and chinchillas. *Tijdschr v. Diergeneesk*, **12**, 6–10.

Wiggs, R.B. & Lobprise, H. (1991) Dental and oral disease in lagomorphs. *J. Vet Dent.*, **8** (2),11–17.

Wolbach, S.B. & Howe, P.R. (1933) The incisor teeth of albino rats and guinea pigs in vitamin A deficiency and repair. *Am. J. Pathol.*, **IX**, 275–93.

Woods, C.A. (1976) How hystrichomorph rodents chew. *Am. Zoo Soc.*, **16**, 215.

Zeman, W.V. & Fielder, F.G. (1969) Dental malocclusion and overgrowth in rabbits. *J. Am. Vet Med. Assoc.*, **155**, 1115–19.

Index

Page numbers in *italics* refer to illustrations; those in **bold** refer to tables

abrasion 14–15
  tooth growth relationship 15
abscess *see* intranasal abscess; jaw abscesses;
    retrobulbar abscess
alveolar bullae, exposure of 156, 161, *171*, 174, 175
alveolar nerve block 106
ameloblasts 8
amelogenesis 8
amelogenesis imperfecta 18
amoxicillin 238
ampicillin 238
anaesthesia 90–97
  accidents 96–97
  conductive anaesthesia 106
  drugs used **92**
  infiltration anaesthesia 105
  local anaesthesia 104–105, **105**
  monitoring 93
  performance of 93–96
  perioperative control of 91–93
  postoperative care 97
  reversal 94
  sedation 91
  stages **95**
  triple anaesthesia 93, **93**
analgesia 97–104
  metamizole 103–104
  nonsteroidal anti-inflammatory drugs (NSAIDs) 103
  opioids 99–103
anatomical crown 6
anelodont teeth 10
anisognathy 14
antibiotic therapy 236–239
  antibiotic impregnated polymethyl methacrylate (AIPMMA)
      beads 227–230
  chinchilla **268**
  guinea pig **268**
  hamster **269**
  mice **269**

rabbit **267**
rat **269**
apical orientation 7
apicoectomy 212
aradicular teeth 6
assisted feeding 260, *261*
azithromycin 237–239

benzathine penicillin G 239
bilophodonty 26
bioactive ceramic material (BioGlass®) 230
bone resorption 115, *116*
brachygnathia superior, rabbit 118–121, *119, 120, 131, 137, 142*
  treatment 120–121
brachyodont teeth *6,* 10–11, 182–184
bruxism 14, 23
buccal surface 7
bulb protrusion 38–39
bupivacaine 104–105
buprenorphine 102
burs 113–115
  thermal damage prevention 114
  use of *114,* 191–193
butorphanol 100–102

calcium hydroxide therapy 226–227
calcium requirements 16
  deficiency effects 18, 123, 153
campylognathia 121
caries 250–253
  aetiology 252–253
  brachyodont cheek teeth 182–183
  herbivorous rodents 251–252
  lagomorphs 250–251
  omnivorous rodents 252
  prophylaxis 253
  treatment 251, 253
  see also specific species
carprofen 103

Dentistry in Rabbits and Rodents, First Edition. Estella Böhmer.
© 2015 John Wiley & Sons, Ltd. Published 2015 by John Wiley & Sons, Ltd.

cefazolin 237–238
cementum 9
cephalexin 239
cephalosporins 238, 239
cheek dilators 107–108, *109*
cheek teeth 5, *6*
  examination 43–48
  extraction 195–211
    aftercare 207–209
    complications 209–211
    including jaw osteotomy 201–207
    indications 195, *196*
    intraoral extraction 197, 199–201
    problems with 196–198
    tooth socket management 197–199, 202–203
  lagomorphs 24–27
    malocclusion aetiology 153–155
    pathogenesis 155–162
  radiographic appearance 63, 65–66
  retrograde growth 39
  rodents 28, 31–34
    brachyodont teeth *6*, 182–184
    herbivorous rodents 162–182
  teething 13
  see also molar teeth; premolar teeth; *specific species*
chinchilla
  analgesic dosages **101**
  antibiotic therapy **268**
  caries 179
  cheek teeth 31–32
    extraction 204–207
  cheek tooth pathology 165–175, 176–181
    buccal spurs *169, 214*
    elongation *32, 117*, 165, 166, *169, 178, 187*
    intraalveolar rotation *116, 169*, 171, *178*
    malocclusion *32*, 46, *115–117*, 135, *178–181, 186–187, 208, 214*
    tooth resorption 180–181
  dietary recommendations 262
  hypersalivation *36*
  incisor malocclusion *36, 135, 168*
  jaw abscesses 170–171
    mandibular abscess 219
    maxillary abscess 220
  malocclusion reference lines 75–79
  mandibular osteolysis 178
  nasolacrimal duct compression *166, 172–173, 177–178*
  normal occlusion reference lines *74*, 75
  periodontal disease 242, *243*, 245–246
  prognosis 263
  radiographic examination 52, 53
    intraoral radiography 85–86

isolated views of the mandible 59–60
isolated views of the maxilla 60–61, *62*
  normal radiographic anatomy 74–75
retrobulbar abscess 170, 233
  therapy 235
stress reaction 165
teething 13
tooth growth 16
tooth trimming *115*, 178, 187–188, 193
chipmunk
  cheek tooth pathology *184*
  intraoral radiography *81*
  normal occlusion *34*
chloramphenicol 238, 239
chlorhexidine 248–249, 253
  PeriChip® 249
ciprofloxacin 238
clindamycin 237–238
clinical crown *6*
clinical examination
  documentation of findings *47*, 48
  general examination 37–38
  history 35–37
  intraoral examination 41–48
    incisors 42–43
    oral cavity and cheek teeth 43–48
    restraining the patient 41–42
  palpation 39–40
  visual inspection 38–39
collagen defect 163–164
composite bridge 256–257
computed tomography (CT) 88–89
conductive anaesthesia 106
congenital malformations, incisors 118–121
conjunctivitis 160
coronal orientation 7
crown *6*
  enamel folds 12
  loss *40, 183*
cryotherapy 212
cytotoxic therapy 212

dacryocystitis, rabbit *37, 39, 132, 160*
deciduous dentition 12–13
degu
  analgesic dosages **101**
  cheek teeth 33
    extraction 204–207
  cheek tooth pathology 166–170, 172, 181–182
    dental spurs *168*
    malocclusion *129, 169*, 181, *182, 220*
    step mouth *166*, 182

degu (*cont'd*)
    tooth bridge formation 169
    tooth resorption 182
  dietary recommendations 262
  incisor malocclusion 127
  mandibular abscess 219
  normal occlusion *33, 79*
  odontoma-like lesions *129*, 182
  prognosis 263
  radiographic examination 59–60
    intraoral radiography 85
    normal radiographic anatomy 79
  retrobulbar abscess 233, 235
demineralization 153, *154*
dental cementum 9
dental formula 13, **13**
dental spurs
  chinchilla *169, 214*
  degu *168*
  rabbit *22, 23, 110*
dental unit 112–113
dentin 8–9
  hypoplasia 19, *22, 40, 244*
dentinogenesis 9
dentoalveolar syndesmosis 10
desmodontium 9–10
dietary recommendations 261–262
diphyodonty 12
documentation *47*, 48

elodont teeth 6, 10
elodontoma 128, *129*, 258
enamel 7–8
  changes 17–20
  hypomineralization 18
  hypoplasia 18–20, *22, 40, 244*
  lagomorphs 24, 27
  ridges 12, *12*, 26
    lophs 33, 34
endoscopic examination 44–45, 111
enrofloxacin 238, 239
epiphora, chinchilla 177
erythromycin 238
euthanasia 63, 139, 178, 241, 262, 263
evolution of teeth 5
examination *see* clinical examination
exophthalmos 50, *52*
  critical anaesthetic situations 96
  retrobulbar abscess 39, 170, 230–232
  stress reaction 41
exposure keratitis 39
extraction

cheek teeth 195–211
  aftercare 207–209
  complications 209–211
  extraoral extraction 197
  including jaw osteotomy 201–207
  indications 195, *196*
  intraoral extraction 197, 199–201
  problems with 196–198
  tooth socket management 197–199, 202–203
  incisors 121, 135–141, 144–149
    iatrogenic fractures 141, 144, 147–148
  jaw abscess treatment 221–226
    aftercare 208–209
  peg teeth 144–145, 147
  periodontal disease 247, 250
eye removal 233–236, *237*

fentanyl 102
fluoride 253
follow-ups 262
forceps 115–116, 193
formaldehyde, halting tooth growth 16

gentamicin 238
gerbil
  cheek teeth 33, 34
  periodontal disease 250
giant cell granuloma *258*
gingival hyperplasia *186*
gingival hypertrophy 259
gingivitis 242
  aetiology 243–244
gnawing, rodents 28, 30
  lack of provision for 124
guinea pig
  analgesic dosages **100**
  antibiotic therapy **268**
  apicoectomy *212*
  caries *251*, *252*
  cheek teeth 31
    extraction *200*, 204–207
  cheek tooth pathology 162–176
    aetiology 162–165
    elongation 166, 167
    excessive mineralization 165–166
    malocclusion *11, 31, 46, 59, 140, 187*, 194–195
    retrograde growth *39*
    splitting 173–174, *175*
    tooth bridge formation *28*, 168–169, 175
  computed tomography (CT) *88*
  dietary recommendations 261–262
  hypersalivation 38, *42*

incisors
    fracture *123, 220*
    malocclusion *42, 124, 125*, 133–134, *140*
    splitting *124, 125, 134, 151*
jaw fracture 209
lockjaw *255*
malocclusion reference lines 71–74
mandibular abscess *2, 58, 60, 108, 152*, 175, *217*, 218–219
    delayed wound healing *152*
maxillary abscess 220
nasolacrimal duct 173, 175
    irrigation 172–173
normal occlusion *32, 61, 62*
    reference lines *70*, 71
osteoarthritis of the temporomandibular joint *254*
osteodystrophy *50*
periodontal disease *2, 243, 244*, 245–246
prognosis 263
radiographic examination 52
    intraoral radiography *83*, 85–86
    isolated views of the mandible 59–60
    isolated views of the maxilla 60–61
    laterolateral skull view 53
    normal radiographic anatomy 69–71
    oblique views 56–57
    positioning *54*
retrobulbar abscess *173*, 175, *205*, 233, 235–237
    therapy 235
teething 13
tooth growth 16
tooth trimming 187–188, *193*, 194–195

hamster
    analgesic dosages **101**
    antibiotic therapy **269**
    cheek teeth 33
        crown loss *183*
        pathology 182–184
    maxillary abscess *183*
    normal occlusion *34, 81*
    normal radiographic anatomy 80, *81*
    periodontal disease 250
    tooth growth 16
hand files 116–117
history taking 35–37
honey, wound management 239–240
hydroxyapatite crystals 8
hypersalivation 36
    chinchilla *36*
    guinea pig 38, *42*
    rabbit 38, 158
hypodontia 13, *17*

hypomineralization 18
hypothermia 93
hypovitaminosis C 162–164, 245
hypsodont teeth 10
Hystricomorpha 14, *15*, 27
    classification *28*

incisal orientation 7
incisors 5
    congenital malformations 118–121
    eruption 17
    examination 42–43
    extraction 121, 135–141, 144–149
    fracture 121–122, *123, 220*
        iatrogenic 141, 144, 147–148
        treatment 122
    growth 16–17, **16**
    infections 125–126, 136–138
    malocclusion 118–142
        acquired, non-trauma-related 122–127
        aetiology **119**
        primary malocclusion 118–129
        prognosis 264
        secondary malocclusion 129–142
        trauma-related 121–122, *123*
        treatment 120–121, 122, 126–127, 135–142
    mobility 137, *138*
    peg teeth 21, 23, 24
    pseudo-odontoma 127–129
    rodents 29–31
        pigmentation 30
    sharpening 14
    teething 12–13
    trimming 136, 142–144
        pulp cavity exposure 142–144
    see also specific species
infection
    incisors 125–126, 136–138
    nasolacrimal duct 38, 39, 50
    temporomandibular joint 107, *108*
    see also jaw abscesses; retrobulbar abscess
infiltration anaesthesia 105
infraorbital nerve block 106
instruments
    dental treatment 112–117
    intraoral examination 107–112
intermediary plexus 10
intranasal abscess 49, 50, 131, *133*, 160, *162*, 225
intraoral examination 41–48
    incisors 42–43
    instruments 107–112
    oral cavity and cheek teeth 43–48

intraoral examination (*cont'd*)
  restraining the patient 41–42
  see also clinical examination
intraoral radiography *see* radiographic examination
intrathoracic abscess, rabbit *38*
intrauterine diphyodonty 13
intravenous drug administration 94, **94**, 96–97
intubation 93
isognathy 14

jaw abscesses 63
  abscess surgery 149–152
    local wound treatment 239–240
    radical excision 221–226
    wound healing complications 240
  aetiology 213–214
  aftercare following tooth extraction 208–209
  antibiotic therapy 236–239
    antibiotic impregnated beads 227–230
  calcium hydroxide therapy 226–227
  clinical symptoms 215–216
  debridement 224, 226
  diagnosis 37–38, 214
    differential diagnosis 214–215
  formation 159–161, 170
  lower jaw 216–219
  palpation 40
  periodontal disease relationship 244
  prognosis 240–241, 264
  radiographic examination 49
  therapeutic issues 221
  upper jaw 220
  wound marsupialization 226
  see also specific species
jaw angle injury 184–185
jaw fractures 121–122, 254–256
  iatrogenic 209, 255–256
  mandibular fracture 255
  maxillary fracture 254–255, *256*, *257*
jaw muscles *15*
jaw neoplasia 258–259
jaw relationship 14

lagomorphs 21–27
  caries 250–251
  cheek teeth 24–27
    malocclusion aetiology 153–155
    pathogenesis 155–162
  classification **22**
  enamel 24, 27
  incisors 23–24
  periodontal disease 242–249

prognosis 262–263
  temporomandibular joint 21, *22*
  tooth trimming 189–192
    technique 191–192
  see also rabbit
lamina dura, loss of *117*, 243, *244*
laryngeal mask 96
lidocaine 104, 105
lincomycin 238
lingual surface 7
local anaesthesia 104–105, **105**
lockjaw *255*
lophodont teeth 11
lophs 33, 34
luxators 145–146
  use of 200–201

malocclusion 4
  cheek teeth 153–184
    brachyodont teeth 182–184
    herbivorous rodents 162–182
    lagomorphs 153–162
  enamel/dentin hypoplasia relationship *19*
  incisors 118–142, 264
    aetiology **119**
    primary malocclusion 118–129
    secondary malocclusion 129–142
    trauma-related 121–122
    treatment 120–121, 122, 126–127,
      135–142
  intraoral findings 45–46
  prognosis 262–266
    staging **265–266**
  symptoms **154**
    early symptoms 1
  tooth growth and abrasion relationship 15
  see also specific species
mandibular abscess 216–219
  see also jaw abscesses; *specific species*
mandibular fractures 255
marsupialization of abscess wound 226
masseter muscle 14, *15*
masticatory muscles 14, *15*
maxillary abscess 220
  see also jaw abscesses; *specific species*
maxillary fracture 254–255, *256*, *257*
maxillary nerve 99
mental nerve block 106
metabolic bone disorder 153–154
  indicators of 155
metamizole 103–104
metronidazole 238

mice
  analgesic dosages **101**
  antibiotic therapy **269**
  cheek teeth 33
    pathology 182–184
  incisor malocclusion *125, 126, 129*
  odontoma *129*
molar teeth
  growth 17
  hypsodont 10
  lagomorphs 26
  lophodont 11
  rodents 28, 31–34
  teething 12, 13
  see also cheek teeth
monophyodonty 13
mouth gags 107, *109*
  risks of 43, 107
mouth mirror 111
Myomorpha 14, *15,* 27
  classification *27*

naloxone 102–103
nasal discharge *38*
nasolacrimal canal 207, *208*
  dilation *163*
  narrowing 160
nasolacrimal duct *166*
  infection 38, *38,* 39, 50
  irrigation 39, 131–132, 172–173
  obstruction *130,* 131–133
  opening *162*
neoplasia of the jaw 258–259
nerve block 106
nonsteroidal anti-inflammatory drugs (NSAIDs) 103
normal occlusion
  chinchilla, reference lines *74, 75*
  chipmunk *34*
  degu *33, 79*
  guinea pig *32, 61, 62*
    reference lines *70,* 71
  hamster *34, 81*
  rabbit *10, 21, 25, 26, 56*
    reference lines *65, 66–67*
  rat *11, 80*
  see also malocclusion

occlusal orientation 7
occlusal surface discoloration 45
occlusion *see* malocclusion; normal occlusion
odontoblasts 8, 9
odontological terms **8**

odontoma 127–129, 131, 182, 258
opioid analgesics 99–103
oral cavity
  cleaning 45
  examination 43–48
orientation terms 7, **7**
osteoarthritis of the temporomandibular joint *254*
osteodystrophy 49, *50*
osteolysis, chinchilla 178
osteoma 258
osteosarcoma 258
osteosclerosis 166
osteotomy 149–152, 201–207
  postoperative care 202–203
otoscopic examination 44

pain 97
  signs of 97, **98**
  see also analgesia
palpation 39–40
parathyroid hormone 153
peg teeth 21, 23, 24
  extraction 144–145, 147
penicillins 237–239
periodontal diseases 242
  aetiology/pathogenesis 242–246, 249–250
  diagnosis 246–247
  herbivorous rodents 242–249
  lagomorphs 242–249
  omnivorous rodents 249–250
  treatment 247–249, 250
periodontal ligament 9–10
periodontal probe use 110–111
periodontitis *133,* 242
periodontium 9
plaque formation 242–244
polyodontia 13, *13*
  polyodontia falsa 23
  polyodontia vera 23
postoperative care 97, 260
  anaesthesia aftercare 97
  extraction 207–208
    jaw abscess treatment 208–209
  osteotomy 202–203
power drill 113
premolar teeth, lagomorphs 26
  see also cheek teeth
procaine penicillin G 239
prognosis 262–266
  jaw abscess 240–241
  staging **265–266**
pseudo-odontoma 127–129

pterygoid muscle 14
pulp 6, 9, 10
    removal 144, 146

rabbit
    analgesic dosages **100**
    antibiotic therapy **267**
    assisted feeding *261*
    brachygnathia superior 118–121, *119, 120, 131, 137, 142*
        treatment 120–121
    caries *251*
    cheek teeth 24–27
        extraction *197–204, 208–209*
    cheek tooth pathology 153–162
        aetiology 153–155
        curvature 158–160
        elongation *44, 52, 56, 68, 69*, 154–160, *160, 185*
        malocclusion *22, 40, 45, 51, 130, 133, 141, 157*
        pathogenesis 155–162
        retrograde displacement *52*, 156–159
        splitting/fracture *3, 51*, 157, *158*, 203
    critical anaesthetic situations 96
    dacryocystitis 37, 39, *132*, 160
    demineralization *154*
    dental spurs 22, 23, *110*
    dietary recommendations 261–262
    end-stage malocclusion *40, 163*
    giant cell granuloma *258*
    hairy mucosal fold *6*, 24
    hypersalivation 38, 158
    incisors *6*, 23–24
        extraction 121, 135–141
        malocclusion 21, *43*, 129–133, *136–138, 141*
    intranasal abscess 50, 131, *133*, 160, *162, 225*
    intrathoracic abscess *38*
    intubation 93
    malocclusion reference lines 67–69
    mandibular abscess 2–3, *56, 109, 138–139, 158, 210, 214*, 216–218
        antibiotic impregnated bead therapy *228–229*
        formation 159–161
        rostral abscess *150*
        surgical excision *222–223*
    maxillary abscess *130, 163, 198, 206, 215*, 220
    maxillary fracture *256, 257*
    maxillary nerve *99*
    molar attrition 23
    nasolacrimal duct infection *38*
    normal occlusion *10*, 21, *25, 26, 56*
        reference lines *65*, 66–67
    odontoma *131*
    osteotomy *202–204*
    periodontal disease *3, 133, 244, 247*, 248

polyodontia *13*
prognosis 262–263
radiographic examination *51*, 52
    dorsoventral skull view *54, 55*
    intraoral radiography 82–84, *85*
    laterolateral skull view *53*
    maxillary cheek teeth 67
    normal radiographic anatomy 64–66
    oblique views *51*, 55–56, *57*
restraint 41–42, *44*
retrobulbar abscess *39*, 110, 161, *230–232, 234–235, 241*
    pathogenesis 230–233
    therapy 233–235
step mouth 161–162, *163*
stress reaction 41, *42*, 92
symphysiolysis *256, 257*
teething 12–13, *12*
temporomandibular dysplasia *255*
tongue lesions 158, *159, 185*
tooth growth 16
tooth trimming 189–192
    incorrect *112*
    technique 191–192
radicular teeth 11
radiographic examination 49
    indications 49–50
        cheek tooth pathology 170, 172
    interpretation of radiographs 61–63
    intraoral radiography 81–87
        exposure values 84–85
        film processing 86–87
        film-focal distance 84–85
        intraoral films 81–82
        positioning 82–84
        requirements for 87
        X-ray technique 85–86
    positioning 51
    projections 51–61
        dorsoventral and ventrodorsal skull view 54–55
        isolated views of the mandible 59–60, *61*
        isolated views of the maxilla 60–61, *62*
        laterolateral skull view 53–54
        oblique views 55–57
        rostrocaudal view 57–58, *59*
    reference lines 64, **64**
        chinchilla *74*, 75–79
        guinea pig *70*, 71–74
        rabbit 66–69
    techniques 51
rat
    analgesic dosages **100**
    antibiotic therapy **269**

caries 252–253
cheek teeth *6*, 33
   pathology 182–184
incisor malocclusion *11*, *124*
intraoral radiography *82*
mandibular abscess *127*
maxillary abscess *184*
normal occlusion *11*, *80*
normal radiographic anatomy 80
periodontal disease *11*, 249–250
teething 13
tooth growth 16
recurrence prevention 261–262
reference lines *see* radiographic examination
reserve crown 6
restraining the patient 41–42
   intraoral examination *44*
retrobulbar abscess 230–236
   pathogenesis 230–233
   therapy 233–236
   see also specific species
rhinitis, unilateral 38, 130, 146, 160, *220*, *221*
rodents 27–34
   caries 251–253
   cheek teeth 28, 31–34
   classification **22**, 27, *28*
   gnawing 28, 29, 30
   incisors 29–31
      pigmentation 30
   masseter muscle types 14
   mastication 28–29
   periodontal disease 242–250
   prognosis 262–263
   teething 13
   tooth trimming 192–195
   see also specific species
root 6

Sciuromorpha 14, *15*, 27
   classification *27*
sedation 91
   drugs used **92**
selenium requirement 164
self-cleaning of the dentition 242, 253
Sharpey's fibres 9, 10
slobbers *see* hypersalivation
squirrels 184
   cheek teeth 34
step mouth
   degu 166, 182
   rabbit 161–162, *163*
streptomycin 239

stress reaction 41, *42*, 90, 165
sugar, wound management 239–240
symphysiolysis 256–258

teeth
   abrasion 14–15, 16
   anatomy 5–6
   classification of 10–12
   eruption 17
   evolution of 5
   growth 15, 16–17, **16**
      abrasion relationship 15, 16
      halting 16
      stimulation 16–17
   nomenclature 6–7
   structure 7–10
      dental cementum 9
      dentin 8–9
      desmodontium 9–10
      enamel 7–8
      pulp 10
   see also cheek teeth; incisors
teething 12–13, *12*
temporomandibular joint 14, 107
   disorders 254, *255*
   hyperextension 169–170
   infection 107, *108*
   lagomorphs 21, *22*
   radiographic view 57–58
   rodents 28
tetracyclines 237
thimethoprim-sulfamethoxazole 238–239
Tomes' fibres 8, 9
tongue
   lesions 158, *159*, *185*
      ulceration *45*
   management during intraoral examination 109
tongue spatula 109, *110*
tooth bridge formation *28*, 168–169, 175
tooth extraction *see* extraction
tooth resorption 76, 115, *116*, 165
tooth trimming 112–116
   cheek teeth 184–195
      lagomorphs 189–192
      proper trimming 187–188
      rodents 192–195
   iatrogenic fractures 142
   incisors 136, 142–144
   pulp cavity exposure 142–144
   subtle versus radical trimming 185–187
   see also specific species
trilophodonty 32, 34

triple anaesthesia 93, **93**, 95
tumor palpation 40
tympanic bulla, radiographic view 57–58

vascular access 94, **94**, 96–97
vasoconstrictors 105
vitamin A deficiency 164
vitamin C deficiency 162–164, 245
  supplementation 245, 249

vitamin D deficiency 123
vitamin E deficiency 164

wound management 239–240
  marsupialization 226
  wound healing complications 240

X-rays *see* radiographic examination

Printed and bound by CPI Group (UK) Ltd, Croydon, CR0 4YY

16/04/2025

14658503-0003